PAUL STRATHERN is the internationally acclaimed author of books on science, history and philosophy, including *The Medici: Godfathers of the Renaissance*, *Dr Strangelove: A Brief History of Economic Genius* and *Mendeleyev's Dream: The Quest for the Elements*, shortlisted for the prestigious Aventis Prize.

Other titles in this series

A BRIEF HISTORY OF

MEDICINE

from HIPPOCRATES
to GENE THERAPY

PAUL STRATHERN

ROBINSON
London

Constable & Robinson Ltd
3 The Lanchesters
162 Fulham Palace Road
London W6 9ER
www.constablerobinson.com

This edition published by Robinson,
an imprint of Constable & Robinson Ltd, 2005

A copy of the British Library Cataloguing in Publication Data
is available from the British Library.

ISBN 1–84529–155–7

Printed and bound in the EU

1 3 5 7 9 10 8 6 4 2

To Mandy

Illness is the night-side of life, a more onerous citizenship. Everyone who is born holds dual citizenship, in the kingdom of the well and the kingdom of the sick. Although we all prefer to use only the good passport, sooner or later each of us is obliged, at least for a spell, to identify ourselves as citizens of that other place.

Susan Sontag

One reason why medical history is not much taught in medical schools is that so much of it is an embarrassment.

Lewis Thomas

CONTENTS

ILLUSTRATIONS

Every effort has been made to clear copyright on these images, any
queries regarding the use of material should be addressed to the
publisher.

PROLOGUE

READING AMID THE BATTLE

The discovery of the circulation of the blood by William Harvey in the early seventeenth century marked the beginning of modern medicine. Harvey was recognized throughout Europe, even in his lifetime, as the founding father of a new physiology: the scientific understanding of how the body actually works. When Charles I succeeded to the throne, Harvey was appointed as his 'Physitian extraordinary', and he attended his royal master through most of his turbulent reign. According to the contemporary writer John Aubrey: 'When Charles I by reason of the Tumults left London, [Harvey] attended him, and was at the fight of Edge-hill with him.' This was the opening battle of the Civil War between the Royalists and the Parliamentarians in 1642. Aubrey went on to describe how 'during the fight, the Prince and Duke of York were committed to [Harvey's] care.' This was no small matter: these were the king's young sons, heirs to the throne. The

Prince of Wales, who was twelve, would later become Charles II. His nine-year-old brother, the Duke of York, would succeed him as James II. Despite this great responsibility, Aubrey records how Harvey 'told me that he withdrew with them under a hedge, and tooke out of his pockett a booke and read; but he had not read very long before a Bullet from a great Gun grazed on the ground neare him, which made him remove his station.'

This image of Harvey absorbed in his book, heedless even of his royal charges, while the battle raged around him, has become emblematic of the bemused intellectual engrossed in his cerebral pursuits. It is a tradition which stretches back as far as the philosophers of Ancient Greece: Socrates is said to have exhibited similar behaviour whilst serving as a hoplite (conscripted private soldier) in the Athenian army. Harvey's absorption during the battle particularly epitomizes the medical mind, and makes a fine image of the profession as a whole. The pursuit of learning, amid the everyday battle against illness and disease, is how medicine has proceeded throughout its long history.

Harvey appears to have been capable of bouts of intense concentration until late in life. During his seventies he lived at Cockaine, the London mansion of his brother Eliab Harvey, a succesful merchant. Here, according to Aubrey, Harvey 'was wont to contemplate on the Leads [lead roofing] of the house, and had his severall stations, in regard of the sun, or wind.' By this time: 'He was much and often troubled with the Gowte, and his way of cure was thus; he would then sitte with his legs bare, if it were a frost, on the leads of Cockaine-house, putt them into a payle of water, till he was almost dead with cold, and betake himselfe to his Stove, and so 'twas gone.'

Aubrey, who met Harvey many times, describes him: 'He was not tall, but of the lowest stature, round faced, olivaster complexion; little Eie, round, very black, full of spirit; his hair was black as a Raven, but quite white 20 yeares before he dyed.' In contrast to his frequently otherworldly manner, Harvey appears to have been a difficult character when he came back to earth. Aubrey notes: 'He was very Cholerique; and in his young days wore a dagger (as the fashion then was), but this Dr. would be too apt to drawe-out his dagger, upon every slight occasion.' He held his fellow men in low esteem. 'He was wont to say that man was but a great mischievous Baboon.' He suffered on account of his overactive mind, but once again had his own chosen remedy for his afflictions: 'He was hott-headed, and his thoughts working would many times keepe him from sleepinge; he told me that then his way was to rise out of his Bed and walk about his Chamber in his Shirt till he was pretty coole, i.e. till he began to have a Horror.' The shivers, presumably.

It was not until 1628, at the age of fifty, that Harvey published the work which secured his fame. This is usually known by its abbreviated title *De Motu Cordis* (Concerning the Motion of the Heart). Harvey begins by describing how when he first studied the heart: 'I straightwayes found it a thing hard to be attained, and full of difficulty, so . . . I did almost believe that the motion of the heart was known to God alone.' But he persisted, carrying out dissections on human corpses and those of various animals.

Prior to the publication of *De Motu Cordis*, medical orthodoxy had clung to the medical teachings of the ancient classical masters. According to these, the blood was continuously created in the liver. Pulsations in the walls of the veins and arteries squeezed the blood so that it was distributed throughout the body, where it was consumed by the flesh.

Harvey demonstrated the errors in such theory by using a method which had recently been introduced by Galileo in the new physics. He applied mathematics to medicine. For the first time, measure was introduced in the study of the body. Harvey calculated the amount of blood that passed through the heart. He found that in the course of an hour a volume of blood which was more than three times the weight of the entire body flowed out of the heart. If the liver had continuously produced this amount of blood, the body would simply have exploded! He then showed that if an artery was restricted with a ligature, the side towards the heart began to bulge with blood. This suggested that in the arteries the blood flowed away from the heart. When he restricted a vein, the side away fom the heart bulged with blood – suggesting that in the veins the blood flowed towards the heart. This indicated that the arteries and veins formed a circular system, allowing the blood to circulate throughout the body. Harvey also demonstrated that this circulation was maintained by the pumping motion of the heart (this was *de motu cordis* itself, the motion of the heart).

Initially, many were sceptical of Harvey's revolutionary discovery. Although even the sceptics were forced to concede that it did account for one anomaly which had puzzled anatomists for centuries: Why did poison kill so quickly? Evidently, once ingested it passed into the bloodstream and rapidly circulated throughout the body.

On the other hand, there was one thing which Harvey was not able to explain. How did the blood pass from the ultimate branching limits of the arteries into the similarly branching limits of the veins, so that it could flow back to the heart? He noted that the branching network of the veins and arteries became ever tinier, until their traceries became too small to be detected by the eye. This led him to conjecture that the connections between the limits of these two systems were too minute to be seen. Yet he could find no proof of this with which to confound his critics. In the strictest scientific terms it remained a theory which could not be proved.

In 1661, four years after Harvey's death, his hunch concerning the link between the arteries and the veins was confirmed by the Italian physiologist Marcello Malpighi. Using a microscope Malpighi detected that the tiniest branches of the arteries were linked by fine hairlike blood vessels to the system of the veins. These minute links would later be named 'capillaries', from the Latin *capillaris* meaning 'like hair'.

Harvey's discovery of the circulation of the blood laid the foundation for the scientific study of the body. He showed how its main organism (the heart) worked, and how this distributed the essential blood throughout the body. This discovery showed how the body maintained itself, and kept itself functioning. It showed how the body kept itself alive.

The secret of the heart was no longer 'known to God alone', but was instead a matter of scientific study. Life, in its corporeal aspect, was no longer a spiritual matter beyond our understanding. It could be determined, experimentally and rationally, in terms of flesh and blood.

I

OUT OF THE DARKNESS: FIRST LIGHT

The practice of medicine is as ancient as humanity itself. The first illnesses, the first accidents, literally cried out for the first cures. In that distant age the world itself was a vast and threatening mystery. Protection could only be sought by means of superstition: the invocation and casting out of spirits, the performance of spells and rituals. Some rituals proved more efficacious and persisted. This was the beginning of medical lore.

When the nomadic hunter-gatherers settled among their domesticated animals, new ills began to afflict humanity. Diseases endemic to dogs, cattle and poultry jumped to the humans in close proximity: measles from dogs, salmonella from poultry, parasitical worms from cattle. As settlements grew into towns, which expanded into cities, so illnesses expanded into epidemics. As civilization grew, so medical practice became more formalized: shamans and village witch-doctors gave way to specialists in divination and necromancy. Almost a thousand tablets listing diagnoses and cures survive from the Babylonian era. Many of these depict recognizable diseases: 'The patient coughs frequently, and what comes from his mouth is viscous and may contain blood. His breathing makes a noise like a flute. His hands are cold, his feet are warm; he sweats and his heart flutters.' Today such a patient would be diagnosed as having tuberculosis (which humans originally caught from cattle). Travelling to Babylon during the early fourth century BC, the Ancient Greek historian Herodotus recorded a quaint custom which was prevalent in the city during this period. The sick would be laid out in the street in front of their dwellings, so that any passer-by could offer his medical advice. Yet such casual medical diagnosis was not without its dangers. If a patient died as a result of a misdiagnosis, the diagnostician was liable to have his hand cut off.

Yet all this should not be mistaken for the beginnings of scientific medical practice. It was still accepted without question that the cause of all illness could be traced to the influence of the gods. Such a belief precluded, or at best undercut, any hint of a scientific approach. The same was true in Ancient Egypt, which also had established medical sorcerers and healers, many of whom even specialized in different afflictions. Bone fractures were bound and set between ox-bones. Evidence of trepanning has been found – along with evidence that the patient even survived this early surgery (some skulls have separate holes, drilled on different occasions). But the reason this pioneer surgery developed was to allow evil spirits to escape – or to allow more beneficent spirits to do their work, in the case of the ox-bone splints. Meanwhile, alongside this more advanced practice were all manner of quack cures, including such hardy perennials as remedies for baldness. A typical Ancient Egyptian cure for this depressing affliction (one of whose most persistent side effects seems to be gullibility) was a concoction containing an extraction of the vulva and the penis, together with a black lizard. Such cures hinted more at the socio-sexual perception of the ailment they sought to cure, rather than at any empirical approach.

Much the same was true of Ancient Greece, where medical practice traced its origins back to the quasi-divine Asclepius, son of Apollo, who may have been an actual miracle-healer around 1200 BC. (Zeus, the ruler of the gods, is said to have killed him with a thunderbolt, because he feared that Asclepius' healing methods might prove so successful as to make human beings immortal.) Nearly a thousand years later, Asclepius was the centre of a flourishing cult. Patients would be brought to sleep at his shrines, which were situated in peaceful rural surroundings. Here, in a dream, the patient would be visited by the god, or his emissary in the form of a snake, who would give advice on the correct cure. The Ancient Greek sign of Asclepius, a staff entwined with a snake, remains to this day the emblem of medicine, as seen adorning modern pharmacies.

It was not until the birth of the scientific outlook in Ancient Greece during the sixth century BC that medicine first took on a rational aspect. Only then did the accumulated body of ancient medical wisdom first become infected with the germ which would eventually destroy it. The passage of this disease would ebb and flow through the body of medical knowledge during the coming centuries, until eventually the spiritual content of this knowledge would wither, leaving in its place a body of purely scientific understanding. Even so, the ghost of that earlier spirituality continues to haunt medicine. We still recognize the power of psychology alone – having faith in a particular doctor, or an ineffectual prescription, can itself bring about a cure. But prior to the advent of medicine as a science there was nothing else: only faith, and more or less fantastic ways of inducing it. This was all the witch-doctors, the healers and the shamans knew. They had a power, and certain practices, which appeased the gods in the heavens and the spirits which inhabited the world all around. The earliest Greek practitioners of scientific medicine would be the first to locate medical practice entirely in the body. The affliction and its cure were to be sought here, and nowhere else. From henceforth, they decreed, medicine should be a scientific rather than a religious practice. Yet at the outset this was only the initial inkling, the way forward.

This change in medicine was part of a more widespread process. Why this crucial development in human evolution took place, and why it took place where it did, remains a matter of conjecture. The loosening of religious autocracy, diet, climate, cultural diversity, individualism and leisure for speculation – all probably played their part. The Ancient Greeks first began to liberate the western mind from the superstitions and myths of previous metaphysics around the middle of the sixth century BC. The Greek scientific mindset would be optimistic rather than fatalistic: the unpredictable gods would gradually be dethroned in favour of purely human endeavour. The Ancient Greeks' belief in reason and an essentially materialistic functional approach would be the belief upon which our western civilization has grown: the belief in rational scientific practice. It is difficult to overstress the enormity of that great advance made over two and a half thousand years ago. No less than the hitherto unthinkable – the wilful ignoring and defiance of the gods who ruled the earth – was necessary for humanity to come into its own. The new outlook first manifested itself in the origins of Greek philosophy, which included 'natural philosophy', or what we now call science. Yet it would take almost a century before this outlook permeated the more peripheral practice of medicine.

Hippocrates is generally regarded as the father of medicine as we now understand it. He was born on the Aegean island of Cos around 460 BC. To this day, in the square of the island's main town, there is a large and very ancient gnarled plane tree, in the shade of which Hippocrates is said to have conducted his practice. Like this tree, much else related to Hippocrates is legendary. Little is known for certain about his life, though a few stories recur in the different sources. He probably visited Egypt and Babylon, where he became acquainted with ancient medical wisdom. According to another story, he was summoned across the Aegean by the worried citizens of Abdera, who were concerned that their local philosopher, the celebrated Democritus, had finally succumbed to madness. Hippocrates was led beyond the gates of the city, where he found Democritus sitting alone beneath a tree roaring with laughter. After talking with Democritus, Hippocrates returned to inform the citizens that their philosopher was not mad, he simply could not stop laughing at the folly of the world.

Around seventy treatises have survived which bear Hippocrates' name. These are in a variety of styles, and date from a period stretching over a hundred years. Many of these may well be authentic, but the majority were evidently written by the pupils of Hippocrates' renowned school. By the time Hippocrates died around 377 BC he was famous throughout the Greek world. He is mentioned twice by his contemporary Plato, who describes him as having a philosophical approach to medicine. This is only true in so far as Hippocrates was a 'natural philosopher': his attitude was strictly scientific, rather than what we would call philosophical. Hippocrates specifically sought to disengage medicine from the influence of religion and the theoretical speculations of philosophy. In his own words: 'The first thing to remember is that the study of wisdom [philosophy] is a separate discipline from medicine.' What Plato may well have implied was that Hippocrates treated the human body as a whole, and studied it in the context of the world it inhabited.

Besides being holistic, Hippocrates' approach was founded on the treatment of the patient, rather than dealing with specific illnesses. This is an important distinction: the emphasis is on active cure, rather than the conceptualization of disease as a specific entity. The emphasis on practice, rather than learning, would prove crucial in the characterization and development of medicine as a whole. Its influence is still evident to this day. (It is quite possible that medicine could have evolved very differently. Imagine, for instance, if it had proceeded with the same methodology as the law, with its inclination to precedent rather than practitioners relying upon their own judgement.) Despite this emphasis on practice, Hippocrates favoured refraining from intervention with the patient. Where possible, the curative powers of nature should be allowed to follow their course. In fact, the treatment of the body as a whole, rather than any emphasis upon investigating particular illness, made a virtue of necessity. Medical knowledge was still far too scant for specific diagnosis and the prescription of particular remedies. Such practice also took into account the reality of the physician's precarious social role. For the most part, a practising physician in Ancient Greece was little more than a travelling wise man, who took up temporary residence in one place before moving on to another. Under such circumstances, failure could prove fatal to more than the patient. In his writings, Hippocrates firmly counsels against treating any patient whose overall state is deemed beyond cure. The physician had to recognize the right moment to continue hastily on his travels.

Aside from such diplomatic niceties, the great innovative aspect which defines Hippocrates' approach – and that of his pupils and followers – is his appeal to reason, rather than to supernatural powers. In this aspect, all medical treatment prior to Hippocrates can be considered prehistoric. (Though inevitably, aspects of this irrational era would linger on.) It was Hippocrates who introduced the new Greek method of thinking to medicine. One of the central tenets of the Greek world was: 'Nothing in excess.' Hippocrates taught that illness was caused by an imbalance in the body, caused by some excess. Disease was literally 'dis-ease'. This was why the body had to be treated as a whole. Disease was caused by an imbalance of the body's fluids, which had to be rectified. Yet surely this was just another unfounded belief?

On the contrary. Here Hippocrates was not just replacing one set of metaphysics with another. Like the earlier Greek philosophers, his theory was deduced from practical observation. A century or so previously, the first philosopher Thales had deduced that the world was made of water. He was led to this conclusion by seeing water in springs literally springing from the earth, from whence it flowed to the sea where it condensed into clouds, the clouds then deposited rain, which was in turn absorbed by the earth. This cyclical process provided convincing reasons for Thales to believe that ultimately all things consisted of water.

Similar careful observation led Hippocrates to a similar conclusion: liquid was the source of life. He theorized that all living things owed their life to the fluids or sap they contained. Without sap, plants died – they withered and dried up. The same was true of human beings: rotting cadavers leaked liquids and eventually became dry skeletons. But the human body was more complex than a plant; it contained a variety of fluids. These he called *chymoi*, from which our word 'humour' derives. The human body contained four 'humours', all of which flowed from its orifices as part of its natural functioning. These were blood, phlegm, black bile and yellow bile. They could appear when the body was healthy (menstruation, nosebleed); or they could spill out when the body suffered from imbalance and excess, becoming ill (vomited bile, runny nose). The illness was caused by an excess of one particular fluid accumulating in one part of the body. Of the humours, bile and phlegm were particularly associated with illness, and soon flowed as an indication of sickness.

The humours were also affected by the seasons. Cold wet winters produced an excess of phlegm, which caused colds. Hot summers produced more bile, which could lead to diarrhoea. Excessive heat could even cause the bile in the brain to boil, resulting in mania. According to Hippocrates: 'The blood in the body reaches its lowest level in autumn.' This is when bile is liable to predominate, causing its own characteristic diseases, such as melancholy or apathy. At all times, hot fever may be caused by an excess of blood. Such imbalance can be remedied by drawing off some blood from the body. This was the origin and justification for a tradition of blood-letting which would persist for over two millennia, with the use of medical leeches only dying out just over a century ago.

Illness often arose from excessive behaviour: overindulgence in wine, overeating, exhilaration, sloth, and so forth. The balance of the body could be restored by regulated diet, exercise, gentle bathing, sleep or sex. In common with Greek thinking (ancient and modern) Hippocrates placed great emphasis on sex. Participation in this activity should be varied according to age and season. 'During the months of winter sexual activity should be more frequent.' Also: 'Older men should have sexual intercourse more often than younger men,' according to what is probably one of his later writings.

All diseases had material causes, and could thus be cured by material means. Hippocrates even sought to diagnose and suggest a cure for epilepsy, which was known as the 'sacred disease'. Previous accounts diagnosed the victim as suffering from 'possession' by spirits – a highly plausible explanation, given the symptoms of the disease and the belief system of the period. Hippocrates boldly proposed his own account, in line with his humoral theory. He conjectured that epileptics suffered from an excess of phlegm. This blocked the passages where air was transmitted in breathing. An epileptic fit was nothing more than the body struggling to free its passages from this strangulating effect. Hippocrates' explanation is as poetically convincing as the previous spiritual explanation – but significantly it provides a material explanation which indicates a possible cure. It also lays itself open to material disproof: a vital element of the new scientific thinking. Metaphysical explanations could never be *proved* wrong (any more than they could be proved correct.) With a material explanation, wrong answers could be *shown* to be wrong, and eliminated. Crucially, such thinking allowed for progress. In the origins of western thinking lay the seeds of its vast development.

On the other hand, Hippocrates' approach to medicine also contained certain crucial defects. For a start, it relied upon surface medicine: the health of the body was judged by its appearance and the fluid it emitted. This was an understandable shortcoming, when physicians were unable to practise exploratory dissection on cadavers, which was regarded as violating the sanctity of the human body. Similarly, Hippocrates' concentration upon bodily imbalance took no account of infectious disease. Here was a surprising omission. The historian Thucydides, writing of the plague which devastated Athens in 430 BC, was well aware that this disease was contagious. He even gave a highly accurate description of the symptoms – authenticated by his catching the disease himself – which he recorded expressly 'so that it may be regarded by medical men if it recurs'. Hippocrates certainly visited Athens during the following century, and must have been aware of this record. Indeed, one legend even has him saving Athens from a plague in 340 BC – using preventative measures which betray a knowledge of its contagious nature. However, this tale is probably just that. The fact is, Hippocrates' humoral theory takes no account of transmitted diseases.

Another severe defect relates to the humours themselves. Hippocrates conjectured that each of the humours was produced by a particular organ. Blood was produced by the heart, phlegm by the brain, yellow bile by the liver, and black bile by the spleen. An excess of black bile was said to darken the blood and the faeces, and to appear in vomit. (To this day, we still speak of feeling bilious.) Its appearance was invariably ominous of disease. But the fact is, black bile does not exist, whether produced by the spleen or any other organ. So how did Hippocrates account for it? Curiously, he even describes it in some detail. He speaks of it frothing when it fell to earth; it was also said to burn things with which it came into contact. Such reports suggest an acidic content. These mythical properties ascribed to black bile outside the body are presumably just an exaggeration of genuinely felt internal experiences.

Hippocrates' central medical theory sought to redress humoral imbalance by treatment with opposites. The nature of acids and neutralizing alkalis had yet to be discovered; yet the sensation of burning juices in the stomach (now known to be acidic), and their cure by certain specific substances, especially plants (now known to be alkaline) had been understood since *Homo sapiens*' upright stance first encouraged indigestion. (Animals often instinctively gravitate towards such curatives –

as seen when cats experience the need to chew grass.) The effectiveness of these cures would presumably have confirmed Hippocrates in his erroneous notion of black bile. And if black bile had simply been a conceptualization to account for a number of unpleasant internal effects, this would not have mattered so much. However, it was a lot more than this. It was a central concept in his whole idea of bodily health: it completed the necessary balance in the humoral scheme of things. In this aspect, Hippocrates' humoral theory is severely flawed and falls short of his embryonic scientific approach.

However, Hippocrates is best remembered today for his celebrated Oath, which for many centuries had to be taken by all medical students before they could qualify as doctors. This contains many features which remain to this day definitive of the medical profession. (The very name profession originally referred to someone who 'professed' to an oath.) As part of the Hippocratic Oath, the future doctor swore 'to use my power to help the sick to the best of my ability'. Unlike other professions, doctors are still expected to give readily and freely of their abilities if they are present at an emergency. (Imagine a theatre where there is a dispute between an actor and the management over his contract, and someone appears in front of the curtain to ask: 'Is there a lawyer in the house?') Conversely, it must indeed have been a sobering moment for many hell-raising medical students when they were required to swear: 'I will be chaste and religious in my life and in my practice.' The Hippocratic Oath also instituted the notion of professional secrecy: 'Whatever I see or hear, professionally or privately, which ought not to be divulged, I will keep secret and tell no one.' It goes on: 'I will not cut, even for the stone, but I will leave such procedures to the practitioners of that craft.' Such practical tasks were considered inferior: the true physician used only knowledge and thought. This formalized the separation between physicians and surgeons. The very word surgeon derives from the Greek words *cheiros* meaning 'hand', and *ergon* meaning 'work'. For centuries to come, physicians would consider themselves superior to surgeons. Although this imbalance has now been redressed, it still accounts for certain anomalies. For instance, in Britain a physician is granted the title 'doctor', whereas a surgeon, who must also be a qualified physician, likes to distinguish himself from a mere doctor by being addressed as 'mister'.

Somewhat more controversial contemporary effects of the Hippocratic Oath are seen in the declaration: 'I will not give a fatal draught to anyone if I am asked, nor will I suggest any such thing. Neither will I give a woman means to procure an abortion.' However, just because the founding ethos of scientific medicine forbade euthanasia and abortion, is no reason why these practices should remain anathema. After all, how many doctors over the past two thousand years have chosen to disregard the 'chaste and religious' clause without feeling the need to abandon their calling?

In many ways as interesting is Hippocrates' *Aphorisms*. This begins with resonant wisdom: 'Life is short, art is long; opportunity elusive, experience fallacious, and judgement difficult.' Artists putting their trust in posthumous fame are particularly fond of the opening assertion. In fact, the art referred to here is the art of medicine: 'science' would be a more accurate translation. The *Aphorisms* are mainly confined to medical remarks, and contain the usual mixture of the insightful, the insipid and the idiotic, which is common to the aphoristic form. Each reader will find his own favourites. 'A woman is never ambidextrous.' 'People who lisp are especially prone to prolonged diarrhoea.' And the inevitable topic: 'People who are bald do not suffer from varicose veins, while should someone who is bald develop such veins, then his hair grows again.'

Hippocrates marked a distinct new start in medicine. Yet the metamorphosis from magic to the beginnings of a real science would continue over two or three centuries. The shrines to Asclepius flourished alongside Hippocratic practice. Even the Hippocratic Oath opens with an appeal to the gods and Asclepius: 'I swear by Apollo the healer, by Aesculapius [sic], by Health and all the powers of healing . . .' Surprisingly, in the light of Hippocrates' warning against philosophy, the next major contribution to medicine would come from a philosopher.

Aristotle's philosophy was to dominate all spheres of western thought for almost two thousand years to come. Initially an inspiration to scientific method, it would eventually become a stranglehold, restricting innovative thought while reducing speculation to empty formalism and appeal to his 'authority'. But Aristotle should not be held responsible for the sins committed in his name. Such domination could only have been achieved by one of the supreme intellects of all time, whose thought ranged through almost all spheres of learning known to the ancient world. In many cases, Aristotle's treatises were the founding works in new fields, ranging from aesthetics to zoology. However, his consummate contribution is generally taken to be the invention of logic.

Aristotle was born at Stagira in northern Greece in 384 BC, just seven years before the death of Hippocrates. Aristotle's father was court physician to the king of Macedonia, and may even have learned his trade at the feet of Hippocrates. Aristotle's initiation into higher learning was almost certainly through the Hippocratic works in the possession of his father. As a young man, Aristole travelled south to Athens, where he studied at Plato's Academy, quickly establishing himself as Plato's most distinguished pupil. Following Plato's death in 347 BC he left Athens in a huff, after being passed over for the post of principal of the Academy. Later, he was employed at the court of the benign eunuch tyrant Hermias, who ruled over the city of Assos on the northwest coast of Asia Minor. Hermias was so impressed by Aristotle that he even offered the middle-aged philosopher his sister Pythias as a wife. This was presumably an offer which Aristotle could not refuse: despite this he remained happily married to Pythias for the rest of his life. In a treatise on marriage he even covertly used his own marriage as an exemplar of how this often difficult institution should be conducted.

Aristotle may have been Plato's best-known pupil, but his interpretation of Plato's philosophy to all intents and purposes turned it upside down. Plato had believed in the supreme reality of abstract ideas, with the world as mere appearance constructed out of these ideas. Aristotle rejected this essentially oriental metaphysical approach; for him, it was the world which was reality. His philosophy would always remain grounded in scientific fact. His early reading of Hippocratic texts had laid the foundations of his thought: every symptom implied its own form of illness. Out of this approach came his invention of logic. Likewise, it led him to believe that everything in the world had its own specific purpose. As he put it: 'Nature does nothing in vain.' From the petals of plants, to the antennae of animals, to the organs of human beings – each had its allotted function, its purpose. These could be classified in groups according to distinct resemblances. The hoof looked like a simple claw, which in turn became more complex in the form of the hand. (It is fascinating to watch Aristotle edging uncannily close to the idea of evolution.) All this could be discovered by patient observation and rational pondering. In the same way, it could be surmised that each organ in the human body played its part in the purpose of the whole. Logic and function were the key to much of his philosophy, and this also characterized his approach to medicine.

Like Hippocrates, Aristotle was a great believer in observation. But unlike Hippocrates he also carried out dissections, though these appear to have been conducted largely on animals. In this way, Arisotle discovered the network of veins which extends from the heart throughout the body. Unfortunately he discerned no difference between the veins and the arteries, an oversight which would severely handicap later investigations that relied upon his authority. Aristotle's study of how the embryonic chick develops inside the egg led him to a further vital, but flawed, conclusion. He noted that the first sign of life within the embryo was the appearance, after four days, of the beating heart. From this he deduced that the heart was the life-giving organ of the body. Here evidently was the location of the soul, which registered all sensation and was the instigator of thought and movement in the body. He concluded that the heart and its orifices 'are the springs of man's existence; from them spread throughout his body those rivers with which his mortal habitation is irrigated, those rivers which bring life to man as well, for if they ever dry up, then man dies.'

At this point Aristotle's explanation becomes unclear. He states that the heart produces life-giving heat, which is carried by the blood, suggesting that heat rather than moisture is the vital provider of life. And his consequent physiology appears to support this latter view. He then goes on to state that the near-boiling turbulence of the blood produces the pulsing of the veins. Meanwhile the air inhaled by the lungs serves to cool the blood. This accounts for why the air exhaled by the lungs is invariably warmer than the air inhaled. Such ingenuity is marred by yet another serious oversight. His dissections evidently failed to detect the presence of the nervous system, which extends from the brain throughout the body to the nerve-endings. However, if all organs had a purpose, as he believed, what was the purpose of the brain? Aristotle concluded that 'it tempers the heat and seething of the heart': the brain also cooled the blood, and served to regulate its turbulence.

Aristotle's natural philosophy was based upon the four elements theory, which had already been current for almost a century. According to this theory the world, and everything in it, consisted of a mixture of earth, air, fire and water. This theory was less simplistic than at first appears. Aristotle's early acquaintance with Hippocratic medicine had led him to be more concerned with the qualities exhibited by bodies, rather than their ultimate constituents. For him, all things appeared to contain a mixture of solidity (as exhibited by earth), airiness (air), heat (fire) and liquidity (water). In terms of tactile and visual experimentation this classification makes considerable sense.

Unfortunately, this error was further compounded when Aristotle adopted an idea which Greek culture had inherited from oriental metaphysics. This was the idea that the microcosm reflected the macrocosm: the inner world, the smaller world, echoed the larger world around it. The elements of the body echoed the elements of the world. According to Aristotle, the workings of the human body could be explained in terms of the basic four elements which constituted the natural world. The heart contained heat and liquidity. The cooling brain was made up of cold earth and moist water. This even appeared to be confirmed by scientific experience. In the course of a somewhat gruesome experiment, Aristotle discovered that when the brain was heated in a pot it gave off steam (water), and solid matter (earth) remained.

The idea of the microcosm mirroring the macrocosm would recur frequently through the ensuing centuries. It was invariably a sign of theory overcoming practice, tying up loose ends in an aesthetically pleasing symbolic picture. In science, such comparisons *can* yield imaginative insights, but the extension of this method of thought into a coherent system belongs to religion and art, rather than science. Science never manages to tie up all the loose ends in any particular detective story. Indeed, it is the discovery of these loose ends which leads to the next detective story.

In 342 BC Aristotle was summoned by the king of Macedonia to become tutor to his teenage son Alexander. Upon completing one's education, one should be prepared to confront the world. Aristotle's headstrong pupil appears to have taken this somewhat literally, and set off to conquer the world. As a result of this megalomaniac enterprise he would become known as Alexander the Great. Aristotle now returned to Athens, where he founded his own school, the Lyceum. The facilities at the Lyceum soon began to outshine those at the rival Academy, which was being run by Plato's followers. Eventually the Lyceum even had its own zoo, containing exotic animals sent to Aristotle by Alexander during his campaigns. The vast collection of scrolls which Aristotle had collected – and written – during his lifetime formed the Lyceum's library, generally acknowledged as first great library to be assembled in a private (rather than royal or temple) collection. After Aristotle's death in 322 BC, these scrolls would become the core of the greatest library in the classical era at Alexandria.

The Library at Alexandria and its attached Museum (literally 'place of the muses') is estimated to have contained nearly 70,000 scrolls at its prime. Scholars from all over the Greek world, and later the Roman Empire, came to study here. This was where Euclid compiled his *Elements*, which would remain the definitive work on geometry until the nineteenth century; this was where Archimedes, one of the supreme mathematicians of all time, first learned the rudiments of

his subject. It would also produce two great medical figures –
Herophilus and his pupil Erasistratus.

Previously Greek learning had inherited a number of historical oriental concepts; in Alexandria it encountered some of the
darker oriental and African arts which continued to flourish.
These included *khemeia*, practices derived from the Ancient
Egyptian embalming of the dead, which centuries later would
evolve into the practices of *al-khemeia* (alchemy). Another,
related, practice included a heritage of expertise in substances
which affected the living body – from poisons to narcotics.
(The lotus, so prominent in Ancient Egyptian wall carvings, is
now thought to depict an ancient narcotic strain of this plant
which produced beatific hallucinations.)

Allied with Greek medical understanding of the body, such
knowledge often became adapted to scientific use. This produced a significant advance in the understanding of medicine.
But the biggest factor in the advance of Alexandrian medicine
was largely fortuitous. Embalming involved operating on
cadavers, of which the Greeks had no knowledge because
such practice was taboo. But Plato's idealist philosophy was
becoming increasingly pervasive, especially amongst mathematicians and some natural philosophers. According to Plato
it was only the soul which was sacred – not the body, which
was mere appearance. As a result, in Alexandria dissection was
eventually permitted, for the only brief period during the entire
classical era. And, aided by the anatomical knowledge and
preservative practices of *khemeia*, it flourished. The dissections
carried out by Herophilus and Erasistratus would enable them
to discover secrets of human anatomy which could have been
found in no other way. Such discoveries would lead them both
to profound theoretical speculations about how the human
body worked.

Quite what these dissections involved remains problematic.

The Roman encyclopedist Celsus, writing some three centuries later, is quite certain that Alexandrian physicians 'cut open the bodies of the dead'. But he goes on to mention claims that 'Herophilus and Erasistratus did this in the best way by far. They cut open criminals received out of the King's prisons, and they studied, whilst the breath of life remained in them, the things which nature had hitherto concealed.' Whether this involved actual vivisection, or simply dissection of the recently executed, remains unclear.

Herophilus was born around 330 BC at Chalcedon on the Asian shore of the Bosphorus. He appears to have studied at the Hippocratic school in Cos before moving on to Alexandria. The pioneering investigations he carried on here have led many to regard him as the father of anatomy. In the course of detailed dissection of the eye, he discovered and described the light-sensitive inner coating of the eyeball which we now call the retina. He identified the section of the small intestine which leaves the stomach, naming it the duodenum because it was twelve (Greek *duodeka*) finger-widths in length. He also discovered the gland at the head of the male sexual organs, which he named the prostate (from the Greek for 'stands before').

Even more importantly, he questioned Aristotle's view that the heart was the centre of feeling and perception. Herophilus' careful dissections led him to discover that the nerves led to the brain. He also recognized the importance of the pulse in diagnosis. He is said to have measured the pulse with a portable water clock, taking account of four different aspects: rate, rhythm, size and strength.

His pupil Erasistratus was born on the eastern Aegean island of Chios around 300 BC. According to one tradition, he was the grandson of Aristotle, but this seems unlikely. He extended Herophilus' investigation of the nervous system, noting that there were in fact two different types of nerve, which entered the spinal cord at separate points. In this way, he established the difference between sensory nerves (which relay impressions from the senses) and motor nerves (which are reponsible for bodily motions). Like many of Herophilus' followers he believed that the nerve was hollow, and conducted 'nervous spirit'. Acting upon Herophilus' recognition of the importance of the brain, he carried out a series of careful anatomical examinations. These led him to discover that the brain consisted of the large cerebrum, which enclosed the smaller cerebellum. Studies of human and animal brains prompted him to the highly perceptive conclusion that the more complex folds of the human brain were indications of its greater intelligence. He also surmised that the lungs absorbed *pneuma*, or air (as in pneumatic), which then passed into the arteries. He believed that only the veins contained blood. He likened the heart and its motions to the bellows used by a blacksmith. When blood spurted from a severed artery, the air first escaped, and then the blood rushed in, forced on by the bellows of the heart.

Further investigations led him to conclude that the stomach digested food by grinding it into fragments. This prompted him to tackle the problem of digestion, which he did with a series of carefully controlled experiments on chickens. He noted that the chickens consumed a greater weight of food than they excreted, and suggested that this loss of matter was due to 'insensible perspiration'. He is also credited with the invention of the catheter (from the Greek 'to probe'), the slender tube-like instrument used for drawing urine from the bladder.

From all this it is easy to see with hindsight that Erasistratus was on the brink of a number of important discoveries – especially with regard to circulation, respiration and digestion. His further understanding was hampered by the current primitive notions of biological process. Nonetheless, he might in time have overcome even these difficulties had he not taken his own life around 250 BC, when he discovered he had incurable cancer.

Not long after this the tide of opinion turned against the use of human bodies for medical investigation, and once again dissection became taboo. After a brief period of great scientific advance, medicine was once again forced to adopt an essentially behaviourist stance. What went on inside the human body could only be conjectured from its external behaviour, or by analogy from animal anatomy. As a result, theory would return with a vengeance, severely hampering medical science for the next one and a half millennia.

2
A TRADITION IS BORN

One man, more than any other, was responsible for the medical theory which would establish a stranglehold over practice during the coming eras. Ironically, he was also the greatest clinical practitioner, pioneer and medical thinker of his age, gathering and systematizing much of the medical learning that had accumulated during the classical era, as well as making untold vital contributions of his own.

By the time Galen was born in AD 129, the Greek world had been absorbed into the Roman Empire for almost three centuries. His birthplace, the city of Pergamum on the western hinterland of Asia Minor, was one of the most prosperous and beautiful in the entire eastern Mediterranean. At its height, it had a population of nearly a quarter of a million, over a dozen pillared marble temples, a famous altar to Zeus, and a library second only to that at Alexandria. (The latter, jealous of its rival, eventually banned the export of Egyptian papyrus for making scrolls. To overcome this, the Pergamum librarians invented *Pergamena charta*, which became known by a corruption of this name as parchment.) To this day, Pergamum's steep hillside amphitheatre, once capable of seating 10,000 spectators, offers a breathtaking view out over the littoral plain towards the distant blue Aegean. Below, beside a river amidst the fields, stand the ruins of the shrine to Asclepius, at whose renowned medical school Galen was educated.

Galen was born into the family of a rich architect, who according to his son was 'a calm, wise and kindly man'. His mother, on the other hand, 'would sometimes become so enraged that she bit her serving maids, and was always shouting at my father'. From an early age, Galen was educated impartially in the four leading philosophies: Platonism, Aristotelianism, Epicurianism and Stoicism. In view of life at home, the latter was probably the most useful. According to legend, when Galen was 16 his father was visited by Asclepius in a dream, and informed that his son should study medicine. Galen was duly enrolled at the school attached to the local shrine of Asclepius. At the time, this shrine and its medical school had such a reputation for healing that it attracted rich and famous figures from all over the Roman Empire. The sight of these distinguished visitors would have a lasting effect on the impressionable young Galen. He quickly grasped that there was an even larger and more powerful world far beyond the dreams of provincial Pergamum. Galen proved an exceptionally gifted student, and soon knew all that his masters had to teach him. He then travelled across the Mediterranean to Alexandria, still the magnet of learning. But the city proved a disappointment, and Galen soon became contemptuous of his lecturers, especially their chief Julianos, whom he referred to as 'the leader of a pack of braying donkeys'. Modesty and reticence would never feature high on Galen's list of qualities.

In AD 157, at the age of 27, he returned to Pergamum determined to demonstrate his exceptional talents to the full.

The shrine of Asclepius at Pergamum had become so prosperous that its high priest even kept his own troupe of gladiators, who staged contests at the great city amphitheatre. (On other occasions, the valley floor would be flooded, and great naval battles between triremes, rowed by hundreds of galley slaves, would be staged.) Galley slaves were dispensable, but gladiators were a different matter. A prize gladiator took years of coaching, and would often become a star in his own right. Galen was appointed chief physician to the high priest's prize gladiators, a post with considerable prestige and opportunity. Healing the gruesome wounds of his patients would require all his skills, yet the experience he gained here would prove invaluable. Dissection of human bodies was still banned, but this would prove a useful substitute. Not often does a physician have a chance to treat patients who obligingly perform their own dissections on one another.

Galen honed his technique, at the same time covertly extending his understanding of human anatomy. His job also required him to nurse his 'gang of brutes' back to a state where they could return to the arena. As a result, he quickly built up an expertise in healing medicines, dressings, dietary formulas and exercise techniques. Although such medical specializations were barely recognized, and it would be centuries before their names were even coined, we can see that Galen was by now gaining an understanding which ranged throughout medical practice. Already he had a grasp of what is now recognized as anatomy, as well as physiology (the function of the bodily organs), surgery, pathology (the changes in the body caused by illness), and pharmacology (drugs and medicines). Here was the consummate physician, quite unhindered by any snobbish Hippocratic distinctions between theory and operational practice.

Yet at the same time Galen had pretensions of his own: he wanted to become more than just a doctor. He dreamed of his medical expertise leading to even greater fame as a philosopher and writer of great literature. In between his heavy duties at the gladiator school he still found time to continue with his philosophical studies, becoming particularly influenced by Aristotle and his wide-ranging scientific ideas. From this period also dates the start of Galen's writing career. He now began composing literary treatises on medical and philosophical topics.

At the age of 32, Galen decided to take the plunge and set off to seek his fortune in Rome. Here, surely, he would be able to give full rein to his ambitions. Rome was at the apex of its glory, the capital of an empire that stretched from northern Britain to southern Egypt, covering the whole of North Africa and stretching as far east as Syria. The statesmanlike, philosophically minded Marcus Aurelius was co-emperor with his incompetent adoptive brother Lucius Verus, and in many ways their joint rule epitomized the strengths and weaknesses of the Empire.

Greek learning had long been fashionable among the Roman upper classes, despite the fact that it was condemned by the influential writer Pliny the Elder as 'effete luxury'. Greek physicians played a prominent role in Roman medical practice. Many were of Hippocratic probity, but there was also a high percentage of flamboyant charlatans and quacks who profited hugely from their antics. In consequence, a popular anti-Greek graffito in Rome during this period expressed the last words of Alexander the Great: 'I am dying from too many physicians.'

Galen's arrival in Rome during AD 162 pitched him into a lucrative but problematic market. Beginning as he meant to continue, he gambled on renting a house of some splendour to impress his future clients; he then set about giving a series of sensational public dissections of animals. At these, he wowed the audience with spectacular demonstrations of his skill and learning, which he was confident none could match. Carrying out a vivisection on a squealing pig, he severed its nerves one by one. He then silenced it by tying off the exposed laryngeal nerve. In this way he dramatically proved his contention that the voice was operated from the brain. His performances – for this is what they were – attracted a number of influential citizens. So impressed were they by his confident expertise that they soon began to employ him.

As Galen's prestige grew, so did his self-esteem. 'It is I, and I alone, who have revealed the true path of medicine,' he declared. At the same time, he launched into a prolific output of treatises, claiming that Hippocrates had 'only given intimations of what I have achieved in reality'. Galen may have been convinced that he knew everything there was to know, but he evidently felt the need for a tactical display of philosophic modesty. So he began attending lectures by the fashionable Aristotelian philosopher Eudemus, who surprisingly took quite a liking to his brash and brilliant pupil. When Eudemus fell ill, Galen devoted his full powers to curing the philosopher, who gratefully introduced him to many of his influential friends, among whom was Marcus Aurelius. Galen responded with alacrity, doubtless displaying his exceptional powers to the full, and was soon established as physician to the emperor's court. In between times he continued to produce treatises, sometimes dictating so long and furiously that he exhausted a succession of scribes. His medical treatises were laced with perceptive philosophical remarks, such as: 'Always be wary when dealing with the philosophical ideas of contemporaries.' However, this high tone was on occasion lowered by diatribes against his medical competitors: 'He attempts in stupid – I might say insane – language, to contradict what he knows nothing about . . . their darling prejudices . . . another piece of nonsense . . . Therefore we must suppose that he was either mad, or entirely unacquainted with practical medicine.' The practices of his rivals are rubbished in some detail, not only on account of their medical ineptitude, but also their logical inconsistencies and moral dubiousness. Not surprisingly, Galen is known to have had few friends outside his own professional practice.

Then suddenly Galen departed from Rome in AD 166. It has been suggested that his long-suffering enemies had endured enough and were about to take matters into their own hands. However, a more likely explanation was an outbreak of plague, which was brought to Rome by Verus' legions arriving back from the war in Mesopotamia. Galen returned to Pergamum, but a couple of years later he was summoned back to Rome. Marcus Aurelius appointed him as physician to his young son and heir Commodius. Galen was to look after him while Marcus Aurelius was away conducting his campaigns against the Germanic tribes beyond the Danube.

It was during this period that Marcus Aurelius – in between butchering barbarians – composed the contemplative musings which were to win him dubious philosophical fame. One cannot help wondering if perhaps he had Galen in mind when he admiringly quoted Epicurus, 'Do not allow physicians to become puffed up with their own inflated opinion of themselves,' adding his own caution, 'When you are ill do not be drawn into gossiping with the ignorant people who attend you, but instead pay close attention only to what is being done to you and the instrument which is being used to do it.' Galen's much-vaunted skill as a public vivisectionist of squealing pigs may not have inspired confidence in all his patients.

In AD 180 Marcus Aurelius fell ill during one of his campaigns. Instead of returning to Rome to be treated by the self-professed 'true path of medicine', he made the mistake of retiring to nearby Vindobona (Vienna). Here he soon died at the hands of an early exemplar of the long line of distinguished quacks from this city. Marcus Aurelius was succeeded by his son Commodus, who was now 19 years old. Commodus is described by Galen's biographer George Sarton as 'an athletic brute, regarding himself as the reincarnation of Hercules, being inordinately proud of his muscular strength in the hunting of wild beasts . . . extravagant and infamous.' One can't help wondering how much Galen had to do with this. He had been in charge Commodus' health and upbringing since he was six years old. Had Galen perhaps applied some of his expertise as a gladiator trainer to the education of the young emperor? This is no idle question, for a few years later Commodus began turning up at the circus in Rome in his capacity as emperor and then insisting upon taking part in the games themselves as a gladiator. Much to the delight of the Roman people, and the horror of their senators, this soon became a regular spectacle. According to the *Cambridge Ancient History*: 'On one occasion he killed a hundred lions with a hundred javelins.' When Commodus took to decapitating ostriches, the senators decided that this was going too far and attempted to poison him. Galen was an expert in toxins, but he was certainly not involved in this plot – for the poison failed, and the conspirators had to bring in an athlete, whom Commodus had recently appointed governor of Syria, to strangle him.

Such details give an indication of the dangerous milieu in which Galen operated, and somehow continued to operate. Yet despite his overweening sense of his own brilliance and his arrogant ability to make enemies all around him, Galen miraculously survived. In the end he would serve as physician to no less than four emperors, during one of Rome's most decadent and treacherous periods. Such an ability speaks of considerable political skills – or luck. Or perhaps he simply managed to convince all parties that he was so pre-eminent as a physician that they just couldn't afford to be without him.

Whichever way, he continued in his post as the emperor's physician, at the same time producing yet further treatises at a prolific rate. Indeed, it has been suggested that Galen owes much of his fame to the sheer volume of his output. This is certainly unjust, but it seems that Galen was taking no chances with posterity. The extent of his extraordinary output can be gauged by the following piece of history. In AD 192 the Temple of Peace in Rome burned down. Galen's nearby house on the Appian Way was also destroyed in the conflagration, and with it much of his collection of scrolls, many of which contained the sole versions of his own works. Yet nearly two millennia later, having survived the consequent sacking of Rome and the Dark Ages, over 350 titles by Galen survive, covering more than 10,000 pages.

What these contain is a priceless legacy. So what exactly did Galen say? What was so important about his work? Galen's anatomical discoveries were severely hampered by the taboo on human dissection. Apart from mutually inflicted gladiatorial dissections, he had little chance to examine the inside of the human body. Such occasions that did present themselves were ghoulish and unpropitious. He mentions examining human bodies 'on the breaking open of a tomb or grave'. He gives a vivid example: 'Once a river, innundating a recently made grave, broke it up and swept away the body of the dead man. The flesh had putrefied, but the bones still held together in their proper relations.'

Otherwise he gained his anatomical knowledge from the dissection of pigs, dogs and goats. He mentions once dissecting the heart of an elephant – presumably after its demise in the circus. But his preferred subject for dissection was the barbary ape, whose anatomy he felt sure must closely resemble that of human beings. Galen's dissections must have been extremely careful and precise, for he made some remarkable discoveries.

His knowledge of bone structure and musculature was un-paralleled in the classical world. This was further enhanced by his belief in Aristotle's teleology: the notion that everything has a purpose. Galen concurred that each part of the body was designed to perform a particular function. Even the smallest bones in the hands and feet were there for a purpose, and every muscle was contrived for its own specific mechanical action. Similarly each organ could be characterized by its function. What Aristotle had largely surmised, Galen actually investigated: what had been a picture in the mind became a picture in the flesh. His investigations banished once and for all the lingering belief in Aristotle's theory that the mind or soul resided in the heart (though neither he nor any of his successors would ever manage to purge this heartfelt belief from our language). Once again using the public dissection of a pig, Galen demonstrated the function of the kidneys. By tying the ureters, the tubes which lead from the kidneys to the bladder, he was able to show that urine is produced by the kidneys, not the bladder, as had previously been believed. His teleological outlook would pave the way to many discoveries, as well as proving highly beneficial to effective treatment.

Galen's examinations of cross-sections of several animal spines enabled him to theorize concerning nervous control of the muscles. During his investigations of various skulls he managed to distinguish seven varieties of cranial nerve. Such discoveries would prove invaluable to his long line of successors. But alas, such would be his authority that his anatomical mistakes would also prove equally influential. Most notable of these was his identification of the *rete mirabile* (marvellous net) of blood vessels, which is situated beneath the brain in hoofed animals – but not in humans, as Galen conjectured. The *rete mirabile* would feature in textbooks of the human anatomy until well into the Renaissance.

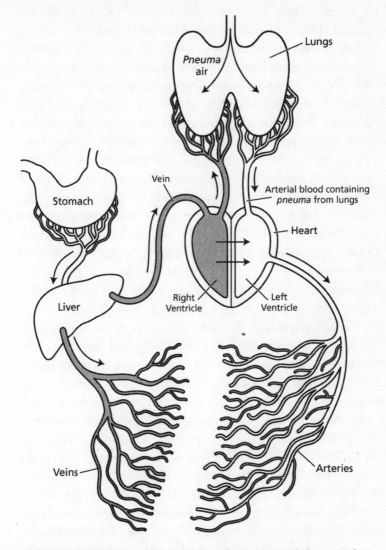

Figure 1. Galen's two blood systems: the venous and the arterial
Dark venous blood is created in the liver and passes through
the central wall of the heart to mix with *pneuma* from the lungs
and become arterial blood. At the ends of the veins and arteries,
the blood is 'consumed' by the flesh.

Galen's other investigations of blood vessels reveal his genius. His explanations for what he found were utterly rational and convincing, as well as being backed by considerable experimental evidence. He discovered that veins and arteries are *structurally* different, and also that arteries carry blood. Erasistratus had claimed that the arteries carried only *pneuma*, or air, absorbed from the lungs. Galen showed that they contained blood, and suspected that the *pneuma* was somehow dissolved in the blood – an astonishingly prescient insight. Of similar importance was his discovery that the blood in the arteries was scarlet, while that in the veins was purplish. But this led him to conclude that the body contained two entirely separate blood systems. Galen was convinced that the blood was formed in the liver, largely because the liver so much resembled congealed blood. This became the cornerstone of his physiology, the first attempt at a truly comprehensive explanation of how the human body worked.

Galen's physiology followed a basic sequence of processes. When the stomach digested food, it produced nutritive juices. These passed to the liver, which created purplish venous blood. This flowed from the liver in two ways. A large amount passed into the blood vessels of the venous system, where it was distributed throughout the body. Here it was absorbed into, and became, the flesh. The rest passed along a vein to the right ventricle of the heart, assisted on its way by contractions in the walls of the vein.

This left Galen with the problem of how the purplish venous blood passed from the venous system to the arterial system and was somehow transformed into scarlet arterial blood in the process. His explanation is both scientific in character and difficult to fault. According to Galen, most of the venous blood in the right ventricle passed through the muscular wall dividing the left from the right ventricle of the heart. A small amount travelled to the lungs, where it also passed into the arterial system. Here in the lungs it absorbed 'vital spirits' from the air, which it carried down into the right ventricle of the heart. These 'vital spirits' (a form of *pneuma*) transformed the purplish venous blood into scarlet arterial blood, which then passed out of the heart and into the arterial system. This blood too was then distributed throughout the body and refurbished the flesh.

The function performed by the venous blood system was to nourish the body. The function performed by the separate arterial system was to give the body vitality by means of the 'vital spirits' it contained. The blood did not circulate, it simply passed one way along the two systems of blood vessels, assisted in its passage by contractions in the blood vessels (the pulse). But one crucial question remained. How did the blood pass through the solid muscular central wall of the heart, the septum, which divided the left side from the right side? Despite meticulous dissections of many animals, including the huge elephant heart, Galen was unable to discover any passage through this muscular wall. As a result, he surmised that there must be minute pores in the septum, which were too small to be detected by the human eye.

The resemblance between this assumption, and Harvey's assumption that the arteries and the veins are joined by minute traceries invisible to the human eye, is uncanny. Both Galen's system and Harvey's system depended upon their different microscopic assumptions. Neither man had any way of telling whether his hypothesis was correct. As history would later demonstrate, Galen's assumption was the incorrect one.

Galen's justifiable belief in two blood systems presented him with substantial problems, but it also provoked him to substantial and ingenious explanations, which could hardly be faulted according to the experimental evidence available to him. In this case, hindsight provides a revealing lesson. Just as Aristotle's teleology brought him recognizably close to an evolutionary theory, so Galen's explanation of the blood carried him to the very brink of Harvey's discovery. These inspired ideas of Galen and Aristotle would last for more than two-thirds of the duration of western civilization. The Roman Empire would fall, the Dark Ages and the Middle Ages would pass, the Renaissance would come and go, before humanity conceived of better explanations.

But Galen and Aristotle were to be linked by more than the astonishing prescience of their two great ideas. Galen also produced a standardized version of pathology, his explanation of illness, which would last almost as long as his physiology. In his pathology, Galen succeeded in incorporating Aristotle's fundamental scientific ideas into Hippocrates' basic medical theory. The resemblance between Hippocrates' theory of the four humours in medicine, and Aristotle's theory that the earth is composed of four elements, suggests that they were both derived from similar ancient sources. They would appear to be microcosmic and macrocosmic versions of the same basic notion. Indeed, several physicians prior to Galen seem to have recognized the resemblance and partially incorporated the two systems. However, it was Galen who brought the melding of these two systems to fruition. In his own modest words, he 'made Hippocrates' idea perfect'.

The figure opposite shows Galen's systematization – or perfection – of the humoral theory. Hippocrates' four humours coincide with Aristotle's four elements at the corners of the tilted square. These are also linked to the appropriate organs. All these in turn exhibit their own dual qualities, which appear at the four corners of the untitled square. The blood, which carries air (*pneuma*) and is hot and wet, is naturally associated with the heart. Phlegm, which was believed to flow down from

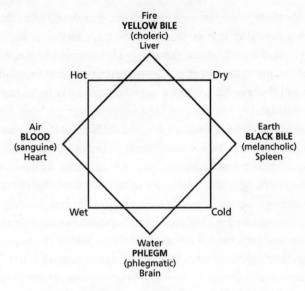

Figure 2. Galen's 'perfected' humoral theory

the brain, is watery: its qualities were thus wet and cold. Such explanations also indicate how this diagram incorporates both medical theory and clinical practice. It outlines how the theory of the humours works, as well as giving an indication of what qualities will prevail when the humours are unbalanced. If a patient is hot and perspiring he is liable to have an excess of blood, and thus bleeding is the appropriate cure. On the other hand, a hot and dry fever, indicating liverishness or an excess of yellow bile (often reflected in a jaundiced complexion), may well be cured by cooling the patient, or inducing him to vomit up the excess of yellow bile.

Surplus humours were prone to accumulate in particular parts of the body, and could result in fever, excessive heat, or even putrefaction. The state of the four humours was equally pertinent when the body was affected by an external accident, a breakage, a wound or such. The balance of the body was just as important when attempting to cure a maimed gladiator at death's door, as it was when treating an emperor suffering from a mild attack of the vapours. (This quaint phrase, which lasted well into the twentieth century, derives directly from the humoral theory: the 'vapours' arose from an excess of hotness and wetness.)

As indicated in the diagram, each of the four humours was also associated with its own temperament. A fiery character was said to be choleric; similarly, we still see splenetic behaviour as characteristic of a melancholic personality. A sanguine character was seen as having a ruddy complexion (excess blood); this became associated with courage and hope – thus sanguine nowadays means hopeful. Likewise, it is easy to associate our present understanding of feeling phlegmatic with an excess of water. This temperamental aspect of humoral theory perists in many aspects of our present linguistic usage. It remains a significant part of our self-understanding. Our word humour orginally derived from the Latin for fluid, and we are still inclined to refer to temperament in terms of liquidity – volatile, fuming, boiling over, even 'wet'. Similarly, the very word humour remains associated with temperamental behaviour (good or bad humour). Whereas a general excess of humour suggests a liveliness of mood, or jolliness: thus, a humorous character.

Over the years, especially during the medieval era, the humoral theory would acquire macroscopic associations. At the very outset, Hippocrates had loosely associated the four humours with the four seasons – colds producing phlegm being more likely to appear in winter, and so forth. Such empirically observed trends hardened into superstitious identification: soon every season had its predominant humour. Subsequently the humoral theory acquired further macroscopic associations with the four ages of man, and even the four points of the compass.

During the Middle Ages the requirements of orthodoxy became paramount, and accepted theory solidified into 'authority' – especially in the case of Galen and Aristotle. Galen's medicine became *the* medicine. With the creative imagination denied original expression, especially in scientific theory, it found outlet in symbolic interpretation and embellishment of the authorities. Rather than original manuscripts, one had illuminated manuscripts; rather than letters forming new words, they were expanded into curlicues and distended into fanciful associated images. But the corpus of Galen's work was essentially scientific: of his great advances in anatomy, physiology and pathology, only the humoral aspect of the latter lent itself to whimsical symbolic interpretation.

Despite its many flaws, Galen's medical theory would play its part in protecting medicine from the worst extravagances of metaphysics which clouded the western scientific mind through the centuries to come. Chemistry would become alchemy; astronomy would become mired in astrology; but despite the inevitable quackery medicine would retain its central core of scientific methodology.

When one considers the handicaps of Galen's era, his achievement is rendered even more exceptional. There is no doubting that he was a medical scientist of superlative quality, and his theorizing from a paucity of fact was often inspired. His ideas always matched, as closely as possible, with the observed facts. This would enable these ideas to endure through the ages, allowing discrepancies to be overlooked. It is unlikely that in two centuries' time – let alone nearly two millennia – many of our present scientific theories will in any way so closely match the scientific knowledge of the twenty-third century. A sobering thought – which can only make one marvel at the longevity of Galen's legacy.

3

FIGURES IN A DARK LANDSCAPE

By the death of Galen around AD 200, the Roman Empire had embarked upon its long, vainglorious and sleazy decline. (With this period in mind, Nietzsche would characterize the ultimate decadence as a combination of sadism and voluptuousness.) Rome's main contribution to medicine had in practice been civic, rather than individual. The cities throughout the Empire contained paved streets with drains. Untainted water was carried in by aqueducts. (Any interference with such a public watercourse was punishable by death.) There were public baths, gymnasiums and public drinking fountains. Yet ironically, lead poisoning from the very pipes which carried this drinking water may well have contributed to the lethargy of the Roman decline.

Other medical factors would also play their part in this decline. The plague which may have caused Galen to flee Rome in AD 166 was just the first of a series which became known as the Antonine Plagues. (Indicative of Greek medical influence, this Roman illness retained the Greek name *plaga*, meaning a 'strike' or 'blow'). The Antonine Plagues swept through the Empire several times over next 20 years. These plagues are now known to have been smallpox, carried by armies and traders from the Levantine provinces. Smallpox was endemic in the Middle East and India, but it was not epidemic – suggesting that the population of this region had built up a partial immunity. With the advent of widespread marine links the disease spread to those populations which were not so protected. At the same time as the Antonine Plagues, China suffered successive waves of the same disease from the same sources.

Demographic historians have noted how population short-age in the wake of plagues tends to be followed by periods of political turbulence. In large empires, such upheavals presage collapse. Midway through the century after the Antonine Plagues, the Roman Empire was swept by a further series of pandemics. (An epidemic is limited to a particular place; a pandemic affects all the people.) In AD 364 the Roman Empire finally split in two, with a twin capital being established at Constantinople (now Istanbul) on the shores of the Bosphorus. Just over 50 years later Rome was sacked by Alaric the Visigoth, and the Dark Ages settled over Europe. Such cities as Londinium (London) and Vindobona (Vienna), once with thriving populations of more than 20,000, now lay in silent ruin. Meanwhile, on the other side of the world, the second great empire of the Orient had also collapsed. The 700-year-old Han Dynasty, which perfected exquisite lacquerwork, invented paper and the seismograph, was also no more.

Disease is at most only partially responsible for the collapse of empires, though it invariably accompanies them. The rise and decline of public health remains an indicative symptom to this day. (During the decade following the recent collapse of the

Soviet Russian Empire, the male life expectancy throughout its former territories, never high, fell from 57 to below 45 years.) A healthy society is more than just a medical institution.

During the Dark Ages the heritage of western learning was preserved in Christian monasteries scattered through Europe – from the remote Atlantic shores of western Ireland to the secluded Alpine valleys of Switzerland. Here this learning inevitably took on a religious tenor, as well as incorporating the corruptions of magic and superstition which had begun to infect learning during the last stages of the Empire. Medical knowledge did not escape this fate. The language of medicine had formerly been Greek, and many mistakes occurred when texts were translated into classical Latin, which now became the pan-European language of learning. The spoken Latin of the Empire had already begun to fragment into what would eventually become separate languages such as French, Italian and Spanish. This influence of classical Latin would remain paramount in medical language until well into the twentieth century, with medicines, diseases and procedures all receiving universally recognized Latin names.

During the Dark Ages scattered texts were copied and combined by a number of serious scholarly compilers. Notable among these was the Venerable Bede, who was born in AD 673 at Northumberland in the northeast of England. Bede is best remembered today for his *Ecclesiastical History of the English People*, the first genuine history of England. He was the first historian to use a dating system based on the birth of Christ, and the popularity of his *History* ensured the widespread acceptance of this system which remains in worldwide use to this day. His scientific compilations contain revivals of certain Ancient Greek ideas, some rare even in their own time. He maintained that the world was a globe, and that the tides were controlled by the phases of the moon. In addition, he proposed original theories on the actual workings of the tides, most notably discovering that high water arrived at successive times at successive places along a coastline. (This was to be described by Jules Duhem, the leading twentieth-century French historian of science, as the only original formulation of nature to be made in the West for some eight centuries.)

Little is known concerning the life of this remarkable man, apart from the fact that he was a monk in the monastery at Wearmouth on the coast of northeast England. He appears to have spent his entire life here, with his only recorded visits being along the coast to Holy Island (Lindisfarne) and the nearby city of York, both within 70 miles of Wearmouth. Even before Bede entered the monastery at Wearmouth it had become a beacon of learning, attracting monks from as far afield as Rome, North Africa and even Tarsus (the home city of St Paul, on the coast of what is now southeastern Turkey.) Bede describes his simple monastic life: 'While observing the discipline and daily round of singing in the church, I have always taken delight in learning, or teaching, or writing.' One of his favourite topics was time, and he himself described how he wrote 'at length about the nature, course and end of time'. (The latter event was confidently expected to occur a few centuries later at the end of the millennium.)

In character, Bede's medical writings are much the same as his celebrated *History*. The latter contains vivid eyewitness accounts and scrupulous attention to the reliability of sources. Yet these are interspersed on almost every page with credulous tales of miracles, visions of prophesying angels, saintly excursions to the underworld and the like (many of which are also given scrupulously attributed sources). In dealing with medical matters, Bede cites Hippocrates and practices related to the humoral theory of medicine. In hot fever or illness caused by an excess of blood he recommends the opening of a vein to permit bleeding. This follows directly from classical Galenic theory. Yet he also recommends 'for the cure of persons bitten by serpents: mix with water scratchings from the pages of books that have been brought from Ireland' (a superstition presumably stemming from the fact that there are no snakes in Ireland). And although he exhibits considerable knowledge of natural remedies from herbs and plants, he was not above recommending abracadabra-type incantations and the wearing of magic amulets against spells cast by pixies. At other places he has sensible dietary recommendations in the Hippocratic and Galenic tradition. Passing medical facts crop up in many of his works – even in his biography of St Cuthbert, who had lived locally as a hermit and died when Bede was fourteen. Bede's mention of a bubonic tumour on the saint's thigh is accepted as reliable evidence confirming the arrival of the plague in this part of England in AD 664.

The important thing is that Bede gathered accurate medical lore as well as metaphysical gossip. His apologist Bertram Colgrave defends Bede's lapses by claiming, 'Science had not yet given men a conception of a universe ruled by unchanging laws.' This is strictly true: even for Aristotle the heavens were subject to different laws from those which pertained on earth. But both these sets of rules were scientific in character. Such was the intellectual darkness into which the Dark Ages had sunk that even a scholar of Bede's calibre could only dimly discern his physics amidst the all-embracing gloom of metaphysics. It is easy to mock his tales of miraculous healing: saint dies, man with leprosy chances to sleep on same spot, wakes cured, etc. Yet the credulous compilations written by Bede and his like during the Dark Ages were all that preserved science in the western world. Amidst the old wives' tales and miracles a kernel of rational medical theory and practice remained. But for Bede, and a rare few writers of similar perception (and

similar supernatural whimsy) the tradition of *scientific* learning might well have vanished altogether from Europe.

During this period, remnant medical science also faced a
very real threat from prevailing Christian beliefs. Formerly, in
later Roman times, Christian compassion had inclined believers to favour medicine as a relief from suffering. But as
Christianity spread over Europe it inevitably began to absorb
many of the more primitive practices and irrationalities of the
earlier religions it overlaid. In place of compassion came
superstition. Common belief now accepted that illness was
a punishment from God, inflicted on account of sins or hidden
transgressions. To attempt to cure such illness thus contra-
vened God's will. Other illnesses were thought to result from
possession by devils, or were caused by witchcraft, or arose as
a result of spells cast by pixies and elves. The only orthodox
way to cure such afflictions was prayer, penitence or calling
upon the assistance of the appropriate saint. For instance, one
prayed to St Anthony for relief from ergotism (known as St
Anthony's Fire). This was caused by fungus-infected rye, and
resulted in such painful internal burning that the sufferers
literally danced with agony, leading onlookers to conclude
that they were possessed by demons. Similarly, one prayed to
St Vitus for relief from chorea, the cause of involuntary
spasmodic movements, which became known as St Vitus'
Dance. (One only has to compare the fatalism of this approach, to Hippocrates' scientific attitude towards epilepsy, to
see how far medical practice had descended into decadence a
millennium later.)

In the climate of such times, religion was often the only
solace. Scientific practice certainly languished, and it is difficult to gauge the precise extent of its ghostly persistence. For
instance, we know that in the ninth century the library of the
famous Benedictine abbey at St Gall in Switzerland contained

over a thousand books. Almost all of these were theological works, a few were forgotten classical texts, and only half a dozen were medical texts. Yet the twentieth-century Italian authority on the history of medicine Arturo Castiglioni claimed that St Gall was 'a famous centre of medical learning'. Our picture of such times remains as clear and fanciful as Bede's.

Around the turn of the first millennium, Europe gradually began to emerge into the more settled medieval era. But the approach to learning remained for the most part religious rather than scientific. Many Christian scholars continued to ignore the scientific sphere altogether, although a few brave individuals would attempt to reconcile the two. In the medical field this task was undertaken by another remarkable figure, Hildegard of Bingen – who is generally regarded as a saint, although her actual canonization never took place owing to a typical medieval muddle over the paperwork.

Hildegard of Bingen was born in 1098, the tenth child of a nobleman with extensive estates along the Rhine valley. At the age of eight she was placed in a convent. This early removal from home may well have been a traumatic event, for soon afterwards she began experiencing migraines and seeing visions. These visions persisted, though only in adulthood did she confide her secret to her confessor. As a result, she was encouraged to write down her visions, which consisted of prophetic and apocalyptic material, as well as divine information on the relation between God and humanity. Hildegard's record of her visions is both pictorial and verbal. The visual images consist of vivid brilliantly coloured designs of stars and waves, also of figures amidst the dawning heavens, jagged flames or spinning stars. Some of the figures are divine; others are part-human, part-beast. Her images were passed on to the ecclesiastical authorities, eventually reaching the pope himself, who became convinced that Hildegard had direct contact with the divine. In her later life, both popes and kings would turn to her for discreet advice from these heavenly sources during times of tribulation.

As one would expect, modern psychology has a sadly mundane explanation of these inspired visions. Reference is made to the 'pseudo-objectivity' of hallucinations experienced by certain types of migraine sufferers. These are often characterized by 'scintillating scotoma', which involve a dizziness and dimming of vision enlivened by flickering sparkly patterns – much as evoked in many of Hildegard's depictions of what she had seen. Such hallucinations would usually be of little interest to medical history except as symptoms; but in Hildegard's case this relationship to the divine informed her entire mental outlook. Once again, this too would have been of no great importance had she not possessed one of the finest minds of her time. Her deeply religious nature, combined with her exceptional interest in medicine, would bring about a unique synthesis.

Hildegard was well aware of her intellectual superiority, and was determined that it should not be stifled. During her late forties, she decided that she had endured enough of her vows. Poverty, chastity and obedience were all very well – but neither poverty nor obedience seemed to fit her character. Making use of the family cash, she decided to found her own convent, where she alone would be in charge. Despite considerable opposition from the Church authorities (male to a man), she eventually succeeded. Her convent was built on Mount St Rupert above the small town of Bingen – on a particularly scenic stretch of the Rhine valley, near the legendary Lorelei Rock, amid a region of steep hillsides covered with vineyards.

Hildegard may have dispensed with poverty and obedience, but she appears also to have dispensed with men and remained chaste. Some have argued against this, pointing to the intimate knowledge of female sexual activities in her writings. These feature largely in her medical works, and in fact cast no aspersions on her virginity. For a start, several of her remarks betray a deep ignorance of actual participation. Other references (also faulty) are traceable to classical sources (invariably male). Where her knowledge is both intimate and correct, it is usually derived from her medical practice.

Established as the abbess of her own convent, Hildegard was able to continue with her exceptional creative activities. Her illustrations of her visions alone established her as a highly gifted artist. Her music, including some exquisite plainsong chants, justly retains its place in the repertoire to this day. On top of this, she produced a stream of religious poetry, theological writings and even drama. More pertinently, she retained a deep and lifelong interest in medicine. Her convent contained its own infirmary, where she practised her medical skills, and she also wrote two important medical treatises. These manage to reconcile the contemporary religious approach to medicine with actual medical theory. This ingenious feat is important as much more than an intellectual conjuring trick. Her ability to jigsaw Galen's humoral theory into existing theological orthodoxy enabled medical theory as such to become part of that all-embracing orthodox picture. Whereas previously medicine had often been seen as an attempt to thwart the will of God, now it became part of his divine providence.

Hildegard's major medical work was *Physica*. (In Greek this word meant 'the things of nature'. Not until around this period did a physician begin to become someone who specialized in that department of natural things which we call medicine.) Like Bede's physics, Hildegard's *Physica* also contained much metaphysics, and not a little plain magic. Indeed, the American medical historian Ackerknecht goes so far as to suggest that 'the therapeutic writings of St Hildegard differ from Cherokee curing spells mainly in the substitution of the names of saints for those of nature spirits.' Despite this, the important thing about Hildegard's medicine is that it has a central core of quasi-science. Hildegard's medicine was based upon humoral theory. By this stage the Galenic theory of the four humours had taken on even further macrocosmic resonances. The humours not only echoed the four elements which made up the world, but also such things as the four regions of the earth and even the four major winds. Everything was being woven into a complex all-embracing overarching tapestry, within which it was becoming almost impossible to disentangle the natural from the supernatural. Everything had its place in this woolly world view, and everything worked in accordance with it.

Despite such distortions and restrictions, the humoral theory still managed to focus on its essential thesis: disease resulted from an imbalance of the four humours. Without interfering with this central mechanism, Hildegard ingeniously succeeded in linking it to biblical requirements. She wrote that the unbalanced nature of the four humours resulted from the fall of man in the Garden of Eden. After Adam ate the apple (the fruit of the knowledge of good and evil), its juices entered his blood and disturbed the humoral balance of his body. As a result, his blood was able to produce the poison of semen. This substance resulted from the foaming of the blood. In women, this same process resulted in the production of breastmilk. Along with human innocence, the humoral harmony of the body was lost forever. The unbalanced humours were thus both the result of sin and the cause of disease. And curing disease could also be seen as helping to ameliorate the inherent imperfection of fallen humanity. Such medieval arguments may appear as mere metaphysical sophistry to the modern sensibility, but they were crucial in their historical context. Only by utilizing these arguments could medical theory *as such* be preserved.

Hildegard also brought her own original interpretation to the four humours theory. In her version, the humours were divided into two pairs, with one pair predominant. These she called *flegmata* (not to be mistaken for phlegm, which confusingly was not one of this pair). The dominant humours were blood and yellow bile, which originated in the heart and liver, and accorded with the 'higher' elements air and fire. The subordinate humours she called *livores* (water and earth, or phlegm and black bile, the humours of the brain and spleen). According to Hildegard, the body could only be healthy when it was ruled by the dominant humours which were 'dry and moist'. Undoubtedly this all meant something to Hildegard, but as her interpreter Margret Berger is forced to concede: 'Attempts to provide a rational explanation of Hildegard's formula have not been convincing.'

Hildegard's actual medical advice is highly varied. Some of it is plain loopy: 'Anyone whose eyesight is beginning to fail because of excessive lust should take the skin of a fish's bladder . . . marinate it in the finest pure wine . . . and place it over his eyes when he goes to sleep . . . but be sure to remove it at midnight.' Other bits are undeniably batty: jaundice is to be cured by tying a live bat to the patient's back, then transferring it to the stomach until the bat dies. Some is heartily medieval: 'No matter whether you are healthy or sick, if when you wake up you feel thirsty you should drink wine or beer, never water.' Parts are gnomically metaphorical: 'Human beings are not hairy for they are rational . . . instead of hair and feathers they cover themselves with reason.' But some of her medical understanding stems from exceptional observation and scientific acumen. She spotted that scabies was caused by itch-mite. Her knowledge of childbirth, menstruation, and many specifically female ailments, though often wayward, helped rescue such matters from folklore and witchcraft. Through her efforts gynaecology and obstetrics would begin to regain a foothold in scientific medicine. In an age riddled with vermin and engrimed with dirt, her infirmary appears to have been a model institution. Her insistence on boiling water must have saved countless lives, while her hot herbal baths for menstrual and other complaints doubtless relieved much pain. Similarly, all must have benefited from her understanding of the importance of diet, and the need for daily washing out of the mouth (at a time when teeth-brushing was unheard of).

Despite all this, it is Hildegard's often tenuous adherence to Galenic humoralism that remains crucial. Here at least medicine continued to resemble a science, its practice guided by a skeleton theory – which Hildegard managed to link to the only body of thought which remained acceptable to this age. Namely, theology.

Yet even this would not prove enough. In 1130 the pope forbade the practice of medicine by those who had taken vows as priests or nuns. Such activity was considered a distraction from their spiritual requirements. However, as was often the case during this period, not everyone paid attention to the pope (not least because there was more than one at the time). Indeed, it seems that many did not even hear about the pope's edict. It is unclear into which category Hildegard fell. Knowing of her high eccelesiatical connections, she would probably have been informed. Yet knowing of her wilful character, she would equally probably have disregarded this information, had she received it. This would be her way, right through to the end. After her clash with the Church in 1178, the local ecclesiastical authorities punished her by strictly banning all singing in her convent. This was publicly observed for only a few months, and when she died the following year her funeral was accompanied by her well-rehearsed chanting nuns, singing just as they had continued to sing privately throughout the ban.

However, the pope's ban on medicine did have an unexpected benefit. Since this was officially forbidden to priests and nuns who took vows, its practice now tended to pass into the hands of lay people. Similarly, the locus of its practice and teaching from this period on began to drift away from monasteries and convents, with the gradual establishment of the 'schools' (early universities) and public hospitals. However, secular establishments for the care of the sick had a long history. Infirmaries of one kind or another had existed since Roman times. Hospitals as such were originally established in Europe to provide 'hospitality' for travelling pilgrims, but these now evolved from simple hostels into public establishments catering for the sick.

Despite these developments, the practice of western medicine as a science had all but died out in most of Europe. Certainly little or no progress was made, and such originalities as appeared were hardly scientific. (Hildegard's 'dry and moist' dominant humours were but one example.) Fortunately, western medicine had long since spread beyond the continent of its invention.

As early as AD 431 the Christian sect known as the Nestorians was declared heretical for maintaining that Jesus had been a human being. The Nestorians travelled east into exile, spreading through what is now Iraq and Iran, bearing with them many rare Greek manuscripts, including works by Aristotle and Galen. Within two centuries they had passed east along the Silk Route as far as China. It was Nestorians travelling back along this route who brought the first barely understood inklings of an entirely different Oriental medicine founded on the yin and yang principle, as well as remedies based on camphor and rhubarb, substances which only now began penetrating westwards. They also brought the closely guarded secret of silk manufacture, transporting live silkworms inside their hollow canes.

Nestorianism somehow managed to survive amidst the religious turbulence of the Middle East. Then in the seventh century came the rapid spread of Islam throughout the Middle East and beyond. Within two centuries the Islamic Arabs had conquered lands ranging from northeast India, through North Africa and up into Italy, across Spain and into France as far as the banks of the Loire. But Islam was not a proselytizing religion, and especially in the Middle East the Syrians, Nestorians, and Jewish subjects of the Arabic Empire were allowed to continue with their culture. The main unifying force of this far-flung empire was language rather than religion. A Christian physician known as Ibn Luqa saw nothing untoward in writing a book on how pilgrims to Mecca should protect their health, any more than Muslim pilgrims found it strange to accept such Christian advice. This state of affairs would only begin to change in 1095 when the Christian Europeans embarked upon a series of crusades to conquer the Holy Land.

By the ninth century the Nestorians had established a great centre of learning at Jundishapur in southern Persia, where they had begun translating the works of Galen and Aristotle into Arabic. The greatest of these translators is known to the west as Johannitius (in the Arab world he is known as Hunayn ibn Ishaq). Johannitius was a Nestorian who was probably of Byzantine Greek ancestry, but was born in Mesopotamia (present-day Iraq) and studied at Baghdad. His particular interest was in the works of Galen. It is said that together with his pupils he translated as many as 130 of Galen's treatises, many of whose Greek originals have since been lost. He even travelled to Alexandria, and undertook a dangerous journey back into the Orthodox Christian Byzantine Empire, in search of works by Galen. Such was Johannitius' profound love for Greek learning that he is said to have walked the streets at night declaiming the poetry of Homer. (One assumes the Islamic prohibition on alcohol did not apply to the Nestorians.)

The Islamic intellectuals of this period had a profound hunger for learning. To them, the way the world worked was the way God worked. All knowledge was 'understanding the mind of God', and thus discovering it was a religious duty, as well as providing a secular benefit. It was also part of their faith that 'God sends down no malady without also sending down with it a cure.' The translated works of Aristotle and Galen, many of which became lost to the West, were now absorbed into Arabic culture. For the next 500 years the most extensive understanding of medicine, and all significant advances in the field, would come from the Arab Empire.

The first great scholar and practitioner in this tradition was Al-Razi (who would become known in medieval Europe by the Latinized version of his name: Rhazes). Al-Razi was born in Rayy in northeastern Persia in 854. He trained at the Baghdad *bimaristan* (literally 'home of the sick'). Like the European infirmaries these were initially attached to religious establishments, in this case mosques. Here medicine was taught in much the same way as religion. The medical text would be read out by the master, who expected his pupils to learn it by heart. The master would then ask questions of his pupils, who were expected to answer by rote. Practical inaccuracies were thus both perpetuated and obscured, although practical experience was gained when the pupils attended the sick. Again, as in European practice, the practical study of anatomy was out of the question owing to a taboo on dissection – apart from exceptional cases of suspected poisoning of influential dignitaries. The large-scale hospitals which were founded in the leading cities of the Arab Empire emerged as important institutions in their own right. The first of these, the Baghdad Hospital, was founded in 805 by Harun al-Rashid (who was immortalized as the caliph in the *Arabian Nights*, where Scheherazade postpones her sentence of death each night by telling him a further fabulous tale). Other great hospitals were established at Cairo, Damascus and Cordoba. All people were treated free at these hospitals, regardless of race, sex or religion. The hospital at Cairo included both a mosque and a Christian chapel, and was still functioning in the early nineteenth century.

Al-Razi eventually rose to become chief physician at the hospital in Baghdad. However, on occasion he would fall from favour at court and find it prudent to return to Rayy, where he would run the hospital there instead. In old age he returned permanently to Rayy, where he became blind, probably from glaucoma. According to one source he died in poverty and obscurity at the age of eighty.

Besides being an exceptional physician, Al-Razi was also known as an alchemist and a philosopher. In the former capacity he made a number of important chemical discoveries, some of which he put to use in concocting medicines. Like Hippocrates, he believed that the study of medicine should be regarded as (natural) philosophy. Illness was nothing to do with religion or evil spirits, and so-called miracles were not cures but simply tricks or illusions perpetrated by unscrupulous 'holy men'. Similarly, the teachings of medicine were not to be regarded as sacrosanct; like philosophy, they should be subjected to criticism where necessary. Medicine was a progressive science. Here he specifically clashed with the Arabic followers of Aristotle, who believed that some scientific knowledge had already achieved perfection, and other scientific knowledge would soon attain this state. Al-Razi was the first to conduct his practical science in a thoroughly modern manner. Each experiment he undertook was written up, with every step precisely described, so that it was possible for others to conduct the same experiment and check its conclusions. He precisely describes a preparation for what is now known as plaster of Paris, showing how it can be used as a cast for holding fractured limbs in place so that they can heal.

Despite disagreeing with the Arabic Aristotelians, Al-Razi had a great respect for Aristotle himself, and shared the Greek philosopher's penchant for classification. Al-Razi was the first to classify substances as animal, vegetable or mineral. This ability to discern and analyse differences and similarities proved invaluable in his clinical work. Until his time, all rashes had been regarded as more or less violent manifestations of the same disease. Al-Razi was the first to make the crucial distinction between smallpox and measles – though curiously he regarded the latter as the more serious disease.

As with his scientific experiments, Al-Razi also precisely recorded his treatment of diseases, in each case giving a diagnosis, prognosis (tracing the course of the malady), and medical prescription (involving drugs, treatment, and so forth). Here he frequently disagreed with Galen, whom he respected but does not seem to have liked very much. He particularly scorned Galen's pretentions to philosophizing; as so often happens, viewing his own efforts in this field as far superior. In several case studies, Al-Razi describes a disease and shows that it often follows an entirely different course from that recorded by Galen. He also shows how Galen's inclination to universal scientific pronouncements sometimes led him astray. For instance, Galen stated the 'rule' that a substance which has the property of cooling down another substance must always begin cooler than that substance.

Similarly, a substance that warms must always initially be warmer than that which it warms. This apparently scientific rule evidently held for the inanimate substances studied by Galen. Yet Al-Razi's superior chemical experience taught him otherwise: cold substances often generate warm reactions. But more importantly, Al-Razi showed that administering a cool liquid medicine to a hot fevered patient can cause a patient to become hotter still as he sweats out the fever. The liquid initiates a process within the body which liberates a potential heat (the malady), causing it to become actual (released from the body in fever). The unseen internal workings of the body could be viewed in this way as a chemical process.

Al-Razi's major work in this field was his *Comprehensive Book of Medicine*. This contains his working medical notes, arranged so as to treat consecutively diseases which affect the body from the head downwards. His speculations concerning bodily functions were ingenious but frequently hampered by his inability to follow through his ideas by performing dissections. He surmised that air containing visual images was transmitted through the hollow optic nerve to the brain. His opinion that there was no place for religion in science led him to believe that the soul was a substance which resided in the brain, the latter being the instrument by which the soul activated the body. This view of the soul bears an uncanny resemblance to the modern materialist conception of mind. Though it should be stressed that Al-Razi was no atheist. He was in fact a firm believer in Islam, who simply objected to ignorant pronouncements by religious authorities – an attitude which won him few friends in this quarter.

In the course of his practical work he improved upon the catheter, the instrument used for internal probing and draining urine from the bladder. Al-Razi had catheters made of lead so that they were more pliable than the original bronze instruments. He also constructed hollow catheters with lateral holes for draining pus from internal infections.

Al-Razi's *Comprehensive Book of Medicine* features a wealth of case histories, including a number taken from Galen. Others come from Al-Razi's medical rounds in the wards of the Baghdad Hospital, as well as case notes from the private practice which he conducted from his home in the busy commercial quarter of the city. Along with prognosis and treatment, his case notes also mention the name and occupation of the patient. From this we can tell that his private practice included a wide range of his neighbours – from craftsmen and labourers to merchants and the nobility.

Al-Razi was one of the first to write about children's diseases. In an age of rampant infant mortality, this subject was invariably ignored: maladies afflicting children were simply regarded as untreatable and left to run their course. Al-Razi also recorded case histories of his own maladies and how he treated them. These include the occasion when he treated himself for a swollen right testicle, which was apparently cured by taking a course of nausea-inducing concoctions of his own manufacture.

The finest genius of the Arabic tradition was undoubtedly Avicenna, who was known throughout the Arabic world as Ibn Sina. (Sadly, our modern standardized spelling disguises the ingenious historical process by which the earlier Arabic name must have become transformed into its European counterpart.) Avicenna's towering intellect established him as a great original philosopher in both the eastern and the western tradition, as well as the most celebrated physician of his entire era. The exceptional quality of his medical thought and practice ranks him alongside Hippocrates and Galen. But this is not all. Avicenna also proved a skilful statesman during a period of extreme political instability. His political skills (devious, verbal and manipulative) enabled him to elude death

on more than one occasion – then, as now, a supreme achievement in Middle Eastern politics. Even his periods in gaol were
suprisingly brief. As if all this was not enough, he was also
renowned as a prolific drinker and womanizer. Wine and
women seem to have encouraged him to song: his poetry
too has survived time, its effect subtly permeating our literature. Most older European literature relied upon alliteration
and rhythm, having no place for rhyme, which was essential to
Arabic poetry. Avicenna's verse would play its part in importing rhyme into the European tradition, and here too Avicenna's contribution is out of the ordinary:

> A rose is like a mule's arse
> with shit at its heart.

Medical students will have no trouble in recognizing such a
poet as one of their own. Avicenna's inability to suffer fools
gladly made him many enemies among this multitudinous and
powerful class. As a result, gossips spread all manner of
seditious stories concerning his character and behaviour:
small-minded tittle-tattle which often fell far short of the
stupendous and outrageous reality. Meanwhile, some saw
him as essentially a theologian, and in the light of this many
of his later commentators came to regard him as a great
mystic, who had lived an appropriately ascetic life. Another
seditious misapprehension which fell far short of the truth.
Either way, Avicenna triumphantly survives all this. In the end
he can be judged by his work alone, which ran to over 250
books. This opus even includes a surprisingly reticent autobiography, which was finished after his death by a pupil.
However, in the words of Avicenna's modern biographer
Soheil Afnan, this latter work is 'obviously neither complete
nor convincing'. Even Avicenna evidently came to the conclu-

sion that there were things about his life which were best left unsaid.

Avicenna was born an ethnic Persian in 980. His birthplace was the legendary Silk Route city of Bukhara (now a shadow of its former self as an oil-drilling centre in Uzbekistan). His father appears to have been a fearsome combination of chief tax collector and wisest man in the city. As a result, Avicenna's home was a magnet for visiting learned men and worried local dignitaries. The child was quickly recognized as a prodigy, and was educated at home by his father. At the age of ten he could recite the entire Koran. By the age of 16 he had read all available philosophical works and mastered all known medical learning. Two years later he was appointed court physician to the semi-autonomous local Samanid caliph. This gave him access to the renowned court library, one of the treasures of this dynasty and the finest collection of books in the region.

Unfortunately, the Persian Samanid dynasty was gradually declining, as Turkic power began to spread through central Asia. When the Samanids were overthrown, Avicenna was forced to flee. This was the beginning of a difficult wandering life. Such was his renown that he was regularly employed at various courts, often as vizier (the equivalent of prime minister for the local prince). Yet because of increasing regional instability these political appointments were dangerous and seldom lasted long.

Eventually Avicenna experienced a period of stability at Hamadan, in southwestern Persia, where he was employed as vizier during two reigns. Though even during this comparatively settled time he narrowly escaped being executed on more than one occasion. It was in these years that he began his five-volume masterpiece *Al-Qanun* (known in the West as *The Canon*). After yet another spell as an itinerant freelance prime minister he found stability at the court in Isfahan in southern

Persia. Here, according to his biographer L.E. Goodman, he was much admired by his prince for cutting a dashing figure 'beautifully dressed in brocaded robes, leather boots, and linen turban'. His appetite for female slaves was also enviously noted. During this period he wrote on subjects ranging from medicine to physics: his understanding of optics was such that he partly anticipated Newton by over half a millennium. Avicenna also saw the indissoluble link between motion and time, realizing that if everything in the world was motionless there would be no such thing as time.

At the age of 57 he was back in the saddle again, attending his caliph on campaigns against the Turkic invaders. As he explains in his autobiography, some of his best work was done while on horseback during military campaigns – as well as in hiding, in dungeons, or in the early hours after a night's drinking. But this time life in the saddle proved too vigorous even for his remarkable constitution. He suffered from a severe bout of colic, which he began treating with his own medicine, and died soon afterwards. However, the strong suspicion remains that one of his servants prepared his medicine incorrectly with the intention of poisoning him.

After Avicenna's death his masterwork *Al-Qanun* would become the most important work in the history of medicine – both in the eastern and the western tradition. This work soon surpassed Al-Razi's renowned *Comprehensive Book of Medicine*. Even during his lifetime Avicenna had been ungraciously scornful of his great predecessor, claiming that he should have confined his activities 'to testing stools and urine'. In *Al-Qanun* Avicenna incorporated much of the learning of Hippocrates, Galen and Aristotle, as well as his own considerable knowledge. Indeed, it was Avicenna's intention that this work should contain *all* known medical knowledge.

In many ways, *Al-Qanun* would live up to its author's

expectations. Too much so. Through the ensuing centuries this would become *the* authoritative medical work in both Europe and throughout the Middle East. As a result, progress in medical thought would be brought to a virtual standstill. Avicenna's *Canon* would still be the standard textbook at the great medical school in Montpellier as late as 1650, well over 600 years after it had been written. Its influence on eastern medicine would be even greater. Avicenna's text remains central to the Yunani medicine which is practised in India and Pakistan to this day. (The very word 'Yunani' is Arabic for Greek, probably deriving from the ancient Greeks of the Anatolian mainland, who were known as Ionians. Yunani medicine regarded its origins as deriving from Ancient Greek (Hippocratic) sources as distinct from Indian or Chinese sources.)

So what is this great work? *Al-Qanun* is a vast compendium of medical information. Its pharmacopoeia (volume on medicines) contains a list of no less than 760 drugs, complete with how they should be taken, their effects, and the maladies they should be used to treat. It is largely through Avicenna's work that the Arabic-based word 'drug' entered European languages. Other pharmacological terms such as alcohol (*al-kohl*), alkali, elixir and syrup also derive from the Arabic – as do such words as sugar, spinach and algebra.

Al-Qanun also deals with a plethora of specific diseases, giving their aetiology (conjunctive and specific causes), diagnosis, prognosis and treatment. Avicenna's interest extended beyond the range of what had previously been considered diseases, going so far as to prescribe treatments for obesity and anorexia. Avicenna's medicine is based upon the humoral doctrine, which is treated with the logical rigour one would expect of the first philosopher to make significant advances in logic since Aristotle. Unfortunately, the logical theory is often at odds with the findings of his actual experience as a physician. Where theory clashed with practice, Avicenna tended to favour the former in his writings. However, the indications are that he did not do so in his clinical practice. In the less theoretical passages of *Al-Qanun* he relies heavily upon his considerable experience and expertise. His description of diabetes, for instance, is the first to note the presence of a sweetish taste in the urine of the patient, a finding which indicates exceptional dedication.

Despite this, Avicenna perpetuated the snobbery which downgraded surgery as an inferior practice: manual, rather than mental. Even so, he treated excessive bleeding by tourniquet: stemming the flow by constricting the veins. Wounds were treated by cauterizing: disinfecting and staunching by burning with a hot iron or caustic chemical. (Both the tourniquet and cauterizing date from ancient Egyptian times.) Al-Razi's catheter was used for draining internal infections. Strict attention was paid to the pulse; bleeding was a constant standby, as were enemas and purges; while urine was scrutinized (and more, on occasion). But otherwise, invasive surgery and anatomical investigation by dissection were frowned upon. The human body was sacred, and as such sacrosanct.

This deficiency in the Arabic tradition was remedied by the work of Albucasis (sometimes confusingly called Abulcasim, and known to the Arabs as Abul Qasim). Albucasis was that Arabic rarity, a great surgeon. It is perhaps no accident that he practised in Cordoba in southern Spain, a caliphate whose distance from the main centres of the Arab Empire gave it a certain freedom from the increasingly restrictive Islamic orthodoxy.

Albucasis was born in 936 in the small town of Zahara in what is now Andalucia. (The first is the Arab name for desert; and al-Andaluz was their name for the whole of Spain.) Little is known of Albucasis' life, except that he became physician to the caliph at Cordoba. This city, more than any other in the Arab Empire, was responsible for the transmission of Arabic learning to the West. While Europe languished in the Dark Ages, Cordoba was a city of fountains and marble courtyards, its multi-pillared mosque one of the architectural wonders of the world. It is from the scholars of Cordoba that Europe first learned of Arabic numbering, thus freeing mathematics from the straitjacket of roman numerals. (Once XLVIII divided by XXIV became 48 divided by 24 arithmetic could take off.) The Greek tradition of learning for its own sake would now return to the Europe of its birth.

Albucasis' major work was *Al-Tasari*, which would be translated as *The Collection*. (Its original full title quaintly encapsulates its author's purpose: 'A Book to Consult for Those Whom Circumstances Prevent from compiling a Medical Book of Their Own'.) *Al-Tasari* was intended as a handbook for surgeons, was the first comprehensive book of its kind in the history of medicine, and would in time become *the* textbook on surgery during the Middle Ages.

Despite its originality, *Al-Tasari* also lifts heavily from the few classical authors who dealt with this disparaged subject. Most notable of these was one Paul of Aegina, a Byzantine Greek who probably copied heavily from lost works of Galen, but also gave original descriptions of mastectomy (from the Greek *mastos* meaning 'breast' and *ektome* 'to cut out') and tonsillectomy. Albucasis himself was the first to describe a number of maladies and procedures. These range from haemophilia, excessive bleeding arising from the blood's inability to clot – to a successful operational method for the removal of blood clots. His work covers such widespread aspects of surgery as dentistry, and trepanning for psychological complaints. The methods he employs are frequently imaginative.

He suggests carving artificial teeth from oxbones. And according to the historian Castiglioni: 'For injuries of the intestine he recommends holding together the edges of the wound and applying large ants.' (This is no misprint. I am assured by an expert formicologist that the jaws of certain large ants do indeed lock closed much like clamps: though presumably the ant itself was detached prior to insertion into the intestines.)

Albucasis also produces a comprehensive account of that Arabic standby cautery. This reveals precisely how widespread the practice was: being used for burning skin tumours, opening abcesses, as well as for the agonizing removal of haemorrhoids. In the absence of genuine invasive surgery, cautery seems to have been regarded as something of a panacea. Albucasis even mentions its use to cure epilepsy and melancholy, although this suggests that its mere mention may often have induced speedy relief from hypochondria.

However, by far the most interesting pages of *Al-Tasarif* are those which contain nearly 200 illustrations of the surgical and dental instruments which Albucasis used. These are both beautiful, ingenious and effective. Several were his own invention: including a tonsil guillotine, an extremely delicate hooked instrument for removing blood clots from veins, and various scalpels for lithotomy (removing stones from the gall bladder). According to Albucasis, these instruments were effectively sterilized by cautery.

Many of Albucasis' aesthetically exquisite instruments have come down to us, and can still be seen in Cordoba. Few artefacts of such grace and beauty were produced anywhere else in western Europe during the entire Dark Ages. They can be compared to the elaborately illuminated Bibles crafted in the far-flung monasteries of Christendom – although Albucasis' instruments were intended to save the body rather than the soul.

4

A FRESH START

The pivotal moment in the return of Greek medical knowledge to Europe was the arrival of Constantine of Africa at the southern Italian port of Salerno, some time around 1075. Little is known for certain about this mysterious figure. He was born a Muslim, probably at Carthage in North Africa. Earlier in his life he may well have travelled as far afield as India and Ethiopia, but certainly visited Damascus, possibly studying at the *bimaristan* there. He later returned to Carthage, but was suspected of being a wizard and forced to flee for his life. This may well explain why he arrived in Salerno.

Constantine's knowledge of medicine was not deep, and the Latin which he somehow acquired was inelegant to say the least. Yet this knowledge, and his arrival at the school in Salerno with numerous Arabic texts, would transform western learning. With Constantine medicine came full circle: it was he who translated Galen from Arabic into Latin, the language of the city where he had flourished (even though he had in fact written in Greek). Constantine also translated Hippocrates' *Aphorisms*, and many minor texts, including possibly some by Al-Razi and Avicenna. The all-but-lost art of Greek medicine was returning to Europe, enriched by its sojourn amongst the Arabs. Constantine would eventually convert to Christianity, ending his days as a monk at the great Benedictine monastery of Monte Cassino in southern Italy. He continued translating Arabic medical works to the last, his texts rendered unmistakable by their wobbly Latin.

According to legend, the medical school at Salerno was founded in the early tenth century by four physicians – an Italian, a Greek, a Jew and an Arab. Significantly, it was a lay school, and thus its learning was not hampered by irrelevant questions of religious orthodoxy. There were even women students and teachers at the school, which is generally recognized as the first university in medieval Europe. Others would eventually follow: at Paris in 1110, Bologna in 1158 and Oxford in 1167 (set up by English students who had been expelled from Paris.) The teaching at Salerno, and in the later schools, would remain strictly in the Hippocratic–Galenic tradition, as it had been inherited by the Arabs. The central guiding principle remained the theory of the four humours: blood, phlegm, black bile and yellow bile. Illness resulted when one of these dominated the body: only when the humours were balanced could the body return to health.

Besides teaching, practical work was also carried out at Salerno. Anatomy was studied by dissecting pigs, and in the course of operations at the attached hospital soporifics in sponges were used to anaesthetize the patients during operations. Early in the thirteenth century Salerno fell under the rule of the Holy Roman Emperor Frederick II, whose brilliant court in Sicily became the focus of a premature minor renaissance. In

1221 Frederick decreed that no one could practise medicine unless they had studied for nine years at Salerno, or passed an examination conducted by the masters of that school. A standard was thus established for the profession, with the schools of Paris and Bologna soon following suit, instituting a qualification recognized throughout France, Italy and beyond.

Despite this, many would study for long periods without apparently bothering to take the final examination. Paris, at the time the largest city in the world, had a mere six qualified doctors in 1296; a century later this had only risen to thirty-two. Population records indicate that this represented just one doctor for every 8,500 Parisians, an astonishing figure in such a malady-infested age. (Men over 50 were a rarity; child-bearing women only had a 50 per cent chance of reaching 30; and infant mortality remained at epidemic proportions.) This suggests that there remained a considerable underclass of unqualified, but more or less patchily educated healers and self-styled 'students of medicine' who made a living from poorer patients. Even within Frederick II's jurisdiction, strict adherence to his decree had fallen into abeyance when its author's attention wandered elsewhere. Frederick became known as 'stupor mundi' (wonder of the world) on account of his great intellect and his equally great achievements. The latter were of such magnitude that he was excommunicated by the jealous pope Gregory IX, who was forced to make an embarrassing rescindment of this edict after Frederick led a crusade which retook Jerusalem. Unfortunately, Frederick had also begun to exhibit symptoms of derangement, which in-cluded blinding his chief minister and exhibiting him in a cage.

Despite the widespread cavalier disregard for medical qua-lification throughout Europe, it is now that the term 'doctor' first comes into use to describe qualified medical practitioners, as well as anyone with a higher qualification from one of the schools. By 1386 Chaucer is referring to a 'Doctour of phisik', which became the usual variant for a medical man.

By this time the mantle of Salerno had passed on to Montpellier in southern France, which would become the most celebrated medical school of the Middle Ages. It is no accident that Salerno was founded at a time when nearby Sicily was under Arab rule, or that Montpellier remained an isolated outpost of the Arabic Empire until the end of the tenth century. In 1277 a graduate of Montpellier medical school known as Petrus Hispanus even became Pope John XXI, the first and only 'doctor of physic' ever to attain this exalted rank. By now a renaissance of learning was beginning to spread throughout Europe. Avicenna's interpretation of Aristotle was causing a philosophical revolution in Paris. And the invention of spectacles was causing an even greater revolution throughout the entire western world of learning. Middle-aged scholars whose fading eyesight had prevented them from reading could now extend their researches into the second half of their life. At a stroke, the intellectual power of Europe was potentially doubled. Even the diet became richer. Rabbits had arrived in Spain with the Arabs, and had quickly multiplied all over Europe, reaching England by the mid-twelfth century. Likewise exotic vegetables such as spinach spread from Arabic Spain into France and beyond. Though popularly known as *herbe d'Espaigne*, this was not in fact the origin of the name spinach, which may well reach beyond its Arabic form to the Indian word *sag*. (Another hidden etymological epic of evolving pronunciation passing by word of mouth from marketplace to marketplace across half the globe.) In the early 1300s the Church even issued an edict calling for abstention by all congregations from flesh-eating on fast days – firm evidence that meat-eating was by now widespread and habitual. At this stage the entire continent of Europe was on the brink of a vast intellectual, economic and social transformation. But it was not to be. In 1347 the Black Death arrived in Italy.

Once again, the bubonic plague had burst out of its Middle Eastern containment. This time it would not pass directly to Europe, instead travelling first across the entire known globe. Carried by flea-bearing rats in the grain supplies it first spread to China. During the 1330s plague and civil war would kill no less than two-thirds of the population. From China the disease spread west along the trading routes through the Turkic regions of central Asia, arriving on the northern shores of the Black Sea in 1346. The Mongol army besieging the Genoese trading port of Caffa (modern Feodosiya) in the Crimea catapulted disease-ridden corpses over the walls. According to the great modern medical historian Roy Porter, this act 'invented biological warfare'. Genoese trading ships carried the disease to southern Italy, and around the shores of the eastern Mediterranean. The Arabs believed that the plague was spread by evil spirits, known as a *djini* (from which derives our word 'genie'). When it spread through the teeming kasbahs of Cairo, by now the world's second largest city with a population of 250,000, it carried away half the population. Its devastating effect in Europe would change the course of western civilization.

European chroniclers record that the plague began with 'a pustule like a lentil'. The contemporary Italian writer Boccaccio described its further course: 'swellings in the groin and under the armpits the size of an apple . . . the contagion then began to turn into black or livid blotches.' Others describe agonizing swollen glands and tell-tale boils circled by black disfigurations spreading over the body, while the tongue swelled and turned black. Within three days the victim died a hideous death, often having turned literally black.

Reactions varied. Milan and Parma simply slammed the city gates shut, barring all travellers. As soon as the pestilence broke out in Marseilles the authorities immediately sealed off the infected quarter, along with its inhabitants, and set fire to the houses. The entire population of the Sicilian town of Agrigento simply ran away. Meanwhile the Adriatic port of Ragusa (modern Dubrovnik) ordered all incoming ships to stay anchored offshore for 40 (*quaranta*) days – thereby originating the term 'quarantine'.

Within three years the great wave of disease would spread throughout Europe, to its very limits, reaching Portugal, Ireland, and even Norway and Russia. Nowhere would be spared – apart from Milan, small pockets in the Pyrenees and Flanders (modern Belgium), and inexplicably almost the whole of Poland. No one knew what to do, as the pestilence swept across the landscape, leap-frogging mountain barriers, rivers and even seas. Eventually it reached Iceland, and from there passed on to the Greenland settlements. Even the qualified doctors of physic had no answer: Galenic medicine did not contain the concept of contagious disease.

Precautionary measures were taken largely on an intuitional basis. With hindsight, we can see that Milan and Ragusa had the right idea. (Though this didn't spare Ragusa, which probably lost a third of its population.) Most turned instinctively to religion. Christianity's concept of disease remained largely unchanged: it was due to sins, demonic possession or witchcraft. Prayer, penance, pleading for intercession by an appropriate saint, or simply flinging oneself upon God's mercy – such were the time-honoured remedies. In this, the Black Death was no different from other afflictions. The waves of lesser epidemics and recurrent minor outbreaks of plague which occurred before and after the Black Death induced many bouts of extreme behaviour. Suspected epidemics could lead to psychic epidemics. Throughout the Middle Ages collective social hysteria was never far below the surface. The most notorious outbreaks included such episodes as the Children's Crusades, the mass murder of Jews in York, outbreaks of 'dancing mania', and the frequent episodes of 'possession by devils' which afflicted closed convents.

Another serious infectious disease which afflicted medieval Europe was leprosy. This pestilence had been known since biblical times, where it was mentioned in Leviticus. A more prevalent form of the disease was probably brought from India by Alexander the Great's returning troops, and consequently spread across the Roman Empire. By the Middle Ages it was firmly entrenched throughout Europe. The Third Lateran Council of 1179 ordered that lepers should be separated from society. Male lepers were subjected to a ceremony in which they were pronounced 'dead unto the world but alive unto Christ'. The victim would be made to stand in a grave while a priest poured earth over his head. He was then deemed legally dead, and his possessions passed on to his heirs. Leper houses were set up in remote spots outside cities. Here the lepers were treated with varying degrees of tolerance: some were compassionately left supplies of food and drink, others were simply left to fend for themselves, some were grimly burned alive.

Leprosy became increasingly prevalent, until in the early fourteenth century as many as 1 per cent of the population were afflicted. Yet by the end of the century it had bafflingly disappeared from Europe. Some commentators suspect that it may have been 'cleared' by the Black Death. Others have proposed more complex and mysterious explanations. They point to the fact that the Black Death may not have been a simple outbreak of bubonic plague. Detailed and seemingly reliable descriptions of the affliction vary greatly. The 'black' bubo was far from being a universal symptom. And if the bubonic plague was spread by fleas migrating to humans when the host rat died, why do practically none of the contemporary reports mention dead rats? Such elements remain unexplained, from a medical point of view.

The most precise and informed description of the plague was penned by the French medieval physician Guy de Chauliac, who graduated from Montpellier and was generally recognized as the finest doctor of physic of his time. His account indicates that the Black Death included two distinct types of plague – the bubonic (buboes, boils: spread by rat fleas) and the pneumonic (lung infection: spread by sputum or contaminated garments). His descriptions also hint at a third variant: septicaemic (blood pouring from nose and mouth: infection injected into bloodstream by rat fleas). Such admirably cool-headed scientific exactitude was rare, though de Chauliac was not alone in suggesting medical treatment for the plague. Measures such as the old Galenic standby of phlebotomy (blood-letting), cauterizing buboes, and cleansing the air with incense or fire were all suggested and tried. But in the end even de Chauliac threw up his hands in despair and gave the traditional advice: *Fugo cito, vade longe, rede tarde.* (Flee speedily, go far away, and return slowly.) By the time the plague, and whatever else it may have been, had passed through Europe over 30 million people had died: more than a third of the entire population.

Some places recovered more quickly than others. As late as 1400 Rome was little more than collections of huts amongst the ruins, a place of outlaws and refuse, with wolves howling into the night around the old St Peter's. Other regions instituted long-overdue reforms in public sanitation, and recovered more speedily. Many suspected a connection between disease and filth. Refuse began to be cleared from the streets of many cities, and their main thoroughfares were cobbled for ease of sluicing. Milan and Paris laid extensive public sewer systems. (In some cases these incorporated disused Roman drainage pipes: civilization was beginning to catch up with itself.) On the other hand, there was widespread popular outrage at many public health measures – such as the edict banning pigs from front rooms giving on to main streets.

The breakdown of civil order which had taken place during the Black Death now led to a loosening of the feudal system on the land, and an erosion of the guilds' stranglehold over city trade. A more general freedom of movement and enterprise soon followed. The merchant banks of Florence gradually re-established trading routes across the Alps to Bruges and east to Beirut. The Greenland settlements may have succumbed to the plague and the encroachments of a mini-Ice Age, but Europe now expanded into warmer climes. The Portuguese rounded the Cape of Good Hope, and in 1492 Columbus recorded that he had set foot in China. Meanwhile the ludicrous decadence of the papacy and general clerical corruption led many thinkers to begin questioning the status of the Church. On 31 October 1517, the German priest Martin Luther hammered his Ninety-five Theses demanding reform to the door of the church at Wittenberg. A movement which would split Europe had begun. This would prove a reformation of more than just religious thought.

Paracelsus was a medical reformer who consciously modelled himself upon Martin Luther. His behaviour within his chosen field would prove not only more radical but also more outrageous. Paracelsus was a heady blend of charlatan and genius. Many Germans, including the present Prince of Wales, still regard him as the founder of modern medicine; elsewhere many regard him as a complete buffoon. There is truth in both views.

Philip Bombast von Hohenheim, who later styled himself 'Paracelsus', was born in 1493. Some claim that his middle name is the origin of the word 'bombast', in the sense of 'blustering blather'. This would be appropriate, but is probably not true. The man we now know as Paracelsus lived his earliest years in Switzerland, but his family soon moved to the Carinthian mountain region of southern Austria. His father was a rare combination of a mining engineer and physician, and his mother was a serf. However, there is no evidence to suggest that his mother displayed the coarse, Rabelaisian behaviour characteristic of a peasant of this era. So whether Paracelsus inherited this trait, or acquired it, is unclear – what is without doubt is that he exhibited the robust manners of this medieval underclass, and persisted in proudly doing so throughout his life.

The young Paracelsus received his first lessons in medicine from his father. At the age of fourteen he left home and crossed the Alps into Italy. As is often the case, when he wished it so, Paracelsus' life at this point becomes obscure. He probably ended up studying medicine at Ferrara. Equally proabably, he did not finish his studies or obtain a degree. He may well have been expelled – for contradicting medical doctrine, ridiculing his teachers, rioting, or drunkenness. Given his character, the possibilities in this instance are legion. Yet one thing *is* certain: he may have exhibited licentious language, but he could not possibly have exhibited licentious behaviour. A childhood illness, possibly mumps, had rendered him impotent. All his life his face would remain hairless, and he would retain an odd high-pitched voice.

Having finished with university, Paracelsus took to the road as a wandering 'student of medicine'. He would pay his way by peddling cures – some bogus, others original and effective. Right from the start there was no doubting his exceptional talent, as well as his exceptional showmanship. If the former didn't succeed, he made sure that the latter did – at least until he had left town. As he travelled further afield, he quickly extended his medical knowledge. He now despised academic learning: 'the more learned, the more perverted.' True medical knowledge

could only be acquired in one way, the way he did it: 'A doctor
must seek out old wives, gypsies, sorcerers, wandering tribes,
old robbers and such outlaws and take lessons from them. A
doctor must be a traveller . . . Knowledge is experience.'

Right from the start Paracelsus' approach would be a
characteristic blend of the scientific (experience) and the
mythical (old wives' tales, etc). Only one thing was not
ambivalent in his method: his belief in himself and his own
infallibility. It was now that he arrogantly took to calling
himself Paracelsus. This means 'greater than Celsus', and is a
reference to the first-century AD Roman medical encyclopedist
Celsus, whose work had only been rediscovered in 1426, and
was then widely acclaimed. Europe was on the brink of the
Renaissance, which would see a huge revival of interest in
classical works of all kinds. Coincident with this was the
technological invention which would revolutionize European
learning. Gutenberg was assembling his prototype printing
press at Mainz in Germany. In 1454 he began his first major
enterprise, printing the so-called 'Gutenberg Bibles' (now the
most expensive books in the world). Just 24 years later an
edition of Celsus' medical encyclopedia would be printed. This
would inspire a European-wide interest in Ancient Roman
medicine whose effect is difficult to exaggerate. The Latin
terminology of Celsus' medical encyclopedia would play a
large part in establishing this as the medical language – for the
naming of diseases, procedures, anatomical features, and so
forth. It was Celsus who bequeathed us such words as abdomen (from the Latin *abdere* 'to conceal', and *adipem* 'fat'),
cartilage, vertebrae, uterus and anus. However, in other re-
spects Celsus' work was hardly original. The excessive regard
it was accorded in Renaissance times would not last. Ironically, Celsus' name is nowadays remembered mainly because
of the name Paracelsus.

So much about Paracelsus is paradoxical. He was inspired to
attack authority by the example of Luther and the Protestant
Reformation, yet he would remain a devout (if highly unorthodox, even heretical) Catholic throughout his life. His
incomplete academic education, and his itinerant gathering of
a wealth of local lore, led him to dispense with all academic
learning. This allowed him to break free from the stranglehold
of Hippocrates, Galen and the humoral theory. Yet in its place
he proposed his own, equally restrictive system. Instead of four
humours, he suggested that there were in fact three basic
substances out of which everything else was made. These were
sulphur, mercury and salt. Sulphur accounted for the inflam-
mability of substances, mercury for their volatility, salt for
their solidity. Fortunately all this did not limit his thought. In
the words of the historian Ackerknecht: 'If Paracelsus' framework of ideas cannot easily be identified as a "system", it is not
because systematic intentions were absent but only because of
his utter confusion as a thinker.'

If anything, Paracelsus' philosophy is essentially mystical.
He believed that the human body contained in microcosm the
macrocosm of the world. Yet this led him to the sensible
approach that Nature was the superior force, and thus the
healer's task was to understand the workings of the natural
world, which eluded the academic doctors of physic. Nature
should, where possible, be encouraged to follow its course.
(Here the echo of Hippocrates is unmistakable, if typically
unacknowledged.) But this in turn led Paracelsus to adopt the
folkloric 'Doctrine of Signatures'. This had long been the
major, and often only, medical resource of the peasantry.
Its knowledge had been passed on by word of mouth through
generations of old wives, witches and other esoteric figures.
According to the Doctrine of Signatures, healing plants visibly
manifested the specific provenance of their healing properties.

For instance, the orchid resembled a testicle, and was thus to be used for curing venereal complaints and diseases. Yellow celandine was the remedy for jaundice, heart-shaped lilac leaves should be used to treat heart disease, and so forth. This was Nature's superior wisdom, and the healer's task was to learn how to recognize these 'signatures' in plants.

Paracelsus' interest in medicine led him into deep waters. From an early age he had been interested in the practice of alchemy, the first rudiments of which he had probably been taught by his father. This would confirm Paracelsus' mystical streak. Alchemists saw their 'dark art' as a means of tapping into the invisible spiritual powers through which the world was governed by God. The alchemists' famed quest was to discover how to transmute base metals into gold. This was both a practical pursuit in search of real gold, and a mystical pursuit which sought to transform the 'base metal of humanity' into golden spiritual purity. As usual, Paracelsus accepted only what he wanted of this doctrine. The pursuit of metallic gold was dismissed as a shallow materialistic heresy. Paracelsus was more interested in the spiritual aspects. Yet even here he insisted upon his own interpretation. If alchemy was a predominantly spiritual pursuit, what was the point of the alchemists' actual experiments? Paracelsus decided that the alchemists' experimental aim was to discover medicines which would cure diseases.

During this period, alchemy was the early form of chemistry. It was the only way of investigating the properties and constituents of matter. Already it had perfected many of the techniques which would become central to chemistry. The basic experimental methods and instruments of scientific chemistry were developed by the dark art of alchemy in pursuit of its unscientific aims. Distillation, the distinction between acids and alkalis, instruments such as the crucible and the alembic (for distilling) – all these would pass unchanged into chemistry, when alchemy shed its mystical pretensions and its obsession with gold.

Paracelsus' deep involvement with alchemy led him to acquire considerable chemical expertise. Yet he abhorred the haphazard and secretive methods of the alchemists. In his experiments he insisted upon using pure chemicals in precise quantities, and following the stages of an experiment in the required order. He understood that particular chemical subtances had particular properties, and compounds containing these substances were liable to retain a vestige of these properties. This knowledge would prove invaluable in the preparation of medicines. Paracelsus believed that a particular disease required a particular remedy, which could be effected by chemical medicines. (Presumably this was in cases where no plant was found to resemble the part requiring treatment.) This insight that a specific disease required a specific treatment of its own was a great step forward for medicine. It directly contradicted the notion of balancing the four bodily humours. Paracelsus was responsible for several important discoveries here. During his preparations of ether, he noticed how this substance made chickens swoon. (Such a discovery conjures up a picture of highly medieval laboratory conditions.) He also noticed that tincture of morphine, which he christened laudanum, had the effect of reducing pain. Each chemical had its effect, which could be used for medical purposes. This recognition would become one of the foundations of modern medicine.

Yet once again Paracelsus would insist upon his own particular variant. Although he derided the alchemists' search for gold as trivial, he remained nonetheless committed to the search for that other holy grail of alchemy, 'the elixir of life'. This was the magic potion, of popular legend, which bestowed 'eternal youth'. Paracelsus would devote long hours in his alchemist's den attempting to produce this elusive elixir. On one occasion he even became convinced that he had found it. After imbibing the finished product, he declared to all and sundry that he would live for ever. For once the academic authorities and the old wives were of one accord: Paracelsus' claims were greeted with deep scepticism. Even his most enthusiastic tavern colleagues remained doubtful, deciding that they would wait and see. Yet Paracelsus remained undaunted. Faced with universal doubt, he coined the saying: 'In the country of the blind, the one-eyed man is king.'

During his years of wandering, Paracelsus would travel the length and breadth of Europe on foot. He is known to have reached as far north as Scandinavia, and probably visited Britain. He certainly stayed in Constantinople during 1522. This must have required considerable powers of persuasion, for by then the city had long fallen to the Ottoman Turks and was ruled by Suleiman the Magnificent. Infidels and foreign visitors were customarily flung without further ado into the notorious Yedikule dungeons, where they rotted until they died. (Visitors sent from their country as ambassadors were usually accorded the diplomatic status of being tortured before being flung into the dungeons.) Yet Paracelsus lived to tell the tale, and indeed brought back with him some unlikely treasures. These included a book containing lost secrets of Byzantine alchemy, and the recipe for the poppyseed-based elixir which he named laudanum. This was after the Latin word *laudare* meaning 'to praise', presumably on account of its pleasant narcotic effects. Paracelsus would keep secret the ingredients of laudanum for many years; only rarely would he allow a wealthy patient to purchase a small bottle of it to relieve suffering. On such occasions he would frequently drop in fragments of gold leaf for added effect, to put any would-be analyst off the scent, and to add to the price. During the eighteenth and nineteenth centuries laudanum would become a medical standby. This was the 'opium' to which De Quincy and Baudelaire would become addicted. Every doctor's medical bag would contain a bottle, and it would be readily available at pharmacists until the late nineteenth century.

During these wandering years Paracelsus acquired his famous sword, which appears in so many depictions of him. This vast phallic substitute would be worn at all times, and was frequently waved above his head during boisterous sessions at the tavern. Paracelsus was so enamoured of his sword that he took it to bed with him at night and even gave it a name – Azoth, the alchemical term for the creative force of Nature. How he acquired this sword remains shrouded in the mystery of at least a dozen conflicting anecdotes, all probably from his own mouth. On one day it might be the gift of a grateful vizier in Constantinople, on the next it might have been stolen from a giant he had bewitched with laudanum in Transylvania, on others he would relate how he had found it on a mountaintop in the Alps.

In the end the years of wandering the highways and byways, the heroic drinking bouts, and the clashes with authorities in town after town, all began to take their toll. By the time Paracelsus was approaching thirty he was balding, had the tanned visage of a vagabond, his coarse faintly hermaphroditic features softened by his lack of beard, and was customarily dressed in 'beggar's garb'. Only his self-belief remained undaunted.

Then in 1527 he arrived at Basle in Switzerland. The great Dutch Renaissance humanist and scholar Erasmus happened to be staying in town. Erasmus was renowned for his open-mindedness in matters of learning and expressed an interest in meeting Paracelsus. When they met, Erasmus was so impressed by Paracelsus that he even asked him if he could cure his recurrent kidney complaint, as well as the gout from which he had begun to suffer. Paracelsus duly effected cures for both Erasmus' ailments.

There is no doubt that Paracelsus could be a highly charismatic figure when the opportunity arose. He evidently charmed Erasmus, who upon being cured told him: 'I cannot offer thee a fee equal to thine art and learning.' This was no small compliment, coming from arguably the most learned man of his era. Erasmus now set about getting Paracelsus a job. As a result of his influence, Paracelsus was appointed town medical officer and professor of medicine at the University of Basle.

Paracelsus began as he meant to go on. Consciously modelling himself upon Luther, he nailed the programme of his lectures to the great wooden door of the university for all to see. In this he declared that contrary to tradition his lectures would be open to all, and would be delivered in the language of the people (i.e. German, rather than academic Latin). The local alchemists and barber-surgeons were specifically invited to attend – as were the staid and prosperous local pharmacists, who were in for a shock.

Dispensing with formal academic robes, Paracelsus appeared for his first lecture dressed in his alchemist's leather apron. He opened by announcing that he would reveal the great secret of medical science. Whereupon he dramatically uncovered a pan of excrement. Immediate uproar – followed by the physicians and other respectable members of the audience indignantly making their way to the exits. Paracelsus harangued them: 'If you will not hear the mysteries of putrefactive fermentation, you are unworthy of the name physicians.' As ever, there was more than a grain of truth in Paracelsus' display. His alchemical studies had led him to understand that the human body was in fact no less than a chemical laboratory. Fermentation was the most important process that took place in that laboratory.

But worse was to come. Just three weeks later, in the middle of the St John's Day celebrations, Paracelsus led a band of cheering students into the marketplace. Here he triumphantly burned the works of Galen and Avicenna (just as Luther had publicly burned the missive from the Pope threatening him with excommunication). Paracelsus had now taken on a young secretary, John Oporinus, who has left us a firsthand description of his master's modus operandi:

> He spent his time on drinking and gluttony, day and night. He could not be found sober an hour or two together . . . Nevertheless, when he was most drunk and came home to dictate to me, he was so consistent and logical that a sober man could not have improved upon his manuscripts.

Surprisingly, the university authorities tolerated this behaviour for almost two years, before despatching Paracelsus back down the road from whence he had come. He remained undaunted: his task was to awaken the world to a new medicine, free from the irrelevant prejudices of the past. Yet perhaps his most unforgivable behaviour was his mockery of all other medical innovators. Paracelsus was only in favour of his own discoveries. Those produced by others were derided. He even dismissed dissection as mere 'dead anatomy'. Yet his practical talents were unrivalled. The most illustrative example is his interpretation of gout. Previously, humoral theory had characterized gout as a 'defluxion in the foot' (*gutta* is Latin for 'liquid' or 'flowing'). Balance the humours by correcting their 'flow' in the foot, and the patient would be cured. But Paracelsus recognized that the cause of gout was in fact chemical. This was a 'tartaric disease', caused by 'seeds' of salts (tartar) coagulating at the joint. He saw that it was similar to other deposits that form in the body – such as gall and kidney stones, and the deposit which forms on the teeth (which we still call tartar). The tartar which caused gout was derived from food and drink, and was released into the body by the digestive process. Those unable to excrete the 'spirit of salt' suffered from deposits. Paracelsus had observed that in Switzerland 'there is no gout, no colic, no rheumatism, and no stone.' He realized that this was due to the purity of the mountain water. 'Tartaric salts' in the water supply were the cause of gout, gall stones, and the like.

Paracelsus was one of the first to understand that chemicals, or lack of them, could cause disease. He also understood their role in curing disease. For this reason, many see him as the father of modern iatrochemistry (medical chemistry: from the Greek *iatros*, meaning 'one who heals'). Interestingly, his understanding that disease could be caused by 'seeds' in the body would open the way to future recognition that germs could cause disease.

Fortunately, later in his life Paracelsus found time to set down his vast accumulation of medical knowledge in several hefty tomes. His *Die Grosse Wundartzney* (The Great Surgery Book) was published in 1536. But he never abandoned his lifestyle. Five years later, at the age of 44, he died after a tavern brawl at Salzburg in upper Austria.

Paracelsus would have a profound effect on medicine. He straddles two ages: the medieval and the Renaissance. His rejection of authority and reliance upon experience was modern, his belief in esoteric mysticism belonged to a departing age. It is his concentration on the aetiology of specific diseases, and the search for their specific cures, especially by means of drugs, which would carry his influence down the centuries. Yet even this continues to be controversial. To this day, homoeopathic medicine recognizes him as a pioneer. The renowned historian of medicine Charles H. Talbot assessed him as follows: 'The problems he discovered are not solved yet . . . They make us realize how primitive and sketchy our present theory of medicine is. We have accumulated a large number of scientifically established facts . . . But we need a philosophy to connect these facts. This is where Paracelsus . . . can teach us a great deal.'

Is modern medicine really in such a primitive state? As with all things concerning Paracelsus, there is another side to the story. Paracelsus liberated medicine from a 'philosophy' – the humoral theory. As a result, subsequent medicine often appeared piecemeal, and as such lacking in any overall philosophy: a state which is frequently associated with the primitive beginnings of a science. But does medicine really need a theoretical systematic approach? Some would argue that the human body itself is medicine's 'system' – or that the scientific approach is sufficient 'philosophy'. Such arguments and counterarguments will recur, with varying justification, throughout the long history to follow.

Towards the end of his travelling life, in 1529, Paracelsus arrived one day in the prosperous German city of Nuremberg. By now his reputation had begun to precede him, and before he could set up shop the local physicians decided to challenge him to a public debate, and let the audience decide between them. Paracelsus wisely chose to turn down this opportunity to expose himself to tricky public questioning before an unknown audience. Instead, he suggested that the resident doctors should present him with a patient they had been incapable of curing, and see what Paracelsus could do for him. He even went so far as to suggest they let him try out his talents on a patient who had contracted syphilis, a disease that was widely regarded as incurable and fatal. Paracelsus was directed to the 'leper colony' outside the city walls, where no less than fifteen syphilitics were incarcerated. To the astonishment of the city

doctors, Paracelsus duly appeared to cure nine of these patients. In fact, we now know that he merely alleviated the
symptoms by using a mercury ointment. This medication he
almost certainly learned from Girolamo Fracastro – better
known to us by his Latin name Fracastorius – the celebrated
Italian physician who first named syphilis.

The grotesque and painful sexually transmitted disease
syphilis was in some ways the AIDS of the period from the
Renaissance to the mid-twentieth century. It was for centuries
all but incurable, it could be passed on in the womb to the next
generation, and in its final stage could result in the slow rotting
of limb and brain prior to death. Syphilis is said to have arrived
in Europe when Columbus first returned from the New World.
It is known that his navigator Pinzon was treated for syphilis
as early as 1493. Three years later it passed from the Spanish
garrison at Naples to the French troops who were besieging the
city. During the French army's long march home the disease
was spread throughout the Italian peninsula, causing it to
become known as the 'French disease'. From here it quickly
spread through Europe. Strong historical evidence suggests
that this particular pandemic was so virulent that its spread
was not limited to sexual contact. It also appears for some
reason to have been particularly prevalent amongst the upper
classes. By the early decades of the sixteenth century the
disease had penetrated to England, forcing Henry VIII to close
down the London 'stews' (brothels). Indeed, it has even been
suggested that Henry himself may have contracted the disease,
which could have been responsible for his rapid mental and
physical decline prior to his death in 1547.

But did syphilis really originate in the Americas? Scholars
have discovered references to a remarkably similar sexually
transmitted disease in writings of ancient China and India.
Suggestions have been made that it was mentioned in the Bible

– as one of the afflictions of Job. Similarly, certain variants of earlier medieval 'leprosy' are known to have been transmitted sexually. Despite close scrutiny of these literary references, as well as scientific examination of early bone fragments, any final answer to this controversy remains as elusive as ever. (The distinguished British astronomer Fred Hoyle even went so far as to claim that syphilis resulted from 'bacterial seeding from a passing comet'.)

One reason why syphilis was so widely detected in Europe in the decades after Columbus' return was due to the work of Fracastorius and his pioneering theory of contagious diseases. Fracastorius was born in Verona in 1478, the scion of an upper class family with a long medical tradition. He went to the nearby University at Padua, then emerging as one of the finest in Europe, where he studied biology, mathematics, logic and astronomy, as well as medicine. Here he encountered the young Copernicus, with whom he remained in contact after Copernicus returned to his native Poland. Fracastorius was said to have been a burly fellow with a large bushy beard and a bluff jocular manner. He appears to have been a typical product of the Renaissance. Besides being a fine poet, he also excelled in scientific fields beyond medicine. Along with Leonardo, he was one of the earliest to understand the true nature of fossils, and he was the first to describe the magnetic poles. After graduating from Padua, Fracastorius returned to Verona, where he set up in medical practice.

It was not until 1530 that Fracastorius finally published the work which brought him Europe-wide fame. This was *Syphilis Sive Morbus Gallicus* (Syphilis or the French Disease). Following in the Ancient Roman tradition of the philosopher-poet Lucretius, this work was composed in stylish Latin verse. In the course of its 130 stanzas it tells the story of the shepherd Syphilis who insulted the God Apollo, and was punished for this by a 'pestilence unknown' which appeared in the form of 'foul sores'. This disease 'arose in the generative region' and was able to 'eat away the groin'. It could produce agonizing pain in the joints, rot the bones, and disfigure the body and face with hideous scabs. And its spread appeared unstoppable:

> Through what adventures this unknown Disease
> So lately did astonish'd *Europe seize*,
> Through *Asian* coasts and *Libyan* cities ran,
> And from what Seeds the Malady began . . .

Fracastorius recommended that the disease should be treated with quicksilver (mercury) ointment, which helped alleviate the sores (as Paracelsus seems to have learned from an early manuscript of Fracastorius' poem which was circulating prior to his 1529 arrival in Nuremberg).

Fracastorius did not invent the mercury ointment, but the many printings of his *Syphilis* throughout Europe ensured widespread knowledge of this treatment amongst physicians, as well as fixing the name of the disease. Here Fracastorius proved effective, if not original. In his other claim to medical fame he would be original, but not effective. Fracastorius was one of the earliest to display a truly Renaissance attitude towards medical studies. His all-round learning was humanist, accepting neither superstition nor ancient authority. Disease was neither God-inflicted nor the result of humoral imbalance. Observation, and a scientific attitude, prompted Fracastorius to theorize with astonishing originality concerning the nature of contagious diseases. His ideas were so in advance of their time that it would be three centuries before they were confirmed by experiment. Though despite such prescience he was unable to effect cures for the contagions he described – these too would require centuries.

As Fracantorius suggested in his poem, he shared with Paracelsus the view that disease was caused by 'seeds' entering the body. But Fracastorius' more rigorous scientific approach led him to a much deeper understanding of disease than Paracelsus. He suggested that contagious diseases were caused by tiny entities which were too small to be visible with the naked eye. These he named *seminaria contagiosa* (disease seeds). They entered the body of the host, where they multiplied rapidly, causing the disease itself in full-flowering form. The seeds, or minute invisible entities, could be transferred to the host by direct bodily contact, by fomes (soiled clothing or bedlinen carrying the infection), or simply through the air. He went even further, suggesting that the seeds which carried infectious disease were specific. That is, each disease was caused by its own specific seed. Here we can see the germ theory of disease in all but name. (The word 'germ' – closely associated with the Latin for 'seed' – would not be used in the medical sense until the early 1800s, and its function not properly understood until Pasteur, over half a century later.)

As a result of Frascatorius' theory, he viewed his medical practice through new eyes. This led him to observe and analyse contagious diseases in some detail. Previously, many physicians had tended to regard contagions and plagues as more or less virulent variants of the same disease. In the heat of the moment – amidst so much hysteria and mortal danger – there was little time or place for analysis. Fracastorius' more clear-eyed investigations led him to understand that there was a whole range of contagious diseases. This prompted him to distinguish clinically between such diseases as plague, leprosy, measles, smallpox and syphilis – providing accurate observations which supported, but could in no way confirm, his theory of invisible specific 'disease seeds'. He was also among the first to describe typhus; as well as this, he has left an intriguing description of a disease, prevalent during the Renaissance, known as the 'English sweat'. This affliction, which could lay a patient low within a day, caused copious sweating, shivers, nausea, cramps and blinding headaches. These frequently led to delirium, unconsciousness and finally death. Henry VIII once suffered from a bout of this disease, but at the time his constitution was sufficiently robust for him to survive. Despite considerable investigation, modern medicine has been unable to identify the English sweat, which may simply have vanished or become latent. Either way, this remains one of the unsolved mysteries of medical history.

Fracastorius' fame, as well as his undoubted medical expertise, ensured that his practice at Verona achieved considerable renown, attracting patients from all over Italy. Eventually he was appointed personal physician to Pope Paul III. In 1545 Fracastorius accompanied the pope to the Council of Trent (now Trento), which had been called to answer the doctrinal criticisms posed by the Reformation. Fracastorius would have a decisive, if unexpected, effect on the Council. When cases of typhus were reported in Trent, Fracastorius advised the pope to leave the city. Forthwith, the entire Council was transferred to the healthier climate of Bologna.

Unfortunately, Fracastorius' pioneering theory of contagious diseases was to prove less effective. Despite its recognition by many humanist doctors, this theory was soon eclipsed by less rational medical notions, such as the popular mysticism perpetrated by Paracelsus. The idea that the body was a microcosm of the world had deep resonances in philosophy, religion and the arts. Such profundity gave reassurance and meaning to life: it would not easily be shed. Medicine was simply not yet ready to go it alone. Even its more thoughtful and honest practitioners were often unwilling to embrace a more scientific approach. Having an inkling of just how blindly they were moving in their treatment of the human body, they clung to some framework with which to justify their actions (to themselves, as well as others). With the benefit of history, we can see that medicine was still piecemeal, lacking any genuine coherent basis. Even Fracastorius' astonishingly far-sighted theory of contagious disease could not yet be justified in any scientific sense. (Seeds invisible to the human eye are no less mystical than a humanity whose parts echo those of the world around it.)

Ironically, the quasi-effective mercury ointment treatment for syphilis, recommended by Fracastorius, would also eventually serve to undermine any more modern approach. Mercury is a poison, and its absorption through the pores produces toxic effects: painful ulceration of the gums, teeth dropping out, even crumbling of the bones. For many this only confirmed Hippocrates' famous aphorism, 'Desperate diseases require desperate remedies', reinforcing his ancient authority. Other side effects of mercury poisoning, such as prolific heavy sweating and salivation, endorsed for many physicians the humoralist diagnosis. According to this, syphilis was caused by an excess of phlegm. Mercury ointment helped correct this imbalance, which could be further corrected by steam baths and other measures aimed at draining the body of excess phlegmatic liquid. Such humoralist explanations were further reinforced by time-honoured religious attitudes. Syphilis was an exemplary case of God punishing the victim for his sins. (As contemporary AIDS has amply demonstrated, epidemics of sexually transmitted disease invariably stir ancient irrationalities and prejudices.) It would be centuries before medicine caught up with Fracastorius' thinking.

5

BLUEPRINT FOR A SCIENCE

The need for a firm scientific foundation on which to base the practice of medicine would eventually be answered in the most obvious and practical fashion. So simple in hindsight, but no less than a revolution in its time. This was the work of the great Flemish physician Vesalius, whose book depicting the anatomy of the human body is widely recognized as the finest of its kind in medical history.

Andreas van Wesele (now known by his Latinized name Vesalius) was born in Brussels on the last day of the year 1514. His father was the illegitimate member of a renowned medical family, and became pharmacist to the Holy Roman Emperor Charles V. The maiden name of Vesalius' mother was Crabbe, indicating that she may have been of English extraction. The father was away much of the time, travelling with the emperor's entourage to Spain, and young Vesalius was brought up by his mother, a superstitious woman. In 1529, at the age of fifteen, Vesalius entered the provincial University of Louvain. His medical studies began four years later when he became a student at the University of Paris. Here he studied under one of the leading physicians of the day, Jacob Sylvius. Unusually for the time, Sylvius recognized the growing importance of the study of anatomy for physicians. Yet like so many others he retained a belief in the teachings of Galen, which were often anatomically incorrect, being based as they were on the dissection of animals.

Despite the intellectual stirrings of the Renaissance, the authority of Galen and Aristotle was still widely taken as the holy writ, especially in Paris. This was the absolute truth, and any denial of it might be regarded literally as heresy. (Copernicus would hold back from publishing his revolutionary heliocentric theory, which contradicted Aristotle, until the day before his death in 1543.) But Vesalius seems to have been driven from the earliest by an obsession with anatomy and the discovery of its secrets. He records how he 'spent long hours in the Cemetery of the Innocents in Paris turning over bones'. This morbid pursuit of learning was not without its dangers: it laid him open to a charge of heretical behaviour, and more besides. As he would later recollect, 'when once with a companion, I was gravely imperilled by many savage dogs.' The religious authorities were not the only ones who wished to protect their collections of bones from unorthodox scrutiny.

In 1536 Paris was threatened by the army of the Emperor Charles V. As a citizen of his empire, Vesalius found it expedient to hurry back to Louvain. Here he persisted with his risky anatomical pursuits. On one occasion Vesalius had himself 'locked out of Louvain so that, alone in the middle of the night, I might take away bones from the gibbet to prepare a skeleton.' The authorities would occasionally permit an autopsy, in order to determine the cause of death. Vesalius made sure that he became involved. Now for the first time he began working on actual cadavers. In order to understand fully what this involved, it is worth turning again to Vesalius' precise description:

> In the course of a dissection when an uninjured ovary is first compressed, like an inflated bladder it usually squirts forth the humor with a crackling noise to an astonishing height, not unlike a fountain. In women that humor is white, like very thick whey, but I have also found it yellowish like somewhat thickened egg yolk . . .

Vesalius was driven to such activity by a curious combination of motives. There is no doubting his scientific intention. He had spotted certain errors in Galen's anatomical descriptions, and wished to correct them by first-hand investigation. However, the intensity of his obsession with anatomy also hints at pathological impulses. Yet neither of these constituted his prime motive, which was nothing more or less than worldly ambition. From the time he entered the University of Paris at the age of 18, and possibly even before, Vesalius had set his sights upon entering the medical service of the Emperor Charles V. He not only wished to emulate his father, but to do better than him. Rather than becoming a mere pharmacist in the imperial service, he would become physician to the emperor himself. This, and this above all, appears to have been the driving force behind his ambitions. He also decided, early on, how he would set about achieving this aim.

Already Vesalius' anatomical expertise must have been recognizably as exceptional. In 1537 he travelled south to Italy, where at the age of just 23 he was appointed professor of anatomy at the University of Padua. By now the humanist Renaissance attitude was beginning to permeate the universities, and several Italian cities permitted the dissection of a limited number of executed criminals. From the start, Vesalius' teaching methods attracted attention. Prior to this, anatomical lectures would usually be delivered by the professor-physician reading from his notes whilst standing at a lectern, or sitting on a professorial high chair. Directly below him a barber-surgeon would dissect a body laid out on a table, illustrating the professor-physician's words. Physicians did not dirty their hands with such things; and the inferior surgeons were often slapdash in their methods. The words and the practical demonstration hardly matched. Vesalius knew that the only way to investigate the anatomy of the human body was to do it yourself, to learn by first-hand experience and experiment what precisely were the working constituents of human anatomy. Unashamedly, he 'would advise the medical students to observe where someone has been buried or urge them to make note of the diseases of their teacher's patients so that they might later seize their bodies.'

He also continued with his own further researches. He tells how he would 'keep in my bedroom for several weeks bodies taken from graves or given me after public executions'. On occasion, he would even 'petition the judges to delay the day of an execution of a criminal to a time suitable for my dissection of his body'. These researches were all leading towards a definite end. Vesalius intended to create the greatest book of human anatomy ever produced. As a trial run, in 1538 he published *Tabulae Anatomicae Sex* (Six Anatomical Drawings). Accompanying the drawings was a detailed descriptive text by Vesalius. Previously, anatomical illustrations had been schematic, or cartoon-like, usually drawn by the medical author, who was at best an amateur illustrator. Vesalius' *Tabulae* was the first anatomical textbook to contain large and precise pictures of human anatomy, drawn with artistic

verisimilitude so that all the parts could could be identified by
students who were performing dissections. In order to achieve
the level of artistic realism and exactitude he required, Vesalius
conscripted a fellow Fleming whom he had met in nearby
Venice. This was Johannes Stephanus of Calcar, a talented
artist who was employed at the time in the studio of Titian,
arguably the greatest artist Venice has produced. Vesalius
could not afford to pay Johannes Stephanus, so he signed
over to him any future profits which the book might make.

Vesalius' *Tabulae* contained several important corrections
to Galenic anatomy. Among these was his revised description
of the coccyx, at the lower end of the spinal column (given by
Galen the Greek name for 'cuckoo', whose beak it was said to
resemble). Vesalius also contradicted Galen's claim that the
lower jaw was divisible into two distinct sections. But the
Tabulae still does not constitute an outright attack on Galen's
anatomy. Surprisingly, it also persisted in maintaining several
of Galen's errors. The liver is incorrectly given five lobes, and
the diagram of a heart is indubitably that of an ape, such as
Galen had described. Most surprisingly of all, Vesalius also
repeats Galen's famous mistake of including the *rete mirabile*
below the human brain, when this net of blood vessels only
appears in hoofed animals.

So how could Vesalius have made such obvious errors?
Firstly, his experience with human dissection was still comparatively limited. He knew far more about osteology (bone
structure) than he did about the more perishable organs. The
fact is, Vesalius still had a high regard for Galen, viewing him
as 'easily leader of the professors of dissection'. At a loss to
explain Galen's errors, he initially thought that the human
body must have changed in the one and a half millennia since
Galen's day. He even went so far as to suggest that the
discrepancy between Galen's curvature of the femur (thigh

bone) and his own observations might be due to the modern fashion for wearing tight trousers. Although he had detected errors in Galen's work, he still viewed the human body through Galenic eyes. Not until his experience with human dissection uncovered more and more errors did he realize that Galen's entire view of anatomy would have to be overhauled. Only then did he famously exclaim: 'I myself cannot wonder enough at my own stupidity and too great trust in the writings of Galen.'

Vesalius now set about rectifying this with his masterwork *De Humani Corporis Fabrica* (Concerning the Structure of the Human Body), now generally known as the *Fabrica*. This would be five years in the making, and would include more than 200 folio illustrations extending over more than 700 pages of encyclopedic text. The finished work was divided into seven books. The first book included three superbly executed drawings of the complete human skeleton. Here Vesalius understood, as many previous anatomists had not, that the bones not only acted as a support for the body, but also assisted and controlled the movements of the body. Also, some bones 'such as the skull . . . the breastbone and the ribs were constructed by nature for the protection of other parts'. Further bones 'were placed before the joints to prevent them from being moved too freely or bent to an excessive angle'. Vesalius was interested in explaining not only the layout of the human body, but also how it worked. In the latter aspect his attempts would only be a piecemeal beginning. Here Paracelsus was the true pioneer, with his chemistry of the digestive system: a central process which affected the whole body.

Even more important, in this context, was Vesalius' insistence upon Aristotelian teleology, which decreed that everything, and thus every anatomical feature, must have a purpose.

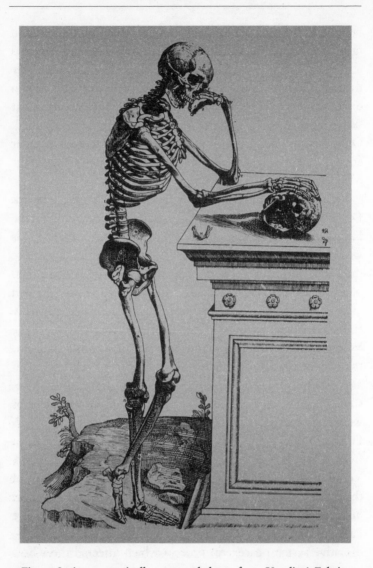

Figure 3. An anatomically correct skeleton from Vesalius' *Fabrica*
The figure of a skeleton studying a skull was a popular medieval
image of mortality. In this example from Vesalius' *Fabrica* the perfect
anatomical detail creates science from art; while the skill of the
illustrator Johannes Stephanus makes art of science.

This would confirm a vital principle: here Aristotle's teaching would not be jettisoned. (Not until Darwin would teleology be turned on its head. Evolution is blind: the fittest elements survive, and are reinforced by natural selection. Strictly speaking, there is no purpose in this scheme of things, though it can still remain useful to regard anatomical features from a teleological point of view. For instance, we say the purpose of the ears is to hear, and so forth.)

The second book of the *Fabrica* contains the series of seven illustrations known as the 'muscle men'. These depict the muscles of the human body in a sequence of increasingly peeled stages of 'undress', each illustration showing a deeper layer of muscles. This would be just how a student dissecting a cadaver would uncover the particular muscles at different depths below the skin. The illustrations of these first two books are works of art. They are almost certainly drawn by Johannes Stephanus of Calcar, but under the strict supervision of Vesalius. He set up the models, posing the skeletons just as they are depicted. For instance, in the seventh 'muscle man', the skull is supported by a noose with the rope threaded beneath the cheekbones. The body is allowed to sag, the better to expose the leg muscles, and the arm muscles are peeled so that they hang from the wrists. No artistic license was allowed. From the initial drawings, exact woodcuts were made so that the plates could be printed with extreme precision. This was a long, difficult and inordinately painstaking process, which must have involved much reworking or starting afresh.

Inevitably, the relationship between the scientist and the artist soon became strained to breaking point. At one point, Vesalius writes of the 'bad temper of artists and sculptors [meaning wood-block cutters] who made me miserable more than the bodies I was dissecting'. (Note how even for Vesalius, prolonged dissection of corpses could be a depressing business.)

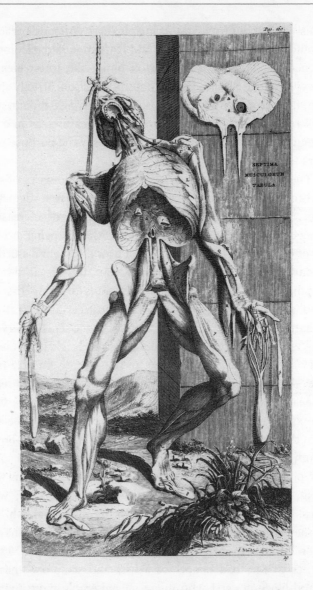

**Figure 4. Anatomical illustration of the seventh 'muscle man'
in Vesalius' *Fabrica***
Drawn by Johannes Stephanus under the author's close supervision.

The illustrations after Book two of the *Fabrica* are no longer works of art. For instance, the amazing 'venous man', which illustrates the structure of the veins permeating the entire body, astonishes only because of its immense complexity, rather than any aesthetic quality. Other illustrations are merely adequate. These ensuing illustrations are certainly not the work of Johannes Stephanus, who presumably quit the project early, in some dudgeon.

Despite this setback, Vesalius pressed on. The quality of the anatomical examination remained unprecedented. His dissection of the heart led him to doubt that 'the blood sweats from the right into the left ventricle through passages which escape the human vision'. This was a vital observation, which would have crucial implications for our understanding of how the blood moved in the body. Book seven contained a brilliant and perceptive investigation of the structure of the human brain. This included a number of important discoveries, and equally important revisions of the previous Galenic model. Vesalius' ever-increasing first-hand experience at the dissecting table had by this stage begun to reveal to him even the errors of his own ways. From now on, the *rete mirabile* vanished from Vesalius' human anatomy. Likewise, Galen's five-lobed liver was dismissed: 'The liver is not divided into fibres or lobes.'

Yet errors did remain. Vesalius' comparative lack of physiological expertise led him to go along with Galen's theory that venous blood was produced by the liver. But if blood did not pass from the right into the left ventricle of the heart, as Galen had suggested, where did the blood for his separate arterial system come from? (See Fig. 1 on p. 31.) Vesalius did not investigate this anomaly, which cast the first serious doubts on Galen's two separated blood systems (the venous and the arterial). Galen's entire notion of how the body functioned was now being called into question.

Other anatomical errors in the *Fabrica* are more curious. Some of Vesalius' descriptions of the visceral organs, such as the kidneys, undeniably belong to pigs or dogs. He also appears to have missed altogether the pancreas and the ovaries. Many of the minor illustrations throughout the work are probably by Vesalius himself. These include depictions of individual bones, and even simple drawings of carpentry hinges to illustrate how particular joints worked. Other illustration are of less certain provenance. For instance, an illustration of a pregnant uterus and its foetus has been characterized as 'medieval in its crudity'. Indeed, his depiction of specifically female organs is particularly weak. The lack of executed female criminals may well account for this lapse.

However, compared with the vast overall anatomical survey presented by the *Fabrica*, these are surely minor failings. This was the first book of its kind. (Leonardo da Vinci's superb anatomical drawings, which predate those of Vesalius by almost half a century, remained hidden in his secret notebooks for several centuries and would play no part in medical history). Never before had the human body been described publicly and in its entirety. Here, with a wealth of detail, was the first intricate depiction of what it is that constitutes a human being in the material and corporeal sense. This was the foundation on which an entirely new *scientific* medicine could be based.

Coincidence and historical significance seldom go hand in hand. Yet it is undeniably more than mere coincidence that Vesalius' *Fabrica* appeared in 1543, the same year as Copernicus' *On the Revolution of the Celestial Spheres*, which displaced humanity from the centre of the universe. Human beings could no longer be seen as a microcosm of the macrocosm. The earth and the planets revolved around the sun. The new science showed the precise location of humanity, as well as the precise location of the contents of the human body. Human knowledge was entering a new era. Observation, rather than authority or metaphoric resonance, would be the key to understanding. Instead of profundity and symbolism, there would be clarity and depth. (The latter in a very real – rather than spiritual – sense, as the Renaissance artists discovered perspective, knowledge explored its ancient classical roots, and anatomists probed deeper beneath the skin).

Vesalius took immense pains over the actual production of the *Fabrica*. He chose the typography, the paper and the binding of the book with as much care as he had taken over the illustrations. The woodcuts were sent across the Alps to Basle in Switzerland, so that they could be set by the one man in Europe who was both a first-class printer and a renowned scholar. This was none other than John Oporinus, who sixteen years previously had been Paracelsus' long-suffering secretary. After escaping from his hectic existence with Paracelsus, he had gone on to become a professor at Basle; though his father had been a painter and engraver, hence his skill at printing.

Vesalius soon crossed the Alps so that he could supervise the printing of his book personally. There were to be no mistakes; everything had to be just as he wanted it. He even went so far as to have the illustrations of the first copy hand-painted. (No other copy would have this feature.) The first book was bound in silk velvet of imperial purple and dedicated to the Holy Roman Emperor Charles V.

In the early months of 1543 Vesalius set out for the German city of Mainz, where he duly presented the first copy of the *Fabrica* to the emperor. The book was received with astonishment and delight. In gratitude, Vesalius was appointed as household physician to the emperor. Vesalius was just 28 years old: the fairy tale had come true. His life's aim had been achieved. From now on, he would accompany Charles V on all his travels throughout his various domains. (Amongst his many other titles, Charles was also king of both Spain and Naples.)

There can be no doubt that gaining this position at the imperial court, rather than causing a scientific revolution, was the true focus of Vesalius' ambition. From now on, he abandoned his researches into anatomy. His obsession became a thing of the past. He never returned to teach at Padua, or any of the other Italian universities where he had conducted his anatomical demonstrations with such success. Though he did sturdily defend his *Fabrica* against the many attacks it provoked. The book presented a direct challenge to Galen, whose authority had lasted for 1,400 years. Vesalius' former professor in Paris, Jacob Sylvius, was so outraged at his pupil's blasphemy that he wrote personally to the emperor. 'I implore His Imperial Majesty to punish severely, as he deserves, this monster born and bred in his own house, this worst example of ignorance, ingratitude, arrogance, and impiety, to suppress him so that he may not poison the rest of Europe with his pestilential breath.' From this time on Sylvius would only refer to Vesalius by the abusive nickname *Vesanus*: Latin for 'madman', whose last two syllables contain an added anatomical insult.

Vesalius now got married, and settled down to the life of imperial physician. He evidently acquitted himself well. When Charles V abdicated from the Spanish throne, he made Vesalius a Spanish count and granted him a generous pension for the rest of his life. Charles' son Philip II succeeded to the throne of Spain, and appointed Vesalius as his court physician. The riches of the New World had made Spain the most powerful nation in Europe, and these were heady times at the court of Philip II (after whom the Philippines were named). When

Henry II, the king of France, was injured in a jousting accident, Vesalius was called in to advise his royal physicians. And when Philip's oldest son Don Carlos cracked his head falling downstairs, Vesalius was despatched to take charge. His duties did entail the occasional autopsy, but his dissecting skills must have become rusty, for this was to prove an embarrassment. According to legend, he dissected the corpse of a nobleman – only to discover that his heart was still beating. Whereupon he was sentenced to death by the Inquisition. In the nick of time, Philip II intervened and personally rescinded the sentence. He decreed that by way of a penance Vesalius should undertake a pilgrimage to Jerusalem.

Vesalius sent his wife and daughter back to Brussels, to live in the large mansion he had built amidst gardens on the outskirts of the city. Then the 50-year-old Vesalius set out on the long and arduous journey to the Holy Land. On his way, he called in at Padua. There is a story that he wished to return to his old post at the university, but it is said that this was forbidden by Philip II. Or did he perhaps just wish to bid farewell to the scene of his former successes? On the return voyage across the Mediterranean from the Holy Land, Vesalius fell mortally ill. In June 1564 he was put ashore at the island of Zakynthos, off the western shore of Greece, and died almost at once.

Vesalius' most revered pupil was Gabriele Fallopius, who made up for his master's few anatomical shortcomings by undertaking a detailed study of the female generative organs. Fallopius would achieve immortality by attaching his name to the Fallopian tubes of the ovary. In the course of his work he also named the placenta, as well as the vagina.

During the ensuing years many lesser anatomists would seek immortality by attaching their names to anatomical features, some of which they had not discovered but were merely naming. Vesalius had selflessly refrained from this practice, giving Latin, Greek and even Hebrew names to the features he described. Alas, Hebrew proved his undoing. At this time Arabic was often written in Hebrew script in Europe, being largely the preserve of Jewish scholars. Several Arabic medical terms had survived the translators of Salerno and Montpellier, and these were occasionally written in Hebrew script. Vesalius would include Hebrew headings in his *Tabulae*, hoping to impress by suggesting that he was fluent in this language. Unfortunately, he knew nothing of Hebrew beyond the alphabet, and was even under the misapprehension that Hebrew and Arabic were the same language. To assist him with his Hebrew he appears to have engaged, perhaps at a cut-price rate, some local Italian-Jewish character who was more conversant with the current street-slang aspects of Hebrew than its purer form. Such is the somewhat faulty Hebrew which appears in Vesalius' early *Tabulae*.

Very little is known for certain about Vesalius' actual personality, and this unfortunate linguistic pretension would appear a harmless foible. Yet the medical historians Singer and Rabin go much further, seeing it as a key to his character: 'The man who intends to deceive in this way is certainly not above some of the less lovable human failings. The most enthusiastic admirer of Vesalius will hardly claim him as a shining example of rigid veracity.' Another fact which is sometimes mentioned in his disfavour is that both his wife and his daughter married a year after his death. It is difficult to tell on such scant evidence, but perhaps the man who in his younger days obsessively haunted graveyards and gallows was not the most savoury of characters. This said, medicine will remain forever in his debt. His work can be seen as a crowning achievement of Renaissance humanism. Likewise, his introduction of practical and detailed anatomy into a medical tradition which had previously disparaged such practice, would further emphasize the scientific attitude in medicine.

After Vesalius' overall anatomy, the next inevitable step was towards detailed investigation of the various body parts. His pupil Fallopius, besides describing the organs involved in human generation and childbearing, would in addition investigate the workings of the inner ear and the kidneys. During a spell in Florence, he is also known to have carried out dissections of the lions at the Medici zoo. Despite accusations of vivisection, it is now known that the lions were dead before Fallopius operated on them. This was fortunate, for according to the renowned medical expert on this period C.D. O'Malley, Fallopius' operations on living human patients were less successful 'as demonstrated by the fatal outcome of a number of his cases'. After this, Fallopius stuck to academic work, eventually succeeding to the anatomical chair at Padua, the position previously held by Vesalius.

6

HARVEY THE CIRCULATOR

Vesalius' star pupil had been Fallopius, and Fallopius' star pupil would be Girolamo Fabricius of Aquapendente, whose anatomical specialization included the human veins. In the course of his work, he discovered flaps in these veins, which appeared to operate as valves. In turn, Fabricius' most brilliant student at the University of Padua was the young Englishman William Harvey. Listening to Fabricius lecture, Harvey became intrigued by this puzzling evidence that the veins had valves, allowing the blood to pass only in one direction.

William Harvey arrived in Padua in 1599, at the age of 21. He had been born at Folkestone, on the south coast of England, where his father had been a wealthy businessman who had prospered in the cross-Channel trade with France. At the age of 15 William Harvey won a scholarship to Caius College, Cambridge. This college had recently been endowed by the celebrated physician and anatomist Dr John Caius, who had studied under Vesalius at Padua. Later, Caius and Vesalius had become friends, to the extent that they had even shared lodgings. But this arangement had come to an acrimonious end when Vesalius began casting doubt on the teachings of Galen, an action which Caius regarded as a form of blasphemy. On returning to England, Caius had been even more shocked by the state of anatomical studies in his country. When he joined the Barbers and Surgeons Company (the professional body of the London anatomists) he discovered that they were allowed by act of Parliament the bodies of just four hanged criminals per year upon which to experiment. He was even more aghast when he discovered that owing to a lack of interest in research even these had not been used.

Caius College, Cambridge specialized in medicine, suggesting that even at 15 Harvey already had inclinations in this direction. However, in other subjects the college was notoriously neglectful. Despite such shortcomings, Harvey's accumulation of knowledge seems to have extended far beyond medicine. This was the age of Shakespeare, whose wealth of reference and popular commercial success speak of a wide and broadly educated audience for his plays. Yet the conservative Cambridge authorities did their best to suppress such 'publicke showes and commen plaies' because of their 'lewd example'. As ever, the undegraduates took little notice of their professors. According to Harvey's biographer Geoffrey Keynes, 'It is notorious that the students in Tudor times were addicted to play-acting.' Yet it soon transpired that even in medicine Caius College 'was not adequate for full training as a doctor'. So in 1599 Harvey set off for Padua to complete his studies and gain his doctor's scroll.

Educationally speaking, Harvey now passed from darkness into light. The University of Padua was at the peak of its brilliance. Fabricius was occupying Vesalius' chair, the enlightened Aristotelian philosopher Zabarella was lecturing on the place of logic in science, and Galileo was professor of mathematics. Padua was the epicentre of the new scientific thinking. Already Galileo had covertly come to the conclusion that Copernicus' heliocentric theory was correct (it would be 30 years before he was tried by the Inquisition for publicly expressing such a view). This was the dawn of the modern scientific era, when the humanism of the Renaissance began to evolve into the rational and empirical approach of the Enlightenment. During the ensuing sevententh century everything would change. Descartes's rationalism would start modern philosophy, and his unification of geometry and algebra would cause a similar revolution in mathematics. First Galileo would lay the foundations of modern scientific method, then Newton would transform our understanding of the entire universe with his work on gravity. Francis Bacon would champion experimental method, Boyle would found modern chemistry, and Leibniz would publicly introduce calculus. Hardly any aspect of European culture would remain unchanged – from the introduction of the muzzle-loading musket (arquebus), to baroque architecture and the music of Bach. In time, Harvey too would take his place amidst this pantheon.

Harvey would remain in Padua until 1602, by which stage Fabricius had acknowledged him as his finest student. According to a contemporary, 'Fabricius was more than a teacher to Harvey, for a fast friendship seems to have sprung up between master and pupil.' Fabricius would conduct his anatomical dissections in a special circular steep-sided lecture theatre, where the tiers of students could peer down over his head (and smell for themselves what it was like to examine a cadaver). The students were often rowdy, especially the Germans, and Fabricius was not a commanding teacher. But in private the power and range of his mind were said to have been inspiring. His intellectual researches ranged throughout the sciences: he observed sunspots some years before Galileo, and was a great believer in comparative anatomy. He felt sure that the dissection of all species could not help but inform our knowledge of our own anatomy. Galen and others had made their mistakes not by comparing anatomies, but by wrongly identifying with them. The simpler organs of animals could only help explain how human organs worked. Harvey hung on Fabricius' words; he would remain forever in his master's intellectual debt. From this time on, Harvey became an avid dissectionist of almost any animal he could lay his hands on: snails, insects, squirrels, frogs, dogs, all were grist to the mill of Harvey's ever-inquiring mind.

It must have been during these years that Harvey took to wearing the dagger mentioned by Aubrey in his *Brief Lives*. In Italy this would have been more than a mere phallic accoutrement. Harvey's willingness to draw his dagger when crossed may well have been a habit which he acquired amidst the volatile atmosphere of Renaissance Italian society. It appears to have been an aggressive-defensive mechanism. There is no record of him actually using his dagger.

On his return to England, Harvey worked at St Bartholomew's Hospital as an assistant physician, becoming physician there in 1609. St Bartholomew's was one of the two main hospitals in London, and had over 200 beds in 12 separate wards. Harvey had 3 surgeons and an apothecary as his junior colleagues, and received the respectable annual salary of £25, plus £2 for his livery. (As a student at Cambridge, he had lived comfortably on less than £5 a year.) This was an important post, though it was not without its dangers. The first man to become physician here, a flamboyant Portuguese by the name of Dr Rodrigo Lopez, had been hung at Tyburn just 15 years previously on suspicion of attempting to poison

Queen Elizabeth (a charge of which he was almost certainly innocent). Harvey's duties at St Bartholomew's were not onerous: he was required to work a minimum of one day a week, though doubtless he put in more. This freedom enabled him to set up a private practice in London, which soon began to prosper.

In 1604 Harvey had married Elizabeth Browne, the daughter of the king's physician, who was also a senior fellow of the College of Physicians. As a result of this tactical alliance, Harvey would be elected a fellow himself in 1607. (Such was the way of the world in those so different times.) Of Harvey's actual marriage circumstances, little is known, apart from the fact that he probably had no children and that his wife kept a tame parrot. Harvey would wax lyrical over this creature, which seems to have absorbed much of the affection that might otherwise have been lavished upon human offspring. 'My wife had an excellent, and well instructed Parrat, which was long her delight . . . If she bad him talk or sing, were it night and never so darke, he would obey her. Many times when he was sportive and wanton, he would sit in her lap, where he loved to have her scratch his head, and stroke his back, and then testifie his contentment, by kinde mutterings, and shaking of his wings.' Yet even this picture of contentment would succumb to Harvey's growing obsession with comparative anatomy. When the parrot died, Harvey conducted a post-mortem – whereupon he was astonished to discover a decaying egg in its oviduct. 'I alwaies thought him to be a Cock-parrat, by his notable excellence in singing and talking.' He concluded that his wife's unsuspected female parrot had died from lack of love.

In 1615 Harvey was appointed a lecturer at the College of Physicians (with no help from his father-in-law, who had died ten years previously). This was a post he would hold for 40 years, and would play a major role in allowing him to develop his scientific ideas. A year later, the year of Shakespeare's death, he began his lectures 'On the Whole of Anatomy'. The notes for these initial lectures are amongst the few of Harvey's papers to survive, and may be seen in the British Library. Like many lecture notes which are used year upon year, they are something of a mess – often comprehensible to the lecturer alone. They are scribbled in a mixture of Latin, English and an inscrutable shorthand of his own invention. This unfortunately owes nothing to his predecessor as physician at St Bartholomew's, Dr Timothie Bright, who invented modern shorthand, becoming so intrigued with this enterprise that he neglected all his duties and had to be dismissed.

Harvey's anatomy lecture notes have several surprising omissions. There is no mention of the skeleton or of several important organs. One can only surmise these have been lost. Yet as one might expect, there is a wealth of references to his comparative anatomical researches. (Though the references to his wife's parrot appear elsewhere, amongst his personal papers.) Inevitably, he also describes clinical observations which he carried out at St Bartholomew's and in the course of his private practice. This was not a time of reticence, and Harvey refers to many of his patients by name and profession, before outlining their often intimate complaints. For instance, he mentions that a certain Lord Clarke (a judge) had such a retracted penis as to encourage the popular belief 'that men can degenerate into hermaphrodites or women'. One can only imagine what his equally unreticent students must have made of all this. Harvey was lucky that he never had the misfortune to appear in court before Lord Clarke.

In the light of such information, it comes as a surprise that Harvey retained any private patients at all. Yet his increasingly lucrative practice continued to flourish. Indeed, he now counted amongst his patients several of the most influential figures in London. The greatest of these would prove to be Harvey's only contemporary English scientific equal – namely Sir Francis Bacon, a giant amongst men who would succeed in a number of differing fields, from philosophy to law, from politics to science, from history to essay-writing. In 1618 Bacon was appointed Lord Chancellor, the senior legal post in the land, which also carried a political power almost equivalent to the modern prime minister. (When the king set off on lengthy trips to Scotland, Bacon would be left in London in charge of the country.) Peacock in dress and extravagant in lifestyle, Bacon was constantly in need of money – to maintain his palatial country house, his many liveried servants and his estates. In 1621 he would be dismissed from his post for accepting bribes. Characteristically unabashed, his defence would be that these bribes had in no way influenced his judgement, as he had always been willing to accept bribes from both sides in any case he tried. After his dismissal, and a brief spell of imprisonment in the Tower of London, he turned to philosophical and scientific enquiries. Bacon maintained a more than passing interest in medicine, experimenting with cures and developing considerable knowledge concerning the effects of various chemicals on the human body. Despite this, he had a rather jaundiced view of the subject: 'Medicine is a science which hath been more professed than laboured, and yet more laboured than advanced, the labour having been, in my judgement, rather in circle than in progression.' He stressed the need for a return to 'Medicinall History' together with 'the ancient and serious diligence of Hippocrates'.

Such views did not go down well with Harvey, who regarded the exotic Bacon as something of a dilettante in medicine, and indeed in other branches of natural philosophy (the name still used for science). Harvey's view of his patient's

intellectual accomplishments was unduly harsh (and mistaken): 'He writes philosophy like a Lord Chancellor.' These two
great minds do not appear to have shared their ideas, and each
would remain blind forever to the accomplishments of the
other. One suspects that Bacon's consultations with his physician were somewhat frosty affairs.

The fact is, the two of them approached science from the
opposite ends of the spectrum. Even so, they were both
scientists in the new mould – believing in experiment, rather
than authority. Yet in the end Harvey was – like Galileo – a
practitioner rather than a philosopher. Writing of the likes of
Galileo, Bacon would say: 'These men spend their labour
working out some one experiment [which may result in certain
discoveries] but because the experiment stops with those few
discoveries . . . many other things equally worthy of investigation are not discovered by the same means.' As has been
pointed out, Bacon was more interested in 'the science of
science' than science itself. In the words of Harvey's biographer Keynes, Bacon 'liked to think that every discovery was
only a link in a chain, the gradual unfolding of which should
be a consciously controlled process'. It is indicative that despite
his polymath intellect, Bacon's original scientific discoveries
were negligible. His originality lay in his understanding of
what science was. Without such thinking, scientific discoveries
– even great ones such as Harvey was to make – are little more
than scattered beacons of light in unstructured darkness. Or,
as the great French mathematician Poincaré would put it
nearly three centuries later: 'Science is built up with facts,
as a house is with stones. But a collection of facts is no more a
science than a heap of stones is a house.'

Harvey would make the actual scientific discovery; Bacon's
discovery would be precisely what the scientist was doing. He
would ask: what is scientific truth? His general answer would

be: induction. As it is tested, again and again, each time proving correct, a truth becomes confirmed. Likewise, one fact leads to another. As one fact is piled upon another, the stone house of science grows. Bacon's contribution was to justify an entire outlook, indicating its validity as well as its method.

It is a sad irony that one of the few actual experiments which Bacon would undertake would result in his death. Returning by coach from London during the bitter snowy winter of 1626, Bacon was suddenly possessed by the idea that the coldness of snow might preserve living flesh from putrefaction. In the words of Aubrey, he immediately 'alighted out of the coach, and went into a poor woman's house at the bottom of High-gate Hill, and bought a hen, and made the woman gut it, and then stuffed the body with snow, and my lord did help to do it himself. The snow chilled him, and he immediately fell so extremely ill.' Within a few days he was dead. Bacon's insight concerning the refrigeration of flesh would, in time, transform the study of anatomy – though this would remain peripheral to his theoretical contribution.

By now Harvey's professional standing had risen still further. In 1618 he had been made one of the physicians to King James I. After James' death in 1625, Harvey continued in his post under Charles I, who would develop an affectionate regard for Harvey. Charles even became interested in Harvey's medical researches into comparative anatomy. As a result, Harvey was given permission to dissect deer carcasses from the royal parks. For his part, Harvey grew extremely fond of Charles, who was known to have been a difficult, often haughty figure. It was a case of like attracting like: Harvey's contentious youth had matured into an aloof and crotchety middle age.

Through his long years of research, Harvey had been developing his ideas. In 1628 he was eventually persuaded to publish these in book form. The result was *De Motu Cordis* (Concerning the Motion of the Heart), which is now regarded as the founding work of modern physiology. The ideas proposed and definitively demonstrated in this book had a long prehistory. As early as the thirteenth century, the Arabic physician Ibn al-Nafis had questioned an important element of the Galenic theory of the blood. Ibn al-Nafis is thought to have been born near Damascus around 1200, and to have been educated at the city's renowned hospital. He ended his life teaching medicine in Egypt some 80 years later. Ibn al-Nafis was the first to pose a serious question about the Galenic theory of the blood, and to come up with a positive answer. He denied the existence of Galen's 'invisible pores' in the wall of the heart, which allowed the blood to pass from the right to the left ventricle. (See Fig 1., p. 31.) In his own words, 'the material of which the heart is made is impermeable, and no blood can pass through its surface. Therefore this must pass by way of the lungs.' Galen had allowed that a small amount of blood travelled in this fashion, but only to carry *pneuma* from the lungs. He insisted that most of the venous blood passed through the septum, the muscular wall dividing the left from the right ventricle. Ibn al-Nafis is generally credited with being the first to suggest the so-called pulmonary transit, the passage of larger quantities of blood through the lungs (Latin, *pulmones*). However, this was ignored – as Galenic theory prevailed and set into unquestionable orthodoxy.

Then in 1553 the Spanish theologian and physician Michael Servetus independently proposed this same lesser circulation by means of the pulmonary transit. He justified his view by pointing to the size of the blood vessels carrying the blood from the right ventricle to the lungs, and from the lungs back to the left ventricle. These were large enough to carry all the blood necessary for the arterial system. Servetus set down this idea at the end of a book dedicated largely to his theological views. Unfortunately, this was the period when Europe was being torn apart by the forces of the Reformation and the Counter-Reformation. Such was the originality of Servetus' theological opinions that he succeeded in antagonizing both the Protestants and the Catholic Church, who concurred in declaring his teachings heretical. Servetus managed to escape the clutches of the Inquisition, but made the mistake of fleeing to Geneva, the home of his Protestant adversary Calvin. As a result, Servetus was burned at the stake, along with all available copies of his book. Fortunately, he had taken the precaution of leaving behind several copies with a book dealer in Lyons.

Somehow, though nobody is precisely sure how, one of these copies must have passed into the hands of Realdo Colombo, who was professor of anatomy at Padua after Vesalius and prior to Fallopius and Fabricius. At first covertly, and then more explicitly, Colombo began introducing the notion of the pulmonary circulation into his lectures. He also confirmed the idea first-hand by the dissection of human cadavers, as well as the vivisection of animals where the passage of the blood could be observed. Harvey would arrive in Padua a good 40 years after the death of Colombo, but it was certainly here that he first heard of Colombo's views. He would refer to 'the very skilful and learned anatomist' Columbo three times in *De Motu Cordis*, citing the importance of his findings on the lesser circulation.

As we have seen, Harvey also learned that Fabricius had discovered the presence of valves in the veins. Fabricius himself remained puzzled by this finding. Ingeniously, he suggested that the veins were to prevent all the venous blood from flowing to the lower half of the body. The young Harvey was not convinced, but for the time being he could come up with no more convincing explanation. It was at Padua that Harvey also learned of Vesalius' doubts concerning the passage of blood through the wall of the heart. The body of evidence against Galen's blood system was growing. Indeed, there is no denying that the idea of 'circulation' was in the air. This is often the case before a major scientific discovery. Great ideas from Darwin's evolution to Watt's steam engine were preceded by strong inklings of what was to come. Few revolutionary scientific ideas come like a bolt from of the blue. Even Einstein's hugely unexpected idea of relativity was preceded by a similar embryonic idea from Poincaré.

Despite the suggestions of a lesser circulation (in the pulmonary transit), valves in the veins, and even speculation that the heart might act as a pump (by Colombo and earlier Arab thinkers), no one took the drastic step of questioning Galen's *overall* scheme. It remained generally accepted that the blood was produced in the liver, that there were two distinct blood systems (the venous and the arterial), and that the blood was somehow *consumed* by the body. These remained essentially one-way systems, apart perhaps from the minor detour of the pulmonary transit. Harvey's ground-breaking originality was to overthrow this system altogether, and to provide incontrovertible demonstration (amounting to proof) that his ideas were correct.

Harvey's overall method was clear, as he announced in his lectures. 'I propose to learn and teach anatomy not from books but from dissections, not from the tenets of philosophers but from the fabric of Nature.' He would proceed solely 'by eyesight inspection and by dissection'.

De Motu Cordis opens by describing the structure of the heart and how it moves. The heart was nothing more or less than an organization of muscle which acted as a pump. Dissection showed that it contained two upper chambers

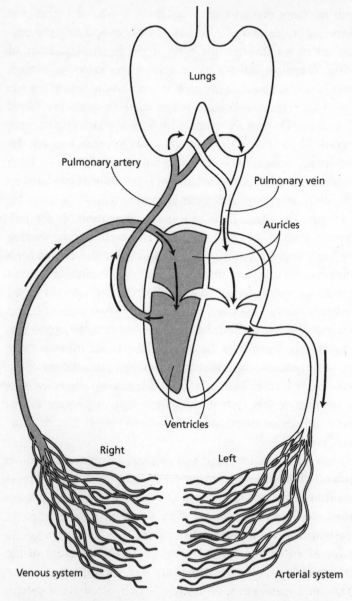

Figure 5. Simplified version of Harvey's circulation of the blood

(auricles) and two larger lower chambers (ventricles). The left auricle and left ventricle were separated from the right auricle and right ventricle by the septum, a wall of muscular flesh which was impermeable. The entire heart contracted (systole), expelling the blood; and it expanded (diastole) drawing the blood in. This accounted for the observable heartbeat: systole, diastole.

Skilled and ingenious investigation had led Harvey to discover the sequence of this mechanism of the heart. In warm-blooded animals the heart beats so fast that it is impossible to discover whether the auricle contracts before or after the ventricle. So he had made use of comparative anatomy, and turned to cold-blooded fish, whose hearts beat more slowly. He had then confirmed his findings here by studying the slowing heartbeat of dying warm-blooded animals. In all cases, the auricles contracted first, followed by the ventricles. And the valves separating these two sets of chambers further ensured that the blood could only flow one way, from auricle to ventricle. Then, as the ventricles contracted, the blood was expelled from the heart. The left ventricle expelled the blood into the arterial system. The right ventricle expelled the blood through the pulmonary transit to the lungs, and back via the pulmonary vein to the left auricle.

Galen had maintained that the blood, created by the liver, passed through the heart and into the arterial and venous systems, then flowed throughout the body, where it was consumed by the flesh. As we have seen, Harvey applied the science of measurement to this one-way system. This he did by studying the amount of blood which passed through the heart of a dog. First he measured the dog's heartbeat, which showed how often the heart contracted and emptied of blood. Then he measured the capacity of the dog's heart. Applying one to the other, he showed the amount of blood which passed through the dog's heart each hour. Extrapolating this to the human heart, he discovered that the liver would need to create, and the body would need to consume, no less than three times the body's own weight in blood each hour. Something evidently didn't add up here.

But there were further problems. Previously it had been thought that the blood was drawn into the heart when it expanded (diastole), but Harvey was able to show that this was not the case. The *active* motion of the heart was systole, the contraction of the heart's muscles, expelling the blood through the ventricles. Galen had taught that the blood was forced on its passage through the blood vessels by the vessels themselves contracting of their own accord, causing the pulse. Harvey was able to show that the pulse was the shock wave from the beat of the heart as it contracted, expelling the blood along the arteries. Galen had also maintained that the blood ebbed and flowed as it passed along the arterial and venous systems. Harvey showed that this was not possible. The valves in the larger veins, detected by Fabricius, ensured that the flow was one-way. And this was the opposite direction to that maintained by Galen. Instead of flowing away from the heart throughout the body, the venous blood only flowed towards the heart. Harvey demonstrated this by compressing a vein, and noting that the blood built up on the side away from the heart. But when he compressed an artery, the blood built up on the side closest to the heart.

What did all this mean? With suitable aplomb, Harvey paused at this point. He was well aware of the sensational effect of what he was going to say. His conclusion was 'of so novel and unheard-of character, that I not only fear injury to myself from the envy of a few, but I tremble lest I have mankind at large for my enemies . . .' After a further page of suspense, he makes his dramatic announcement concerning the blood in the body:

> I began to wonder if it had a movement, as it were, in a circle. This hypothesis I subsequently verified. I finally saw that the blood, forced by the action of the left ventricle into the arteries, was distributed throughout the arterial system to all parts of the body . . . finding, further, that the blood flows back through the veins . . . right up to the right auricle. Which motion we may be allowed to call circular.

Harvey had first begun divulging his views in private lectures to his professional colleagues. It is probable that he began this soon after 1616, when he started lecturing at the College of Physicians. Though in his public lectures to his students he persisted in Galenic orthodoxy, often couched in Aristotelian terms. Only after the publication of *De Motu Cordis* in 1628 would this change. Even then, he would remain strictly orthodox in his actual medical practice. Diagnosis, prognosis and prescription would be conducted on the basis of the four humours. Where medical practice was concerned, he remained highly resistant to innovation.

Harvey seems to have gone out of his way to avoid controversy. He was over 50 years old by the time he made his ideas on the circulation of the blood known to a wider public. Even then, he only 'yielded to the repeated desire of all and the pressing desire of some [of his colleagues]'. The book would be merely 70 pages long: he would make his point, and say no more. His arguments would be succinct, rather than sensational. He chose to have *De Motu Cordis* published abroad in Latin by an English printer called Fitzer, who worked in Frankfurt. This arrangement resulted in an edition published on the cheapest quality paper, which in a few years would often darken to the point of illegibility and begin to crumble. And the book's contents would be littered with misprints. Regardless of such drawbacks, *De Motu Cordis* would in time come to be widely regarded as one of the greatest books produced by an Englishman, standing on a par with the King James Authorized Version of the Bible and the Folio Edition of Shakespeare's plays. Curiously, all three of these books would appear within the space of just 17 years – being published in 1611 (Bible), 1623 (Shakespeare) and 1628 respectively. (Another obvious contender here, Newton's *Principia*, is too technical for the general reader. Harvey may have been no great stylist, but his book is immediately comprehensible – as would become clear to a wider readership when it was translated into English in 1653.)

Despite Harvey's attempts to avoid controversy, *De Motu Cordis* caused widespread public outcry on its publication. As he himself would somewhat testily declare, many years later: 'Since that birthday of the circuit of the blood there has of truth been scarcely a day, or even the smallest interval of time passing, in which I have not heard both good and ill report of the circulation which I discovered.' Harvey's novel ideas soon spread through Europe, causing deep divisions of opinion. In England, according to Aubrey, 'twas beleeved by the vulgar that he was crack-brained; and all the Physitians were against his Opinion.' This is certainly an exaggeration. But Aubrey also noted that 'he fell mightily in his Practize', and it is generally agreed that Harvey's private consultancy suffered seriously as a result of the notoriety his views attracted. Despite everything, the king stood by him and he retained his royal appointment. Amongst his detractors Harvey became known mockingly as the 'circulator', a particularly cutting double-edged epithet (*circulator* is Latin for 'quack').

For the most part Harvey maintained a contemptuous silence, refusing to answer his critics. The facts were evident to anyone willing to carry out an experiment, and open their eyes, rather than appeal to authority. Only 20 years later would he deign to reply, publishing a letter contesting the claims of the celebrated Parisian anatomist Jean Riolan, who persisted in maligning Harvey for daring to attack Galen. In this Harvey refuted Riolan point by point, and with some anger: 'It cannot be helped that dogs bark and vomit their foul stomachs . . . but care can be taken that they do not bite or inoculate their mad humours, or with their dogs' teeth gnaw the bones and foundation of truth.'

In his role as royal physician Harvey was also called upon to investigate other popular fallacies, such as witchcraft. There was still wide belief in this practice, even amongst physicians. One contemporary report tells how Harvey visited Newmarket with the king. Here he was sent to visit 'a woman who was reputed a witch . . . who dwelt in a lone House on the borders of the Heath . . . Hee [i.e. Harvey] said she was very distrustful at first; but when hee told her he was a vizard, and come purposely to converse with her in their common trade, then shee easily believed him [on account of his] very magicall face.' Harvey then asked to see her 'familiar' (the witch's assistant devil, who usually took on the form of an animal, such as a black cat). Whereupon the old woman opened a cupboard and called out a toad, which she gave some milk to drink in a saucer. Harvey persuaded the old woman to fetch him some ale from the pub down the road. The moment she was gone, Harvey leaped on the toad and began to dissect it. 'Hee examined the toades entrayles, heart and lungs.' These observations convinced him that the toad was 'no wayes different from other toades . . . ergo it was a playne naturall toad . . . From whence he concludes there are no witches very logistically.' Unfortunately Harvey became so immersed in his speculations that the woman surprised him bent over her dissected toad. At once she 'flew like a Tigris at his face [so that] he was in danger to have a more magical face than hee had before.' She scratched and clawed and tore at his face and cloak, his hair and his clothes, but fortunately he managed to escape. In some disarray, he returned to Newmarket, where he later told 'the whole story, which was pleasant entertaynment for the King at his dinner'.

Another anecdote of medical interest concerns Thomas Parr, who was reputed to have lived to the age of 152. A contemporary local versifier described Parr in old age:

> He will speak heartily, laugh and be merry,
> Drink ale, and now and then a Cup of Sherry.

Parr was a poor farmer who had lived all his life in a country hamlet outside Shrewsbury. He is said to have married for the first time at 80; at the age of 105 he had to do a penance for comitting adultery; and he married again at the age of 112. Forty years later he was 'discovered' and brought to London. But plentiful rich food and the clamour of celebrity did not suit him, and he died in the same year. Charles I ordered his royal physician to investigate, and Harvey duly carried out an autopsy on Parr. According to Harvey's biographer Keynes: 'This did not reveal any great ageing in the tissues of the body.' Harvey concluded that even at the age of 152, Parr's death had been premature – owing to 'a sudden adoption of a mode of living unnatural to him'. He had suffered especially from the polluted London air and 'the not inconsiderable grime from the smoke of sulphurous coal constantly used as fuel for fires'. Harvey's three-page autopsy report is quoted in full in Keynes' biography, and spares no detail. It even includes a detailed description of Parr's sexual apparatus: this was in full working order until the age of 140, according to his wife, who was specifically questioned on the matter by Dr Harvey. This document, which includes remarks about his diet, as well as his mental and physical habits, remains of intriguing interest to anyone curious about the preservation of life into old age.

By now the dispute between Charles I and Parliament was beginning to split the country. The rising Puritan middle class, supported by the Parliamentarians, was engaged in a power struggle with a king who still believed that he ruled by 'divine right'. Things finally reached the point of no return in 1642, with the outbreak of the Civil War. As we have seen, Harvey faithfully attended his king during the opening battle at Edge-hill, just south of Warwick in the English midlands. Aubrey's story about Harvey's activities on the battlefield were told to him by Harvey himself. Other eyewitness accounts authenticate details included by Aubrey. Harvey certainly retired under a hedge to read a book as the battle raged around him. There is no question of cowardice here: Harvey was a non-combatant, and he was designated to look after the royal princes. The king was more than grateful to Harvey for this dangerous service. Later he would present Harvey with a dual portrait of the royal princes on the battlefield, painted by the court artist William Dobson, who was summoned to the king's new headquarters in Oxford expressly for this purpose.

Harvey himself is not included in this painting, and it seems we shall never know what book he chose to read. Would he have read for instruction, or simply to while away his time, during these hours of mortal danger? Harvey is known to have been a well-read man, conversant with the classics of literature and those of natural philosophy. In his works he quotes Virgil as well as Galen and Hippocrates. But most of all, his language retains an Aristotelian phraseology. He describes the circulation:

All the parts are nourished, cherished, and quickened by the blood, which is warm, perfect, vaporous, full of spirit . . .

> thence it returns to the heart, as to the fountain or dwelling-house of the body, to recover its perfection . . . So the heart is the beginning of life, the Sun of the Microcosm, as proportionably the Sun deserves to be call'd the heart of the world.

The blood being 'perfect', 'full of spirit', the heart as a microcosm of the sun in the solar system – all this remains utterly Aristotelian. Galileo and Descartes had sought to reduce the world to a precise mechanism, whose forces could be measured. The world, for them, was like a gigantic clock. The understanding of the human body, and its more fluent processes, was not amenable to such reductionism. Yet Harvey's Aristotelian language betrays him here. His modern experimental approach had led him to describe, and explain, how the blood circulated through the body. But precisely what happened in the course of this circulation had eluded him. The heart may have been the 'beginning of life'; 'perfect' blood may have 'nourished' and 'cherished' the parts of the body – but such Aristotelian language only obscured the fact that he didn't really know *what* was going on, even if he knew *how* it all took place. And even here there remained a vital gap. How precisely did the blood, which flowed out of the heart into the arterial system, manage to penetrate the venous system in order to return to the heart? Harvey could find no evidence of any connection between these two systems. He was forced to suppose that it existed, but was too small to be visible to the human eye.

Yet these were mere quibbles. Harvey had cleared the way. It is certainly no exaggeration to say that Harvey's discovery of the circulation of the blood was the founding of modern medicine. Others would soon begin to clear up such details as he had left unexplained. In 1667 the English physician Richard Lower noted that the colour of the blood changed from dark purple (venous) to bright scarlet (arterial) after it passed through the lungs in the pulmonary circuit. This transformation did not take place in the heart, as had previously been supposed. The passage of the blood through the left auricle and ventricle was not accompanied by some kind of chemical process which transformed it from dark venous blood into bright arterial blood. Lower speculated that when the blood passed through the lungs it became mixed with some 'nitrous spirit of the air', which then passed on life to the body as it circulated through the arterial system. Lower even managed to prove this by collecting some venous blood in a flask, and then shaking it so that it became mixed with air. The dark venous blood was at once transformed into bright arterial blood. As we have already seen, Harvey's other difficulty would be overcome when the Italian anatomist Malpighi examined human flesh under a microscope and detected the presence of tiny capillaries connecting the arteries to the veins. The missing links in Harvey's system had now been discovered.

7

EXPLORER OF AN INVISIBLE WORLD

Microscopic magnifications were first noticed in drops of water which had fallen onto manuscripts and other dry surfaces. When viewed through a drop of water, what had appeared smooth or featureless was revealed as having an entire geography which had previously remained invisible to the naked eye. A new world – a microcosm – had been discovered. Later, it was noted that globules of glass exhibited the same revelatory quality as drops of water. These were easier to manipulate, and it was soon found that they could be polished to make a lens. This achieved an even greater magnitude and exactness, and was capable of being raised or lowered, focusing it upon the object under observation. As we have seen, one of the earliest to explore this property of glass was the Italian anatomist Marcello Malpighi, who was influenced by the new telescope which had been developed by his fellow-countryman Galileo. Around the same time, the

English physicist Robert Hooke began using a twin-lensed microscope. In 1665 he published his findings in *Micrographia*, which contained illustrations of what he had seen in this newly discovered microcosm. His book was illustrated with monstrously magnified drawings of lice, 'microfungi', and even the eye of a fly. Hooke also noticed that when he examined thin slices of cork under his microscope they were revealed to have 'pores'. He named these structures 'cells', because he thought they looked like small dwelling places, such as prison cells or the pattern of cells within a honeycomb. What Hooke in fact saw were not cells, but when actual organic cells were first observed the name stuck.

These investigations were just the beginning. The first masterful and far-reaching investigation of microscopic objects was undertaken by one of the least likely of the great medical discoverers – a small-town Dutch draper called Leeuwenhoek (his name is pronounced 'Lay-van-hook', which means 'lion's corner', probably after a carved lion on a corner house which gave its name to the district where his family originated).

Anton van Leeuwenhoek was born in the small provincial town of Delft in 1632. His father was a basket-maker, who died just six years later. Young Anton was farmed out to relatives, before being despatched to Amsterdam at the age of 15 to become apprenticed to a cloth merchant. It was here that Leeuwenhoek first came across the glass buttons used by drapers to magnify the surface of cloth, in order to inspect its quality.

At the age of 20 Leeuwenhoek returned to his native Delft and set up his own drapery business. Within six years this was well established, providing him with a reasonable income. More importantly, it also gave him sufficient free time to pursue his increasingly absorbing hobby. This consisted of grinding globules of glass into magnifying lenses, so that he could study minute objects.

Lens-grinding was very much the latest scientific craze in Holland during this period. Dutch commerce, epitomized by the Dutch East India Company (which had a large office in Delft), had made Holland one of the most prosperous countries in Europe. The comparatively liberal democratic conditions prevailing in Holland at the time ensured that this wealth was more evenly distributed amongst the population than in other countries. Besides regularly ordering new clothes from the drapers, the new bourgeois citizens started using the new-fangled spectacles to improve their eyesight. Lens-grinding became a booming cottage industry, requiring only painstaking grinding and immense patience. It was during this period that the philosopher Spinoza supported himself by grinding lenses, just five miles down the road in The Hague.

Leeuwenhoek continued to live an uneventful provincial life in Delft. This is the town of everyday domestic scenes, quiet alleyways and canals, depicted in the paintings of Vermeer, who was born in Delft in the same year as Leeuwenkoek and would continue to live here all his life. Leeuwenhoek married in 1666 at the age of 33, but his wife died, and he remarried in 1671. Now middle-aged, he became almost completely absorbed in his curious hobby. (Others ground lenses for money; but he only seemed interested in keeping his lenses, and looking at things through them.) So things might have continued, if Leeuwenhoek had not made the acquaintance of the celebrated anatomist Regnier de Graaf (who had studied in Paris under Vesalius' old adversary Sylvius). De Graaf was a corresponding member of the recently formed Royal Society in London, an institution set up to record and propagate the latest scientific knowledge. In the wake of Copernicus and Galileo a scientific revolution was now taking place, and such institutions were being set up in several major European centres. Along with a number of other leading scientists, Regnier de Graaf kept in regular touch with the Royal Society, and this continued when he finally took up residence in Delft. Here he established a successful medical practice and continued to extend Fallopius' researches into the female generative system. It was de Graaf who coined the term 'ovary', and the egg-containing sac on its surface is named the Graafian follicle after him.

Leeuwenhoek invited de Graaf to his house and let him peer through his lenses. As soon as de Graaf saw what they revealed he realized its scientific importance. In 1673 he wrote to the Royal Society informing them of Leeuwenhoek's amazing instruments. This intervention was timely, for within a few months de Graaf would perish of the plague.

A letter arrived from the Royal Society inviting Leeuwenhoek to send them his findings. He could only speak and write in the local Dutch dialect, but fortunately he managed to find a translator. Leeuwenhoek wrote a long letter describing what he had seen with the aid of 'mijn nieuw gevonden microscopix' (my newly invented microscope). This was despatched to London, along with Leeuwenhoek's meticulous drawings of what he had seen. These depicted the microscopic revelation of a patch of mould, a bee's sting, and the entire magnified body of a human louse. All this was so amazing that at first the fellows of the Royal Society were sceptical. If Leeuwenhoek was to be believed, the clarity and magnification which he had achieved with his single-lens microscope was even greater than that achieved by their colleague the great physicist Hooke, who had constructed a microscope with two lenses. The secretary of the Royal Society wrote back asking for testimonials from respected local figures who could vouch for the truth of Leeuwenhoek's findings. He duly obliged.

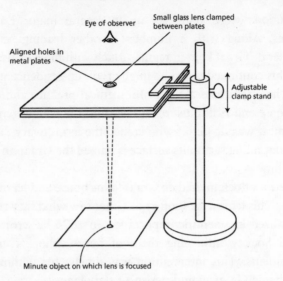

Eye of observer

Small glass lens clamped between plates

Aligned holes in metal plates

Adjustable clamp stand

Minute object on which lens is focused

Figure 6. Simplified version of one of Leeuwenhoek's early single-lens microscopes

Some time later, Hooke followed Leeuwenhoek's instructions and set about building a single-lens microscope of his own. This required two flat plates of brass, each with a small hole. The holes were aligned, and the tiny convex glass lense was clamped between them. The plates were then held horizontally in a stand so that the lens could be raised or lowered, in order to focus precisely onto the surface to be observed.

Hooke found to his surprise that Leeuwenhoek's single-lens microscope was a great improvement on his own dual-lens version. Two lenses may have had potentially greater magnification, but this method suffered badly from globular and chromatic aberration: the image was distorted as if by a fish-eye lens and had disfiguring rainbow-coloured blurs. (This defect would not be fully overcome for another two centuries.) But even with a single lens, Hooke was unable to achieve quite the magnification that Leeuwenhoek had managed. This was Leeuwenhoek's great skill. He not only had seemingly endless patience, but over the years he would develop sufficient expertise to understand precisely what could be achieved with any particular lens. As his lenses became stronger and stronger, he managed to achieve a magnification approaching one hundred times. Leeuwenhoek would jealously guard the secrets of his lens-grinding technique, but it is known that he soon began using lenses which were no larger than a pin-head. How he managed to achieve sufficient light and resolving power for such lenses remains a mystery to this day.

Leeuwenhoek was soon sending regular letters to the Royal Society in London. Many of these were as long as articles, and they began appearing in the Society's magazine *Philosophical Transactions*. His findings caused a sensation. He began examining everything from droplets of water to the fabric of plants, from the scrapings of his tongue and teeth to the anatomy of minute insects. Everything produced wondrous new discoveries. When examining droplets of water he found them to be filled with 'animalcules'. These were bacteria, and he was the first to see them. He examined minute scraps of animal flesh and discovered that muscle tissue consisted of striated fibres. When he scrutinized a flea under his microscope, he found that this tiny parasite even had minuscule parasites of its own. It was this finding which inspired the contemporary Irish writer Jonathan Swift to write his celebrated verse:

> So, naturalists observe, a flea
> Has smaller fleas that on him prey;
> And these have smaller still to bite 'em,
> And so proceed *ad infinitum*.

Leeuwenhoek found himself deeply drawn to the microworld which he observed. This inspired him to vivid, touching, occasionally almost cartoon-like descriptions:

> some animalcules [were] the most wretched creatures that I have ever seen; [when they] hit upon any particles or filaments (of which there are many in water, especially if it hath stood for some days) they stuck intangled in them; and then pulled their body out into an oval, and did struggle, by strongly stretching themselves, to get their tail loose; whereby their whole body sprang back toward the pellet of the tail, and their tails then coiled up serpent-wise . . .

Leeuwenhoek's very lack of scientific learning proved to his advantage. He simply described what he saw, with the minimum of speculation. Only the most basic of principles were applied to his observations. If a thing moved under its own propulsion, he judged it to be alive – no matter how minuscule or curious the object might be. When he observed similarities between plants and animals, this led him to recognize analogous features and functions. In this way, he became highly skilled at interpreting what he saw, and was able to produce ingenious explanations of what was happening to the microorganisms he observed. He understood that they moved, they reproduced, and they died.

This directly contradicted the prevalent Aristotelian theory. Aristotle's careful observations, unaided by the microscope, had led him to believe that many tiny animals simply arose from the putrefaction of organic matter. Others, such as eels, he speculated were generated by dew. Aristotle became convinced that such worms and insects were created by 'spontaneous generation', and over the centuries this had become accepted as orthodoxy. Leeuwenhoek was able to show that his animalcules reproduced like other animals. He had understood the true nature of micro-organisms. They too had a life cycle similar to other living creatures.

Word began to spread of Leeuwenhoek's findings. In 1677 he was visited by an admirer called Johan Han, a medical student from Arnhem. Han told Leeuwenhoek that he had even discovered animalcules swimming in human semen. Not fully understanding the anti-Aristotelian implications of Leeuwenhoek's work, Han assumed that these had arisen from putrefaction. Leeuwenhoek quickly repeated Han's experiment, confirming his observations. But unlike Han, he understood the importance of this discovery. Sperm was alive, but eggs (which did not move) were not alive. After conducting further investigations Leeuwenhoek became convinced that the living creatures in the sperm must somehow penetrate the female eggs and fertilize them. This was in fact mere speculation, as he was not capable of observing such activity. It would be centuries before his conjecture would be proved correct. But such theorizing serves to demonstrate Leeuwenhoek's skill. He may have been an amateur, and lacking in any scientific education, but he had a growing understanding of how the microcosmic world operated.

As Leeuwenhoek's grinding techniques became more skilful, so his lenses achieved even greater magnification. He began observing inside the mouths of insects, discovered protozoa (single-celled organisms), and investigated the walls of blood vessels. Unaware of Malpighi's earlier discoveries in this field, he discovered for himself the existence of capillaries linking the arterial and venous systems. He also rediscovered red blood cells, describing them as being shaped like lentils. Malpighi had identified these as globules of fat; Leeuwenhoek correctly understood that they were blood cells. He did not entirely comprehend the function of the blood, but his painstaking observations led to a considerable advance in this field. It was Leeuwenhoek who observed that the blood moved food particles from the intestines to the tissues of the body. He was also continually extending the field of his investigations. He discovered that so-called 'ants' eggs' were in fact pupae; that mussels and shellfish were not spontaneously generated out of mud but instead came from larvae; and he investigated the nutritional systems of plants.

In the end Leeuwenhoek would produce over 400 lenses, many of which have been preserved in a collection which can be seen at the University Museum of Utrecht. The best of these has a magnification of 266, and a resolving power of $1.4 \times$ (this means that it can distinguish between features separated by just 0.0014 mm!) Though according to Johannes Heniger of the University of Utrecht, 'from his recorded observations it may be surmised that he must have actually made lenses of 500 power, with a resolution of $1.0 \times$.' (Leeuwenhoek could not have achieved such magnification with his known lenses. And it would have been impossible for him to achieve this with the instruments at his disposal. So how did he do it? It has recently been suggested that Leeuwenhoek's 'secret' was that he somehow managed to combine his tiny ground lenses with the magnifying power of a droplet of water. Experts have ridiculed this idea, but so far no better explanation can be found.)

As Leeuwenhoek's investigations probed into ever more minuscule realms, he found it necessary to devise a scale, so that his measurements could be compared with those of the visible non-microscopic world. For standard measurements, he used a grain of coarse sand (which on the modern scale would be around $870 \times$, or 0.18 mm), a hair from his beard ($100 \times$), a red blood cell ($7.2 \times$), and bacteria in pepper water ($2-3 \times$).

As word of Leeuwenhoek's discoveries spread, he began to

attract considerable fame. He was visited in Delft by royalty, including Peter the Great of Russia and Queen Mary of England. He would continue corresponding with the Royal Society throughout his long life – in the end sending them almost 200 letters. Other letters were sent to the national scientific institutions of other countries, as well as replying to the queries of individual scientists. In gratitude for his achievements, his home town awarded him a sinecure for life, installing him as Chief Warden of the City. Though to his chagrin, many of the superstitious locals still considered him to be merely a wizard. In old age he would be looked after by his sole surviving child, his unmarried daughter Maria. She would nurse him until he died in 1723 at the age of 90.

Leeuwenhoek's work had brought to light a new world. Things which it had previously been impossible to suspect even existed were now revealed. These were a source of great wonder – but they were not yet fully understood. Also, Leeuwenhoek's lens-making was centuries ahead of its time. Not for another 200 years would better microscopes be produced. In the light of all this, it comes as no great surprise that Leeuwenhoek's work would gradually be overlooked after his death. Only in time would the importance of this invisible microscopic world become apparent to medical science.

The scientific age had begun, with physics and chemistry leading the way. Both these specialities would have their separate influence on medicine, giving rise to two distinct movements – the iatrophysicists and the iatrochemists (both from the Greek *iatros*, meaning 'one who heals'). In line with Descartes, the iatrophysicists had a mechanical view of the universe, leading them to regard the human body as a machine. It is no accident that Sanctorius, the man who would become the first leading iatrophysicist, studied at Padua while

Galileo was in residence laying the foundations of modern physics.

Sanctorius, whose real name was Santorio Santorio, was born in 1561 at Capodistria (now Koper, in Slovenia), a small port on the Gulf of Trieste in the Venetian Republic. He studied medicine at the nearby University of Padua while Fabricius was professor of anatomy, but graduated in 1582 just a few years before Harvey's arrival. According to a persistent legend, supported by some scant evidence, Sanctorius was so brilliant a graduate that he was soon despatched across Europe to treat the king of Poland. (Around this time Poland's illustrious monarch Stefan Batory died prematurely at the age of 53, though there is no historical evidence holding Sanctorius responsible for this event.) During the ensuing decade or so, Sanctorius practised medicine at various cities along the eastern Adriatic coast, before settling in Venice in 1599.

From all accounts, Sanctorius was a misogynistic introverted character, who never married and lived a life of monastic frugality. His only known vice was a lust for money, which his successful medical practice enabled him to indulge to the full. Despite having all the classic characteristics of a miser, Sanctorius is known to have been a friend of the ebullient Galileo, who was not one to tolerate skinflints or dullards gladly. Apparently Galileo was amused by the dry misanthropy of Sanctorius' remarks. Despite this lack of social attributes, Sanctorius was appointed in 1611 as professor of medical theory at Padua.

By this stage Sanctorius was already confirmed in his iatrophysical approach to medicine, though he took good care to conceal this from the university authorities, who still adhered to Galenic orthodoxy. Despite the pioneering anatomical work by Vesalius, Fallopius and Fabricius at Padua, any deviation from Galenic *theory* was frowned upon. Even so,

Sanctorius could not resist airing some of his iatrophysicist views in his lectures. These would be covertly introduced as mere suggestions, possible alternative explanations to the Galenic norm. In other matters he saw no reason for caution. Sanctorius' firm belief in the machine-like physics of the body, whose quantative nature was open to measurement, led him to invent a number of instruments for this purpose.

Sanctorius would eventually fall out with Galileo over their rival claims to have invented the thermometer. Galileo certainly invented this instrument, but it was Sanctorius who adapted it to practical use. He was the first to make a scale on this instrument. Thus, in pedantic terms, Galileo in fact invented a thermoscope (enabling one to *see* changes in heat, or temperature), while Sanctorius actually invented the thermometer (enabling these changes to be *measured*). The lower limit of Sanctorius' thermometer was the temperature of snow, the upper limit was the temperature of a candle flame. He was also the first to adapt the thermometer for medical use, so that it could measure the temperature of the human body. Sanctorius' other great medical invention was also an 'adaptation' of one of Galileo's ideas. Galileo had used his pulse to measure the swing of a pendulum. Sanctorius reversed this, using the swing of a pendulum to measure the rate of the pulse with his 'pulsilogium' (pulse watch).

However, Sanctorius' most important medical work was concerned with variations in the weight of the human body. Over a period of 30 years, he conducted a series of experiments upon himself and his metabolism. Using a large scale, upon which he placed his chair and desk, his bed, and all he required for his daily needs, he proceeded to weigh himself at regular intervals. In this way, he was able to compare the fluctuations in his body weight with his intake of solids and liquids, as well as the losses resulting from all he excreted. Psychologists will readily recognize that here Sanctorius' obsessive miserliness extended to more than his finances. The body itself was reduced to double-entry bookkeeping, with each of its incomings and outgoings strictly balanced. One result was that Sanctorius was able to detect and calculate the weight loss from his body due to 'insensible perspiration'. This idea had first been suggested as early as 300 BC by Erasostratus, and had been accepted by Galen. But neither had for a moment suspected that such a thing could ever be measured. Sanctorius was able to discover that when the body was cold or asleep 'insensible perspiration' decreased, whereas during fever it increased. Such findings would prove a great aid in discovering the inner workings of the body.

Here lay the crux of Sanctorius's originality. Previously, Galen's medicine had been concerned with qualitative change brought about by an imblance of the humours. Sanctorius sought to introduce *quantative* methods to measure what was happening inside the human body. Harvey would apply measurement to the blood circulation and the capacity of the human heart. Sanctorius applied it to the other great system in the human body, the metabolism. He sought to measure the effects of the digestive process. (As is so often the case, one pioneer would fail to recognize the other. Sanctorius would learn of Harvey's circulation of the blood, but would remain blind to the full significance of this discovery.)

Sanctorius summarized his findings in *De Statica Medicina* (On Medical Measurement) which was published in Venice in 1618. This proved a huge success, and by the end of the century it would be translated into every major European language. The causes of its success are not hard to find. Its jargon-free aphoristic style made for easy reading. Not only did it include observations on health, but also gave medical advice. This was a book for the perusal of patients as well as doctors. It included reassuring homilies:

> If overnight thou tak'st a dose,
>   And find'st thy self amiss,
> Thou must next morn another take:
>   No remedy like this.

As well as simple advice: 'After meat, sleep; after sleep, concoction [digestion]; after concoction transpiration [perspiration] is best.' It also contained a section 'On Venery', which proved of great interest to all: 'The immediate Injury of immoderate Coition, is a refrigeration of the Stomach; but afterwards an obstructed Perspiration; from whence easily arise Palpitations in the Eye-brows and Joints, and then in the more noble Parts.' There followed a number of perceptive observations on the effects of 'immoderate Coition', which doubtless proved as much a caution to those who indulged in this activity as those who refrained from it.

Yet Sanctorius' pioneering approach was not all that it seemed. He certainly believed in experimental method, and his empirical approach was in line with the new scientific outlook, but he also retained a belief in the old ways. He himself summarized his approach: 'One must believe first in one's own senses, then in reasoning, and only in the third place in the authority of Hippocrates, of Galen, of Aristotle, and of other excellent philosophers.' In the end, he still adhered to the system of the four humours. But this he adapted in his own idiosyncratic way to his new iatrophysical methods. For Galen, illness resulted from 'dyscrasia' or imbalance of the humours. Galen recognized that there could be degrees of imbalance, but saw these degrees as blending into one another. Sanctorius chose to view these degrees as discontinuous and discrete, each different measurable degree accounting for its own specific illness. In this way, he calculated all possible distinct degrees of humoral imbalance, with each one accounting for a particular disease. He ended by concluding that the human body can be affected by no less than 80,000 different diseases.

Many felt that Sanctorius' iatrophysics represented nothing less than a dual foundation to the new medicine, alongside that of Harvey. This overestimates Sanctorius' contribution, though there is no denying his importance. Sanctorius' meticulous 30 years of self-observation resulted in a pioneer scientific system of basic human metabolism. He is generally recognized as the first to have introduced a quantative approach to the pathology of the human body. From now on, the measurement of temperature, pulse rate and weight loss would be prominent in assessing health. Other, more probing and precise measurements would gradually evolve. Iatrophysics established medicine as an exact, measurable science.

Other leading iatrophysicists included Giovanni Borelli who was born in Naples in 1608 and would be heavily influenced by the work of Sanctorius. In 1656 Borelli became professor of mathematics at the University of Pisa, a post previously occupied by Galileo. In the same year Marcello Malpighi, whose microscopic researches into anatomy confirmed Harvey's circulation of the blood, was appointed professor of medical theory at Pisa. All this gives an indication of the close links between these Italian pioneers of modern medicine. Borelli's study of the muscles as a mechanical system did much to explain the interlocking mechanism of the musculature and the function of individual muscles. In seeking to understand muscular function he undertook some remarkable studies in comparative anatomy, recording the muscular actions of birds in flight and fish swimming through water. His hypothesis that there was a circulation of nervous fluid (*succus nerveus*) throughout the nervous system, similar to that of the blood, was erroneous. Yet this hypothesis is suggestive of the daring originality of the new medical thought breaking free of Galenic humoral restrictions. Borelli's theory of the nervous system led him to account for the beating of the heart as neurogenic (i.e. controlled by the nervous system). This would gain acceptance throughout Europe for the next two centuries.

The facts of Borelli's life are often obscure. It has been suggested that he lost his post at Pisa owing to anti-scientific persecution launched by the Counter-Reformation. (This had resulted in Galileo's appearance before the Inquisition a few decades earlier.) It seems more likely that Borelli was dismissed for engaging in republican politics. The last years of his life were spent in exile in Rome, where he eked out a poverty-stricken old age tutoring priests in basic arithmetic. He died there in 1679 at the age of 71.

Another example of iatrophysical ingenuity is found in Giorgio Baglivi, who was born in 1668 at Ragusa (Dubrovnik) and practised medicine in Rome, where he eventually became a physician to Clement XI. In the words of the medical historian Castiglioni, Baglivi 'divided the body machine into many smaller machines, comparing the teeth to scissors . . . the heart and blood vessels to a system of water-works, the thorax to bellows, and so on'. At different times he compared the stomach to a grinding mill and to a flask. A few of these comparisons would give clues to understanding the function of various organs, others were colourful or simply wrongheaded. In Rome, Baglivi became a close friend of the ageing Malpighi, eventually ministering at his deathbed and conducting his post-mortem. Baglivi's masterful description of the cerebral apoplexy which caused Malpighi's death is indicative of his exceptional medical skills. Despite his deep commitment to iatrophysics, he insisted that the physician should set aside his theoretical beliefs during his practical encounters with patients. It was possible to see the teeth as scissors, but when examining the pope's teeth it was best to focus on dental reality.

The iatrochemists, on the other hand, viewed the workings of the human body as a series of chemical processes. This was of course directly derived from Paracelsus, who was the first to use the term 'iatrochemistry'. Unlike iatrophysics, iatrochemistry was chiefly practised in northern Europe. The leading iatrochemist here was Franz De Le Boë, often known as Sylvius of Leyden (not to be confused with Vesalius' teacher and opponent, the sixteenth-century anatomist Jan Sylvius of Paris).

Franz De Le Boë was born near Frankfurt in 1614. He was of Flemish extraction, and studied at various German and Dutch universities before graduating as a doctor of medicine at Basle in Switzerland. Later he practised in Amsterdam, where he became a friend of the French philosopher-scientist Descartes, though without being persuaded of Descartes's mechanistic view of the human body. De Le Boë eventually became a professor at the University of Leyden in 1658. He was a formidable but sympathetic personality, who soon became regarded as the finest teacher of his age, his outstanding lectures attracting students from all over Europe. His teaching also included the novel feature of taking his students on regular rounds of the small ward of the university hospital, so that they could witness his diagnostic methods and learn his practical skills.

De Le Boë was one of the first to recognize the importance of Harvey's discovery of the circulation of the blood, and based his theoretical approach on this foundation. Even so, he placed his iatrochemical ideas within a quasi-Galenic framework. Bodily digestion resulted from the actions of three basic substances – saliva, bile and the pancreatic juices. The saliva assisted the digestion in the stomach, a chemical process of fermentation; whilst the pancreatic juices and the bile controlled the ingested food, directing it into the bloodstream or into faeces. Diseases resulted from 'acidosis' or 'alkalosis' in the blood: 'If all the blood is black, that indicates that acid predominates, while if it is red, the bile predominates. In the former case it is necessary to diminish the acid in the body and the blood; in the latter to diminish the bile and weaken its strength.' He condemned Galenic blood-letting, using instead sudorifics (inducing sweat), absorbent dressings (to soak up pus and dangerous fluids) and emetics. He favoured the new chemical medicines such as antimony, zinc sulphate and mercury, many of which had been pioneered by Paracelsus. But De Le Boë's strength was that he used chemistry as a science, ignoring the metaphysical and alchemical aspects which so muddied the waters of Paracelsus' chemical practice. Crucially, De Le Boë understood that the chemical processes which took place within the body were the same as those which could be observed during experiments, where their effects were more plainly visible and could be analysed in some detail. De Le Boë conducted his chemical experiments before his students in the 'Laboratorium' which the university authorities built at his request. This is generally recognized as the first university chemistry laboratory.

The chemistry of the period was undergoing a revolution, chiefly due to the Anglo-Irish pioneer Robert Boyle, who is generally regarded as the father of modern chemistry. Boyle investigated the composition of chemical substances, seeking to discover their properties. His experiments were meticulously recorded, so that they could be repeated by others. Gone was the secrecy of the alchemist's den, with its mumbo-jumbo and 'transmutations' into real or spiritual gold. Chemistry became a pure science, allowing its substances to be used for purely physical effect in the chemistry of the human body.

Instead of elixirs, we now had medicines. Here we can detect the origins of biochemistry.

Boyle resided at Oxford from 1656 to 1668. The brilliant circle which surrounded him during these years included such luminaries as the scientist Robert Hooke, the philosopher John Locke, Christopher Wren, who would become the architect of St Paul's Cathedral, and the physician Thomas Willis, who became the leading English iatrochemist.

Willis was born in 1621 and grew up in the countryside outside Oxford, the city where he eventually went to university. These were troubled times in England, and the Civil War between the Royalists and the Parliamentarians broke out in 1642, the year before Willis graduated. Following the battle of Edgehill, Charles II went to the Royalist stronghold of Oxford, which would later be besieged by the Parliamentarians. During this period the elderly Harvey continued to attend the king as his personal physician. Harvey is known to have given a lecture demonstrating the circulation of the blood in a live dog to the sceptical and conservative academics of Oxford. The young Willis must have attended this, and there is good reason to believe that he came to know Harvey personally. Willis was certainly a great advocate of Harvey's cause from early on. He also believed in the king's cause, and joined the 'Royal Voluntaries' in defence of the city. In 1643 a lethal epidemic of 'camp fever' broke out amongst the king's soldiery, and also killed Willis' father. According to Willis' biographer Hansruedi Isler, 'In several villages around Oxford the old people were completely exterminated, so that many old customs and privileges were lost forever.' From Willis' meticulous description of this fever we now know that it was typhus.

Willis remained in Oxford after the defeat of the Royalists and the execution of Charles I. In 1650 he accidentally achieved wide renown. A woman called Anne Green was hanged for murdering her illegitimate child, and Willis conducted the autopsy. According to an eyewitness report, 'Mr Thomas Willis . . . perceiving some life in her, as well for humanity as for [his] Profession sake, fell presently to act in order to her recovery [sic]'. Willis had all but raised her from the dead, and news of his feat quickly spread throughout the land. This miraculous tale had a suitable fairy tale ending. Willis' students took a collection for Anne Green and she was allowed to go free. Whereupon she married the father of her child, by whom she had further children, and apparently lived happily ever after.

More substantial repute came in 1656 when Willis published *De Fermentione*, in which he set down his iatrochemical analysis of the bodily functions. The digestive system was a process of fermentation. In the stomach, ingested unfermented juices became wine; meanwhile bread and other wheat products became beer. Food was converted into chyme (an acidic pulp) by the action of gastric secretions. This then passed into the upper intestine, where it was absorbed into the blood. In the bloodstream another process of fermentation took place. As the blood carrying the dissolved food circulated through the heart 'accension' (fermentation) produced heat and turned the food into nutrient blood. Fermentation also caused plants and animals to grow, a process which continued after their death, resulting in the corruption of flesh and organic matter.

Around this time Boyle arrived in Oxford, and the circle of progressive scientific thinkers which gathered around him would meet once a week to perform experiments. This group was known as the 'Invisible College': most of the visible Oxford colleges still clung to the old medieval authorities, refusing to countenance any such thing as experiments. Boyle voiced his contempt for the teaching of chemistry at Oxford, referring to 'the Illiterateness, the Arrogance and the Impostures of too many of those who pretend skill in it'.

The 'Invisible College' was the forerunner of the Royal Society, which was founded in 1660. This year marked the Restoration of the monarchy, when Charles II returned as king. Willis was rewarded for his loyalty to the Royalist cause and appointed professor of natural philosophy at Oxford. Four years later he published *Cerebri Anatome* (Anatomy of the Brain), which was expertly illustrated by his friend Christopher Wren. At the age of 45 Willis moved to London where he set up a fashionable practice. This involved 'a great deal of drudgery, that he did undergo in his Faculty, (mostly for Lucre sake) which did much shorten his life.' He died nine years later, worn out – but the wealthiest physician in London. Besides earning hefty fees from his rich patients, he also received royalties from *Cerebri Anatome* and other writings, which went into many editions and were translated into several European languages.

Willis's *Cerebri Anatome* is a pioneer work, especially with regard to the nervous system, which displays Willis at his best and at his worst. His explanation of the nervous system draws on his deep researches into 'comparative anatomy' (a term which he coined). Willis dissected all manner of animals, from dogs to fish, from birds to pigs – all of which gave him insight into the workings of 'neurologie' (another word which he invented, meaning the study of the nervous system). Willis was the first to classify the cerebral nerves, and this work contains the first description of many cranial nerves, including the 'nerve of Willis', the eleventh cranial nerve. He recognized the cerebrum as the organ of thought, and designated specific locations for such activities as instinct (middle brain), perception (corpora striata), memory (cortical gyri) and even imagination (corpus callosum).

Despite the stress on experimental science at the Invisible College, Willis and his fellow members were notoriously prone to theorizing far beyond their experimental findings. Willis' ideas could be highly ingenious, and he was the first to use the term 'psychology' in its medical sense, proposing his own original system. In his view, impressions received by the senses were carried to the corpora striata where they gave rise to our internal perception. When an impression proceeded beyond this to the corpus callosum it gave rise to imagination. If it was conveyed to the cortex, this left a memory. When impressions were merely reflected back to the voluntary muscles, the result was 'reflex action', which was not directed by our volition. Descartes had recognized this automatic process, but Willis was the first to try and explain 'involuntary' and 'volitional' movement in a medical sense. Willis also speculated that many mental effects – such as vertigo, hysteria and nightmares – were neurological in origin, rather than resulting from humoral imbalance or supernatural sources.

Psychology appears to have begun in the freely speculative mode in which it would continue. Yet Willis' imaginings would provoke others to more pertinently argued investigations – medical, psychological and philosophical. Willis was some way ahead of his time. It would be a quarter of a century before John Locke, his colleague at the Invisible College, would publish his ground-breaking *Essay Concerning Human Understanding*. Modern philosophy had begun with Descartes's insistence that all truth was based upon reason. Locke's philosophy was the first convincing progress beyond this rationalism. Taking a lead from his scientific colleagues at Invisible College, Locke would insist that all truth is in fact based upon experience. This arises from the 'simple ideas' we receive from our senses, which pass into our mind where they are combined to form the 'complex ideas' of our knowledge.

His purely philosophical argument appears to draw heavily upon Willis' strictly medical speculations, which the two of them would certainly have discussed together.

Locke is remembered today as the first great English philosopher, the founder of empiricism (the belief in the primacy of experience). His deep involvement with contemporary medicine – both in theory and practice – is often overlooked. In 1667 Locke would become personal physician to Lord Ashley, later Lord Shaftesbury and as Lord Chancellor the most powerful man in the country under the king. Locke had acquired considerable medical expertise (though without ever actually taking a course in medicine), just as Shaftesbury occupied the senior legal post in the land (Lord Chancellor) without legal training. Such were the times. Despite this, Shaftesbury's quack personal physician would save his life. Shaftesbury was suffering from a suppurating abscess on his liver, whose discharge was gradually poisoning his body. With considerable daring, and no previous experience of surgical procedure, Locke decided to operate. A barber-surgeon was summoned and ordered to slice open his lordship at what Locke estimated was the appropriate spot. Locke then inserted a silver tube to drain the ulcer. To the relief of all concerned this worked, and Shaftesbury would continue to wear Locke's tube for the rest of his life.

This case is indicative – and not because it had a successful outcome. The fact is, the balance between knowledge and ignorance in medicine still swung heavily in favour of the latter. Doctors did not fully know what they were doing. Many qualified practitioners were far less knowledgeable than Locke, and unqualified quacks abounded. Despite the issue of medical doctorates by colleges and universities, medicine was not yet a fully regulated profession. And even its greatest practitioners were capable of quackery (Paracelsus was far from being alone); while many who were properly qualified clung to outmoded Galenic beliefs. Some hangovers from the theory of humoral balance, such as blood-letting by leeches, would persist for another 200 years and more. The borderline between inspired insight and sheer wrongheadedness would long remain disputed. Only with hindsight can we see that Willis' speculations were on the right track. Others would prove even more convincing, yet lead into far more questionable territory.

The leading Dutch physician, Cornelius Bontekoe, did much to further the cause of iatochemistry in Holland. In 1720 he published an influential tome entitled *The Theory of Alkali and Acid through the Workings of Fermentation and Effervescence*. This claimed that illness resulted from a thickening of the blood, which was best cured by tea-drinking. The effects of the ensuing tea-drinking craze which swept the country were in fact largely beneficial, and not only because it lessened the vast intake of gin which was customary at this time. However, it was subsequently discovered that Bontekoe was being paid a fat retainer by a leading group of Dutch tea importers. At a stroke, both iatrochemistry and tea-drinking became suspect in Holland, and the national health suffered.

Ignorance and self-interest quickly shelved into avarice, unscrupulousness and outright quackery. In the eighteenth century, there was a growing demand for quacks. The coming of the Enlightenment had seen a decline in witchcraft and alchemy; 'magic' was becoming discredited; and widespread urbanization meant that many 'old wives' remedies' were no longer available. The new urban poor could not afford physicians, and the popularity of cut-price quacks increased accordingly. The 'medicines' which they peddled became good business. Quacks occupied a gap in the market, and the most successful made sure that their medicines did the same. They made claims that bona fide physicians could not fulfil, such as cures for cancer or consumption. Other 'patented medicines' claimed to address complaints which patients might have felt reticent about mentioning to their family doctor, such as venereal disease, premature ejaculation or lack of virility. Quacks may have been entrepreneurs, but they were not always detrimental. Indeed, in the 1790s the medical scholar Isaac Swainson went so far as to claim: 'In physic, all changes . . . have been forced on the regulars by the quacks, and all the great and powerful medicines are the discoveries of quacks.' Yet here too there may well have been a conflict of interest. Swainson started life as a draper, before taking a scholarly interest in medicine. He then bought the rights to 'Velno's Vegetable Syrup', which was claimed to cure consumption. Within a few years he was selling 20,000 bottles a year, the large majority of which he claimed were bought by physicians to pass on to their patients (at extra cost). Swainson quickly earned enough to buy a mansion with extensive grounds to the west of London. The grounds he transformed into a 'physic garden' for the study of the healing and medicinal properties of herbs. As a medicinal research centre this even outshone the Royal Botanical Gardens at Kew, just down the road. If Swainson was a quack, he certainly went a long way to fulfilling his own high opinion of quacks.

However, Swainson's success – as well as his ambiguity of effect – was far exceeded by that of his near contemporary Joshua 'Spot' Ward, purveyor of the celebrated 'Ward's Pill and Drop'. 'Spot' Ward (so nicknamed after a birthmark on his face) was born in 1685 and became a riverside pickle-seller in London. For obscure reasons he then fled to France, where he lived off his wits before returning to England to avoid imprisonment in the Bastille. He was soon demonstrating the confidence of an exceptional conman. In 1617 he presented himself at the Houses of Parliament as the MP for Marlborough, only to be deprived of his seat two months later when it was discovered that he had received no votes.

As is often the case with such ebullient quacks as Ward, his earliest contacts with medicine remain obscure. He almost certainly bought the recipe for his 'pill and drop' from a physician. The pill contained an antimony compound which lowered the temperature of fevered patients, also acting as an expectorant and an emetic. The 'drop' (a tincture) purged the bowels. This combined cure had the effect of calming the fevered brow as well as ridding the digestive system of anything in it. Afterwards, the patient may well have felt better, and would have exhibited a hearty appetite. The recipe 'worked' – after its own fashion. All that was now needed was some determined and successful promotion. For a character of such self-confidence as Ward, this was the easy part.

In no time, 'Ward's Pill and Drop' was being recommended by prominent figures. The writer Henry Fielding, who suffered from dropsy and gout, found his symptoms alleviated and was highly impressed. Lord Chesterfield positively gushed.

> I very early took Mr Ward's drop . . . reaped great benefit from it, and recommend it to so many of my friends that I question whether the author of that great specifick is more obliged to any one man in the kingdom.

Even better was to come. When George II began suffering from intolerable pain in the joint of his thumb, the royal physician diagnosed gout. The king was dissatisfied, and someone seems to have recommended Ward, who even more surprisingly seems to have recognized that the king had merely dislocated his thumb. With a few daring twists, Ward managed to relocate the king's thumb. Ward was rewarded with a free apartment in Whitehall for his services, and from now on his fame and fortune were assured. 'Ward's Pill and Drop' were taken on as standard issue in the medical cupboard of every ship in the Royal Navy. Ward also took the precaution of curing Lord Jekyll, Master of the Rolls, who was so delighted that he granted Ward personal exemption from all legal inspection by the College of Surgeons. Like his fellow quack Swainson, Ward too was grateful for the vast fortune that he had accrued. So much so that he became the leading philanthropist in London. He would end up by personally endowing no less than four hospitals for the treatment of the sick and impoverished. Admittedly, in a characteristic move these hospitals were all required to make liberal use of 'Ward's Pill and Drop'. This would have been good advertising, but little else. Such patients could not have afforded to pay for their treatment.

Like all good conmen, Ward believed in himself. Indeed, he was so persuaded of his enormous benefit to the nation that in his will he asked to be buried in Westminster Abbey. His immortality was more fittingly celebrated by the contemporary poet Alexander Pope:

> Of late, without the least pretence to skill,
> Ward's grown a famed physician by a pill.

Panaceas were all the rage, and the peddling of such medicines was by no means the sole preserve of 'empirics', as the quacks were ironically termed. (They learned by experience.) In 1744, no less a figure than Bishop George Berkeley, the Irish philosopher who succeeded Locke in the empiricist tradition, published a work describing the universal benefits of drinking tar water. According to Berkeley, this was 'a cold infusion [of] resinous exsudations . . . from all sorts of pines and firs whatsoever'. Berkeley's intellect and motives remain beyond question: here was a mind of sufficient calibre to expose the philosophical anomalies inherent in Newton's calculus, and his life was of such blamelessness that he came to be known as 'the good Berkeley'. Yet his advocacy of tar water knew no bounds. He claimed that it could alleviate ills ranging from 'tedious and painful ulceration of the bowels' to smallpox. He even vouched for claims that it cured everything from 'Bleeding cancer' to 'Blotches', as well as 'Hectic Fevers', 'Inflammatory Itch' and 'the most violent Scorbutic Humours'. Such is the human thirst to believe in medicine – ever open to exploitation by empirics of all waters.

8

AN ERA OF MEDICAL ENLIGHTENMENT

The greatest medical figure of the eighteenth century is generally recognized as Albrecht von Haller. His superlative talents and encyclopedic learning also spilled over into such disparate fields as botany, politics and poetry.

Haller was born in 1708 in the Swiss city of Bern. He came from a long-established bourgeois family of no great social standing. Amidst the stifling provincial conformity of this small city, the individualistic behaviour of some members of the family meant that the Hallers had come to be regarded as somewhat odd. Yet it quickly became clear that young Albrecht Haller was no ordinary oddity. By the age of ten he was composing poems in Latin and attempting to unravel the grammar of the ancient Mesopotamian language known as Chaldean (a task which was not fully accomplished until the twentieth century). Haller's father died when he was young, and he was brought up by his step-uncle, who was a physician.

When Haller was 14 his step-uncle introduced him to the philosophy of Descartes, but he quickly rejected this and indicated that he wished to become a physician. Later he was sent to Holland to study under the celebrated Hermann Boerhaave, who had established Leyden as the greatest medical centre in Europe, eclipsing even Padua. Boerhaave was recognized as the supreme teacher of his age, and according to the historian Garrison his 'reputation as a great physician extended even to China'. Yet he passed on little of originality to posterity and his medical reputation gradually 'evaporated'.

At the precocious age of 18, Haller graduated as a medical doctor, presenting a thesis which demonstrated that a salivary duct identified by one of his professors was in fact a blood vessel. Such meticulous experimental work, particularly on blood vessels, tissue, and small organs, would be typical of his future medical researches. His consequent activities also give an indication of the broadness of his other researches. Immediately after graduation Haller embarked upon an academic tour which included London, Oxford, Paris and Strasbourg. He ended up at Basle, in Switzerland, where he studied mathematics with no less than Johann Bernoulli, a member of the famous Bernoulli family whose contribution to mathematics parallels that of their contemporaries the Bachs to music.

Before finally returning home to Bern, Haller set out on an expedition into the Alps, where he collected the first specimens which would form the basis of his vast botanical collection. He then pursued his own anatomical researches, supporting himself by giving lectures, private tuition and running a private medical practice. During this period he also developed into a poet of consummate skill. His 1732 poem *Die Alpen* (The Alps) was arguably the first to celebrate the beauty of Alpine mountain scenery. This would prove one of the forerunners of the Romantic movement, and would directly influence such poets as Schiller and Coleridge. In the midst of all this activity, he also found time to get married, but his wife died in 1736.

In the same year a new university was established at Göttingen by the Elector of Hanover (who also happened to be King George II of England). Haller successfully applied for the post of professor of anatomy, surgery and medicine. He would remain at Göttingen for 17 years, during which time he conducted a wide range of original experimental work (especially in anatomy), established one of the leading botanical gardens in Germany, and produced a steady stream of scientific papers – as well as lecturing in all branches of medicine. He also married again; this wife too died, and he married a third time.

At the age of 45 he returned to Bern. It was said that his departure from Göttingen was occasioned by inconsolable homesickness. Other evidence suggests that he had been tempted by the offer of a political post in his home city. At any rate, on his return the famous professor was appointed city magistrate, a post which he occupied for several years. At the same time his scientific work continued unabated, resulting in a plethora of important discoveries in experimental physiology. In 1759 he embarked upon his massive *Elementa Physiologiae*, producing a fat volume each year for the next eight years. Such was the range of his encyclopedic knowledge that this work included all that was known of the physiology of the human body up to this time. (A generation later, the leading French physiologist François Magendie would observe drily that whenever an ambitious young physician thought he had conducted an original experiment, he was liable to find that it was already described somewhere in *Elementa Physiologiae*.) Learning new languages, composing original poetry, even writing novels expressing his enlightened political views – Haller's activity appears to have known no bounds. At the

same time he also conducted 'the most gigantic correspondence in the history of science' (now collected in 67 volumes).
This included letters exchanged with many of the leading
scientific figures of the day. Typical of these was his correspondence with the great Swedish botanist Linnaeus, who
proposed the system of simultaneously naming and defining
plants by genus and species. Haller characteristically dismissed
Linnaeus's system, proposing his own instead.

Haller was never one to suffer fools gladly – or anyone else
for that matter. His all-consuming drive to work (surely
psychotic in origin) left him famously cantankerous. This
can in part be blamed on illness. Even as a young man he
was sickly, though this did not stop him undertaking energetic
hiking expeditions into the Alps in search of botanical specimens. Yet obsessive overwork soon ground him down, ruining
what remained of his health. He began suffering from insom-
nia, bouts of depression, and spells of dizziness. These were
soon accompanied by pains in his eyes and in his kidneys, as
well as gout. Gamely he stuck to his self-destructive obsession,
ministering to himself with increasingly large doses of veronal
(opium), to which he became addicted. The slight young man
who had strode up the Alpine tracks now became a bloated
240-pound physical wreck, who found all walking painful.

Those who encountered Haller found a Jekyll and Hyde
character. He was now one of the greatest figures of his age,
and not only in the physical sense. In Casanova's *Memoirs*, the
great lover records a meeting with Haller, remarking on his
courtesy and deep learning. Haller may have been notoriously
irascible, yet he could sometimes prove delightful company.
Kindly and modest, he could also be an overbearing boor.
Even in his last raddled years, the genial genius would sometimes unexpectedly shine from within the arrogant misan-
thrope. This cannot entirely be set down to narcotic

consumption: his entire character seems to have been built on inner conflict. His constant industry was selfless in the extreme, yet he was also very ambitious. His correspondence was driven by a need to make friendly contact with his peers throughout Europe, and freely exchange his ideas with them. Yet these correspondences frequently descended into bitter rivalry. He enjoyed passing on his original ideas, but would fly into a rage if anyone pointed out defects or inconsistencies in his thought. Attempts to 'improve upon' his ideas met with a similar response. As a result this masterful scientist, who would have such a long and profound influence upon medicine, would leave no school of followers.

So what precisely were Haller's achievements? Amidst the cornucopia of theoretical insights and experimental discoveries just a few major examples must suffice. By far Haller's most important contribution was his fundamental distinction between the qualities exhibited by nerves and muscle fibre. He understood that the primary quality of muscle fibre is its 'irritability': when it is stimulated it contracts. On the other hand, the primary quality of nerve tissue is its 'sensibility', which is exclusive to the nervous system. Thus when a nerve passes through muscle fibre it can stimulate the muscle to contract. Repeated experiment led him to discover that some muscle fibre was highly irritable and would respond to slight stimulus, whereas other was less irritable and required a stronger outside stimulus. Haller also discovered that irritablity could be stimulated by a variety of means, ranging from the mechanical to the chemical and the electrical. Indeed, when conducting experiments on sensitive muscle fibre he found that this could even be stimulated by blowing gently on its surface. This painstaking experimental research demonstrated that the body was not, as previously surmised, a purely mechanical organization (Descartes), or simply some kind of chemical–physical system (Paracelsus). By carefully tracing the nervous system Haller was able to show that all nerves eventually led to the spinal cord or to the brain itself. This made him conclude that these were the regions in which we were aware of our sensations, and where we originated our responses to these sensations.

Haller's distinction between 'irritable' muscle fibre and the 'sensitive' nervous system marked the beginning of modern neurophysiology. It also marked an important step forward from Harvey's initial discovery of the circulation of the blood. Haller's discovery enabled him to explain that the heart was in fact an automatic unit, which operated entirely through the irritability of its highly sensitive layers of musclar fibre. The venous blood entered the left auricle of the heart (see Figure 5 p. 118), where it irritated the muscles, making them contract (systole). This forced the blood into the ventricle, which in turn caused it to contract; meanwhile the auricle was no longer stimulated and relaxed (diastole), allowing it to fill again. Thus the regular process of systole and diastole continued. This 'irritation' explained how the heart worked by itself, and was not operated by the nervous system – as Borelli had previously led people to believe. Haller's finding was further confirmed by his demonstration that when the heart was removed from the body, it often continued to beat of its own accord for some time afterwards, an action which would have been impossible if it was controlled externally. As Harvey had shown, the heart acts like a pump; Haller had demonstrated precisely how this pumping mechanism took place. Despite this, it would be over a century before Borelli's revolutionary neurogenic (i.e. controlled by the nervous system) theory of the heart was replaced by Haller's myogenic (autonomous muscular control) theory.

Others had previously speculated that the blood carried the *anima* would ' – the individual animating spirit, life force or soul. Haller was able to disprove this when he conducted an ingenious investigation on a pair of prematurely born Siamese twins. These were joined at the chest and abdomen, sharing a common heart, while their other major organs were separate. Most importantly, they also had separate nervous systems, and could thus control their bodies separately. This meant that they would each have had a separate will. However, their blood was thoroughly mixed between their two systems, thus leading Haller to conclude that their individual *anima* could not have resided in their blood.

Although Haller rejected any purely mechanical explanation of the working of the body as a whole, he found such explanations more convincing at the microscopic level. According to Haller the heat of the blood was caused by the friction of the individual red blood corpuscles rubbing against one another and against the walls of the blood vessels. Haller maintained that this happened to such an extent that the red corpuscles were rubbed round, contradicting the evidence produced by Leeuwenhoek and his microscopic investigations, which showed that the red cospuscles were in fact lentil-shaped. Here Haller appeared to be going against his own experimental method and contradicting the microscopic evidence. There was undoubtedly an overbearing streak in Haller: he did not like having his theories contradicted, or even 'improved'. But in this case he probably felt that the evidence confirmed his idea. The laws of physics supported his view, and so probably did his own microscopic investigations. Unfortunately, late in life he suffered from declining vision, and may simply not have been able to distinguish through his microscope that the red corpuscles were lenticular. The human factor has always played, and would continue to play, a largely unacknowledged role in science. Haller was a great experimentalist, yet astonishingly he never conducted a clinical operation in his life (even Locke is known to have conducted at least one!) As we shall see, medicine would on occasion be advanced by inspired investigative scientists like Haller, though its major advances were usually addressed to the more immediate practical needs of pathology (the study of suffering or disease, from the Greek word *pathos*).

The founder of modern clinical pathology is generally regarded as Giovanni Morgagni, another physician who throughout his life applied scientific method in the systematic accumulation of a truly encyclopedic knowledge. Medical science was now in need of such figures if it was to establish itself as a respected profession amidst increasingly bourgeois European society.

Giovanni Morgagni was born in the small northeastern Italian town of Forlì in 1682. At the age of 16 he went to Bologna to study philosophy and medicine, where his mentor was the renowned physician Antonio Valsalva, a pupil of Malpighi. Morgagni would succeed Valsalva, and in 1715 he would be appointed professor of anatomy at Padua, where he would become the last in the long line of medical geniuses to hold this chair. Morgagni quickly established himself as the leading anatomist in Italy, but it was not until he was 79 that he published the great work for which he will always be remembered: *De Sedibus et Causis Morborum*. He would continue to lecture at Padua until he died ten years later during the fierce winter of 1771. At the time, the nearby Venice lagoon had frozen over, and the students at his lectures were said to huddle for warmth in pairs beneath their thick cloaks as Morgagni's mist-wreathed words emerged from his trembling lips.

The idea behind *De Sedibus et Causis Morborum* (On the Location and Cause of Diseases) is contained in its title. Morgagni sought to locate the organs in which diseases originated. He gained much of his knowledge from precise post-mortem examination of bodies, in which he sought to discover the change wrought in organs by particular diseases, which thus accounted for the clinically observable symptoms in the ante-mortem living patient. *De Sedibus* describes no less than 640 post-mortems, some of which were in fact performed by his master Valsalva; he is not afraid to draw on detailed knowledge from trustworthy predecessors. Morgagni's descriptions make use of logical argument to reach their conclusions, and are meticulously thorough, especially in their minute examination of organs and lesions (any abnormality of structure or function within the body, ranging from wounds to chemical imbalances, tumours or abscesses). This approach enabled him to demonstrate that apoplexy was not caused by a lesion of the brain, as previously thought, but was due to abnormalities of the cerebral blood vessels; he was also able to show that this took place on the opposite side of the brain to the ensuing paralysis. Previously it had been thought that blood clots in the heart chamber were a pathological phenomenon, but Morgagni was able to show that this was a regular feature of the post-mortem condition. Likewise he was able to show that cerebral abscess was the result, rather than the cause, of a discharging ear.

Despite his concentration on precise detailed examination of each different organ, Morgagni's work was based upon a comprehensive overall view of the body. This he viewed as a complex organic machine, with each organ contributing to the overall function of the whole. Each organ itself also functioned like a small organic machine, and as such was liable to the same malfunctions as any inorganic machine. Its parts could wear out, or it could break down, disrupting the overall body function and causing disease. However, Morgagni was no rigid mechanist: he understood that the organic workings of the body consisted of a variety of physical and chemical functions. He also recognized that these workings could be affected by outside factors, such as environment, psychology or even occupational hazards.

These last factors feature heavily in the cases he describes in *De Sedibus*, which is composed in the form of 70 letters written to a colleague. In these the patients are introduced both as individuals and as cases, just as any doctor might describe them to a fellow doctor. Here Morgagni brings the Hippocratic bedside manner to fruition, extending it beyond the means available to the great founder of medicine by not only describing the individual case histories but also any subsequent findings of post-mortem examinations. For this reason, Morgagni is generally regarded as the founder of morbid anatomy for clinical purposes. His post-mortem descriptions enabled physicians confronted with similar cases to gauge from the symptoms what was taking place in the affected organs.

Very few clinical works can claim to be as sympathetic, and on occasion as genuinely moving, as *De Sedibus*. Some brief quotations will illustrate why this remains one of the greatest medical books ever written. 'A noble virgin of Verona, of sixteen years of age, having . . . a sparrow which she fed, and with which she played; endeavouring one day to take it from her right shoulder (on which it happened to hop) with her left hand, the mischievous little animal bit her forefinger with a very violent stroke of its beak . . . It was plain, from the appearance of the finger, that some nervous part was wounded . . . and for that reason it became less moveable soon after, when pus formed in the wound, the pain being increased, and the hand also becoming contracted and swollen . . .' He goes on to describe how the case was brought to him, citing similar cases in half a dozen authorities, including Hippocrates and Celsus, and how it was eventually cured. Other cases were less successful: 'A wool-comber quarrelled with another wool-comber, who was, I believe, his uncle . . . Both of them were heated with wine, which they had drunk in great plenty, as most of the common-people are wont to do here on the eleventh of November; for that was the day, in the year of 1745. In the night-time, at length, they went from words to blows. The first happened to fall down, being lame on his right side. The other wounded his thigh, as he lay, with a knife, and even pierced it through. For the point of the knife, entering a little above the knee, on the anterior and internal side, had come out again on the posterior and external side. A great effusion of blood was instantly made from the wound on both orifices: and this haemorrhage . . . could not be restrained by those who were about him.' As a result the man died, and later Morgagni carried out an autopsy: 'Upon opening the wound carefully, the cause of so great an effusion of blood came into sight. For we found that the crural artery, where it goes to the ham, and the attendant vein, were, in great measure, cut transversely.'

But he does not stop there, going on to a thorough anatomical examination of the cadaver. 'In the belly, moreover, the omentum, which was moderately fat, was drawn up to the stomach, both on the left and right side. The stomach was full of wine; yet no chyliferous vessel was found creeping anywhere through the mesentery or intestines . . .' and so on. Later, he suggests: 'If a skilful surgeon had been at hand immediately upon the infliction of the wound, by applying the tourniquet, and constringing the femur, above the wound, he would, at least have preserved the patient so long as to give time to consider amputating the limb.' Here indeed were patients treated as people in the true Hippocratic manner. Morgagni deals with each case on its merits, describing even the more complex cases with a similar step by step simplicity, from initial symptoms to diagnosis, and where relevant the final post-mortem findings. It is no surprise to find that even before Morgagni's death this 600-page work had been translated into English and other major European languages, where it would spread the study of pathological anatomy.

Another great eighteenth-century advance was the full medical recognition of surgery, and the subsequent advances in this field. Nowhere was this more noticeable than in obstetrics, which specializes in pregnancy and childbirth. Owing to taboo, this had largely been the province of female midwives who often had little training; from now on it would increasingly become recognized as a branch of medical specialization. Some feminist historians have seen this as a male invasion and takeover of an essentially female preserve. This is undeniably true, but despite much male insensitivity (and worse) during this transformation, the end result would be a significant medical improvement in the field. The fundamental sexist injustice lay in the fact that women were prevented from training as fully qualified obstetricians, rather than in the tentative, and not always successful, introduction of scientific method in place of folk tradition. However, this transformation was far from uniform. In Britain, the scientific revolution was more advanced and already beginning to inspire an industrial revolution; consequently the transformation of obstetrics into a science was comparatively more advanced, with new birthing techniques, infant care methods and the encouragement of breastfeeding. In France, the teaching of a scientific obstetrics was in many ways even more advanced, with male midwives operating at the royal court and being granted by Louis XIV the official title *accoucheur* (literally 'bringer to bed'). But throughout the rest of the country the old methods largely prevailed and such customs as wet-nursing remained the norm. Many German states were quick to understand the benefits of a scientific approach, and midwives were given training, along with lectures, before being granted licences. Meanwhile in Catholic Italy and Spain, where the

Church prided itself as the defender of female modesty, the advent of male obstetricians was fiercely resisted. Though in Catholic Austria, the Emperor Joseph II took a more sophisticated view: when told that Viennese women were too modest to allow male midwives to examine them, he replied: 'If only the rest of their behaviour was as modest.'

The leading propagandist of the scientific approach to obstetrics in Britain was William Smellie, who was born at Lanark in Scotland in 1697. He is thought to have studied in Paris, whereupon he returned to Scotland and for 20 years was the male midwife for Lanark, then a village with a population of just 2,000, and the surrounding countryside of the Clyde valley. Around 1740 he arrived in London, where he set up as a teacher of obstetrics, giving courses in the house where he lived. He charged three guineas and it is said that in ten years he gave 280 courses of lectures to a total numbering several thousands of students. His lectures made use of a leather-covered mannikin supported by actual human bones, and despite his 'uncultured bearing' these lectures were said to be 'distinct, mechanical and unreserved'. They would launch a generation of male obstetricians throughout the land, and even as far afield as the colonies of the British Empire. But it was not all plain sailing for Smellie, who was voiciferously opposed by the celebrated London midwife Mrs Nihell, who famously referred to him as 'a great horse godmother of a he-midwife', a remark which is said to have referred to his appearance as well as his abilities. Despite this opposition, Smellie would end up making a sufficient fortune for him eventually to retire to a country estate near Lanark.

In 1752 Smellie published *Midwifery*, which set down all his knowledge of this subject. He advocated that women should where possible give birth in airy rooms illuminated by daylight. Newborn infants should not be wrapped up in swaddling clothes, but should be allowed free movement which allowed the limbs to develop and gave strength to their bones. He also encouraged breastfeeding as a natural process which helped the mother and child to bond. Smellie introduced the measurement of the pelvis, as well as attempting to measure the foetal cranium *in utero* (within the uterus, or in the womb). He is also responsible for the first public introduction of an improved forceps to assist difficult births, though he was far from being the inventor of this instrument.

The forceps has a curious secret history, which is illustrative of general medical practice in the sixteenth and seventeenth centuries. The instrument was said to have been invented by William Chamberlen, a French Protestant surgeon who had fled France in 1569 as a result of the persecution of the Huguenots. This forceps consisted of two cupping blades, which held the foetal head as if between two hands. These blades could be inserted separately, and their handles then joined, so that they could attempt to ease out the foetal head. This instrument became a closely guarded family secret, and William Chamberlen, together with his sons, used their forceps to great commercial effect. However, apart from this the Chamberlens appear to have shown little surgical skill, making some suspect that the forceps 'was originally acquired by purchase from some obscure and forgotten practitioner'.

William's son Peter Chamberlen became so successful that he attended Queen Anne, the wife of James I. This appears to have gone to his head, and although he remained only a surgeon he frequently resorted to the lucrative practice of prescribing medicines to his society patients, a prerogative which was jealously guarded by qualified physicians. In 1612 he was summoned before the College of Physicians (where William Harvey was now a fellow); Chamberlen was charged with *malla praxis* (malpractice), and flung into the notorious

Newgate Gaol. Only when the queen ordered the Archbishop of Canterbury to intercede on Chamberlen's behalf was he released. This incident seems to have had little effect on his practice, for he later attended Queen Henrietta Maria, wife of Charles I, using his forceps to deliver her of a miscarriage in 1628. During the course of his duties he would certainly have encountered Harvey, who was now the king's physician. There is no record of them meeting, so Harvey's withering scorn can only be surmised.

The Chamberlen family had now become rich through their secret forceps, and purchased land in Kent, as well as Woodham Mortimer Hall, a country house with an extensive estate in Essex near the North Sea coast. (In 1818, an ancient chest would be discovered hidden beneath the floorboards here, and this was found to contain a box full of antique medical instruments. Amongst these were identified the obstetric forceps which had once belonged to someone called Peter Chamberlen. However, this may have been a relative, sometimes known as Peter Chamberlen the younger, who did in fact qualify as a doctor at Padua, and became a fellow of the College of Physicians, only to be stripped of his fellowship in 1659 'for repeated contumacious acts', i.e. insubordination.)

The forceps would remain a lucrative Chamberlen family secret for well over a century, until it fell into the hands of one Hugh Chamberlen, a self-styled doctor of medicine, though in fact unqualified. In 1685 he published a work entitled *Manuale Medicum: or a small Treatise of the Art of Physic in general and of Vomits and the Jesuits Powder in particular* [sic], which brought him considerable publicity and many further rich patients. In keeping with family tradition, he too would be summoned before the College of Physicians and charged with 'evil and illegal practice of medicine'. Whereupon he was fined ten shillings and threatened with Newgate

Gaol if he persisted. Unabashed, he continued to operate as a society man-midwife who prescribed a variety of medicines on the side, and he too attended at court, this time to Queen Anne, wife of James II. Such was his success that his ambitions now began to extend beyond medicine. Around 1690, he issued a pamphlet entitled 'Dr Hugh Chamberlen's Proposal to make England Rich and Happy'. This outlined his scheme for a Land Bank, which on the security of landed property would issue currency in the novel form of paper notes. Amazingly, this scheme attracted backers, and according to a contemporary report: 'The next nine years found Chamberlen living in an atmosphere of the keenest excitement.' The spectacular collapse of this scheme, and the subsequent flight of its perpetrator, attracted widespread publicity, including the publication of a pamphlet entitled 'Hue and Cry after a Man-Midwife'.

Chamberlen ended up in Holland, where he fell on such hard times that around 1720 he sold the secret of the forceps to a syndicate of Dutch surgeons. In 1735 an Essex surgeon Edmund Chapman published a picture of the forceps, but this seemingly attracted little attention. Not until 12 years later did a Dutch surgeon break his oath and publish the secret. Three years after this, in 1750, William Smellie created an improved version, the straight forceps, which he described in his *Midwifery*. The use of the forceps now quickly spread through the profession, with various improvements being made on the earlier designs, one of which was Smellie's longer forceps in 1754. Soon this instrument would be saving the lives of children and their mothers throughout Europe.

As is so often the case in medical history, one simple discovery would prevent countless unnecessary deaths. Another contemporary confirmation of this truism was the pioneering work undertaken by the Scottish naval surgeon James

Lind in the cure of scurvy, which is caused by lack of vitamin C. This disease had become increasingly prevalent on European ships undertaking ever-longer voyages of exploration. As early as 1498 the Portuguese explorer Vasco da Gama recorded symptoms of scurvy among his sailors after rounding the Cape of Storms (later renamed Cape of Good Hope). In 1602 a priest on board a Spanish ship voyaging up the east coast of South America after rounding Cape Horn vividly recorded how the sailors succumbed, with their whole bodies becoming painful to touch and covered in purple spots. Later their gums became so swollen and spongy that they could not even close their jaws, until 'the teeth become so loose and without support that they move while moving the head'. Others recorded how the joints of those afflicted became swollen and the victims were overcome with apathetic lethargy, heart failure and death. Though the Spanish priest noted that frequently 'they die all of a sudden, while talking'.

The captains aboard the merchantmen of the Dutch East India Company sailing on the long voyage to the Far East noticed that the disease only struck when regular supplies of fresh fruit and vegetables were no longer available. As a result, the Dutch planted citrus orchards on the islands of St Helena and Mauritius, where their ships would put in to replenish with fresh stocks on the long voyage. But few others paid attention, and even this remedy only had effect on merchant ships which undertook regular voyages along this single known route. Voyages undertaken by men-o'-war and fighting ships had no such predictability. The British Navy finally realized that something had to be done after the catastrophic round-the-world expedition led by Lord Anson. This had returned in 1744, having accomplished its mission of capturing the Spanish treasure galleon which set off annually from the Philippines to Mexico. But for the sailors concerned, Anson's voyage had proved less of a success. Of the

1,955 men who had set out, 320 succumbed to typhus and other diseases, whilst a massive 955 died of scurvy. Three years after this, James Lind carried out the first clinical trials in medical history aboard HMS *Salisbury*. Taking a dozen men suffering from scurvy, he divided them into six pairs. Each pair was given a different dietary supplement, ranging from spoonfuls of vinegar to a garlic, mustard seed and horseradish concoction, from a daily quart of cider to a daily allowance of two oranges and a lemon. The last pair were fit for duty again within six days, whilst those who drank the cider showed a small but significant improvement (cider, as then brewed, would have retained a certain level of vitamin C). The other four pairs showed no signs of recovery. Lind had demonstrated beyond doubt that citrus fruit was a cure for scurvy.

Curiously, Lind failed to recognize that scurvy was caused by a deficiency, and remained convinced that it was due to the constant moist sea air blocking the pores of the skin and restricting normal perspiration. He surmised that the lemon juice broke down the retained toxic particles, allowing them to pass out through the constrained pores. But it was Lind's reliance upon his medical survey, rather than his theoretical skills, which would one day prove decisive. In 1753 he published his *Treatise on Scurvy*; however, this book by a minor ships' surgeon was largely ignored, while His Majesty's Navy preferred to rely upon such standbys as Ward's 'Pill and Drop'. Only a few progressive figures like Captain Cook understood the benefits of Lind's recommendations; as a result, on Cook's four-year circumnavigation (1768–71), during which he found and mapped New Zealand and Australia, he did not lose a single sailor to scurvy. Over four decades after the publication of Lind's *Treatise*, this work finally came to the attention of Sir Gilbert Blane, Physician to the Fleet. Blane's bravery under fire had won him friends in high places, and his campaign on behalf of Lind's cure for scurvy resulted in a 1795 Admiralty Order directing the regular use of lemon juice in all ships throughout the navy. Within two years scurvy had disappeared from British ships 'as if by magic'; while other navies, particularly the French, continued to suffer to such an extent that in the words of Roy Porter, 'Lemons perhaps did as much as Nelson to defeat Napoleon.'

Later in his career James Lind would introduce the idea of baking all clothes worn by newly signed-on sailors, many of whom had been press-ganged from vermin-ridden gaols. This had the effect of reducing lice-born diseases, especially typhus. Lind would also introduce a method for distilling sea water for drinking purposes.

Outbreaks of scurvy would continue to occur other than at sea. This disease would in fact account for many of the deaths during the 1845–6 Potato Famine in Ireland, where potatoes had often been the only supply of vitamin C. Other large-scale outbreaks occurred during the 1849 California Gold Rush and the Crimean War of 1854–6. During the nineteenth century there was also a prevalence of infant scurvy, especially amongst the upper classes, where instead of breastfeeding mothers used powdered milk which was lacking in vitamin C. But doubters concerning the efficacy of citrus fruit remained. Arctic expeditions noted that the Inuit survived without fresh fruit or vegetables, but when these doubters ventured forth following the same diet as the natives they invariably succumbed. They had not realized that the Inuit gained their necessary supply of vitamins because they ate their meat raw. In 1850 the British Navy replaced lemon juice with lime juice from the West Indian plantations, unaware that this was in fact somewhat less effective. It was this move which gave rise to the derisive term 'limey' for British sailors and travellers abroad, a word which eventually became synonymous for

British in the United States during the first half of the twentieth century.

It was Lind who maintained that armies lost 'more of their men by sickness, than by the sword'. The man who did much to remedy this was his contemporary Sir John Pringle, who is widely regarded as the founder of military medicine. Pringle, another Scot, was born in 1707 and finished his medical studies under the great Boerhaave at Leyden in Holland. He became a senior military surgeon in 1742, serving with the British Army in the Low Countries during the war against the French. Ten years later he published *Observations on the Diseases of the Army*, which established many principles for public medicine as whole, emphasizing the need for sanitation, ventilation and cleanliness in communal accommodation. Where the army was concerned, he even went so far as to insist that the men and their uniforms should be washed 'from time to time'. (The standard of hygiene prior to this revolutionary suggestion can only be imagined.) Pringle analysed the general medical dangers inherent in large numbers of people being kept in confined spaces such as barracks, prisons and hospitals. As a result, he was able to show that such diseases as 'hospital fever' and 'jayl fever' were in fact the same thing. He pointed to the effects of putrefaction and infection, even suggesting that contagion might be caused by animalcules. Indicatively, he also coined the term 'antiseptic'. Within decades his work had been translated into several languages and his recommendations were being put into effect in all major European armies.

In the preface to his *Observations*, Pringle tells how in 1743 as the opposing British and French troops gathered on the eve of the Battle of Dettingen,

the Earl of Stair [the British commander] . . . proposed to the Duke of Noailles, of whose humanity he was well assured, that the hospitals on both sides should be considered as sanctuaries for the sick, and mutually protected. This was readily agreed to by the French General . . . This agreement was strictly observed on both sides all that campaign.

The proposal almost certainly originated from Pringle himself, and he has rightly been credited with this great humanitarian advance, which despite his hopes he was forced to concede 'has been since neglected'. However, this was the beginning rather than the end of the matter. Just over a century later the Swiss banker and humanitarian Jean Henri Dunant happened to witness the Battle of Solferino, after which some 40,000 dead and wounded were scattered over the battlefield. Many lay dying in unrelieved agony, while others pitifully attempted to drag themselves to nearby villages for help. Dunant was so horrified by what he saw that he set up a makeshift emergency hospital at the village of Castiglione, which had been overwhelmed by thousands of casualties. Here he set about organizing all present to assist, including the women of the village, an Italian priest, some passing English tourists, and a Parisian journalist.

Following this incident, Dunant would press for the adoption of Pringle's idea, and more, at an international convention which was called at Geneva in 1863. The result was the Geneva Convention (the so-called 'rules of war') and the founding of the Red Cross, whose flag, in recognition of the Swiss banker's leading contribution, would be the colour-reversal of the Swiss flag. But this great contribution to humanity would cost Dunant dear; his neglect of his financial affairs ruined him, and after this he lived for years in obscure poverty in the small town of Heiden near Lake Constance. At the age of 67, now with a long white beard, he was 'rediscovered' by a journalist, and justice was done when six years later he received the first Nobel Prize for Peace.

9

A NEW CURE FOR
AN OLD SCOURGE

Evidence of smallpox has been found in the scars of Ancient
Egyptian mummies dating from 1,600 BC, and the disease
certainly reached Ancient Greece before 400 BC. The first
authoritative description of smallpox was by the great Persian
physician Al-Razi, who wrote a treatise on the subject in AD
910. The symptoms began several days after exposure to the
disease, with high fever, aching limbs, vomiting and delirium.
Three days later a rash of red spots appeared, mainly on the
face (and often the eyes), but also in the mouth and other parts
of the body. Within days these spots became blisters filled with
pus. The disease was highly contagious and had a mortality
rate varying from 20 per cent to 40 per cent, while those who
survived suffered from gross disfigurement (the scabs from the
blisters leaving pitted scars in the skin) and often blindness. It
is estimated that between 1600 and 1800, as much as a third of
the population of London had faces disfigured with smallpox

scars, and the disease accounted for two-thirds of those who were blind. It afflicted all levels of society. Queen Mary, who ruled Britain with her husband King William, died of smallpox in 1694. In 1713 the 23-year-old Lady Mary Montagu, who had scandalously eloped with a Whig politician and was widely regarded as the most beautiful and talented woman of her time, was struck down by the disease. As she recorded in a poem:

> In tears, surrounded by my friends I lay,
> Mask'd o'er and trembling at the sight of day.

She survived, but was left with badly disfigured skin and no eyebrows. Despite this, she continued with her literary salon, impressing the poet Alexander Pope with her talents. Later, after she had spurned an amorous advance from the poet, he would satirize her in his poem *The Dunciad*. But Lady Montagu was sufficiently robust to weather such an immortal pinprick, and at the age of 50 eventually eloped once more – this time to the continent with a young Italian writer, who promptly abandoned her. She continued writing the poetry and essays which have deservedly established her in the feminist canon, and at the age of 57 she finally settled down with a 30-year-old Italian count on the shores of Lake Garda.

However, it is arguable that Lady Montagu's greatest contribution lay neither in her literary talents, nor in the considerable qualities of her humanity. Three years after the 26-year-old beauty had been struck down with smallpox, she travelled to Constantinople with her husband, who had been appointed ambassador to the court of the Turkish sultan. Here she came across the practice of 'ingrafting', which the Turkish women used to protect themselves against smallpox. In a long letter to a friend in England she described how 'the old woman comes with a nutshell full of matter of the best sort of smallpox, and asks what veins you please to have open . . . and puts into the vein as much venom as can lie upon the head of her needle.' The ingrafting would be followed by a mild dose of smallpox, which left no disfigurement, and appeared to protect the subject against any further infection from the disease. Lady Montagu went on, 'Every year thousands undergo this operation . . . and you may believe I am very well satisfied of the safety of this experiment, since I intend to try it on my dear little son.'

Lady Montagu was as good as her word, and the ingrafting of her son proved successful. When she returned to London she mounted a campaign to introduce the practice into England. The Latin word for smallpox is *variola*, and consequently this practice became known as variolation. Intent on publicity, in 1721 Lady Montagu invited three members of the Royal College of Physicians, along with several journalists, to witness the variolation of her daughter. News of the success of this operation quickly spread, and eventually the Prince of Wales, the future George II, was persuaded to have his two daughters variolated.

Meanwhile a parallel development was taking place across the Atlantic. In Boston, a local physician called Zabdiel Boylston had heard indirectly of variolation from an African slave. In 1721 there was a virulent outbreak of smallpox in Boston, and Boylston decided to try variolation as a last resort. Out of the population of 11,000, several thousand are reckoned to have fled into the surrounding hinterland. Among those who remained, a massive 5,980 became infected with the disease, of whom 844 died. Boylston variolated 244 patients, of whom only six died. This was the first widespread test of variolation.

Here we see two entirely disparate strands of medical history combining. As with Paracelsus, medicine was learning from a long-established folk tradition, in this case one practised by Turkish women and among some African tribes (though it is now known that variolation of some sort was also practised in many remote regions of Europe, from Transylvania to the Western Isles of Scotland). However, this interchange between medicine and folk practice would always remain problematic. In many fields, such as obstetrics, medicine was seeking to emancipate itself from folk tradition. This directly relates to the second strain which comes to the fore with variolation: the introduction of experimental scientific method with the clinical test. Previously, this method had been tried by Lind, in his experiment with a cure for scurvy. Boylston's 'experiment' on the people of Boston was carried out in desperation, though its widespread involvement (over 200 people, rather than Lind's mere dozen) has led some to see this as the first genuine clinical trial. As well as absorbing ancient practices which appeared to work, medicine was also seeking to establish itself as a science, but this balancing act would prove difficult to maintain, as its originator Paraclesus had shown.

It would be over 50 years before the uncertain pioneer practice of variolation was replaced by the safe method of vaccination. The man responsible for this transformation was an English country doctor called Edward Jenner, who began as an eager advocate of variolation. Early in his medical career he noticed during his rounds of the farms and villages of the Severn valley that for some reason milkmaids seemed immune to smallpox. His observation was supported by popular local lore, and this set him to wondering why this apparently unscientific myth should so invariably turn out to be true. But this was just one of a whole host of intellectual pursuits and pastimes which occupied Jenner's omnivorous mind. Beneath the exterior of this enthusiastic, conscientious, apparently somewhat naive country doctor there lurked a rare scientific brain.

Edward Jenner was born in the small Gloucestershire market town of Berkeley in 1749. His father was a country clergyman and his mother was a country clergyman's daughter, and both would die within weeks of each other when he was five years old. From then on Edward was looked after by an adult older brother, and to all appearances had a happy childhood. However, in later life he would recall, 'I have been through life, almost from the earliest period of my recollection, haunted by melancholy, but yet at times my spirits have mounted to the highest pitch of vivacity.' Throughout his life those who encountered him would frequently be struck by his manner of eager innocence.

At the age of 13, Jenner was apprenticed to a local surgeon, whom he would accompany on horseback as they went on their rounds through the country villages. Upon the completion of his apprenticeship eight years later, he travelled to London to study anatomy and medicine at St George's Hospital. Here he became the pupil of the renowned Scottish surgeon John Hunter, and resided in his house. Hunter was a gruff domineering ogre, who was nonetheless worshipped by his starry-eyed young pupil, to such an extent that even the irascible Hunter soon warmed to his bright young houseguest. Besides being a first-rate surgeon, Hunter was also a keen anatomist and biologist. His pride and joy was his vast biological collection, which contained 13,000 items, including specimens exhibiting symptoms of almost all known human diseases.

Hunter was to be a major influence on Jenner's life. The older man's attitude to science was determinedly down-to-earth: 'Why think? Why not try the experiment?' By now the great Newtonian era of scientific discovery, which had produced such exceptional experimentalists as the chemist Boyle and the physicist Hooke, was over. The path of science was diverging – on the one hand into technological advance (e.g. canals, the spinning jenny), and on the other into theoretical speculation (e.g. atoms, mathematical innovation). The course of medicine lay between these two, and Hunter's insistence upon experiment would prove invaluable in shaping Jenner's approach.

A year after Jenner arrived in London, Captain Cook returned from his first great voyage of exploration, during which he had mapped the coast of Australia and New Zealand. Hunter was asked to assist in classifying the vast array of hitherto unknown biological specimens which had been collected during the course of this expedition. He seconded his young pupil to assist him, and together they set to work with a will. Noting Jenner's enthusiasm for the task, Hunter suggested that he should join Cook on his next voyage; but Jenner was homesick for country life, and in 1773 he returned to take up a country practice in Gloucestershire.

Here Jenner resided in the house of his older brother, living the life of a country doctor and cultured country gentleman. As a result of inheritances, he now owned land and was reasonably well off, with sufficient time and means to pursue a wide range of activities between his doctor's rounds. He played the flute and the violin, developed a deep interest in ornithology, chemistry, and other scientific subjects, and cultivated a talent for minor poetry which he would continue to write all his life. His finest poem 'Signs of Rain' is still anthologized, and demonstrates his keen awareness of nature:

> The hollow winds begin to blow,
> The clouds look black, the glass is low,
> The soot falls down, the spaniels sleep,
> And spiders from their cobwebs creep.

But not all his amateur versifying was confined to rural subjects. Jenner may have lived deep in the countryside, but he did not bury himself there. With the advent of newspapers (*The Times* would be launched in 1788) country gentlemen could now keep abreast with the latest developments in politics and science. When the parliamentarian William Wiberforce began exposing the evils of the slave trade – 18 million black Africans had been transported to the Americas by 1772 – Jenner wrote and composed the music for a series of anti-slavery songs.

His scientific investigations proliferated, and he studied a variety of naturalistic topics, ranging from the growth of feathers in young blackbirds to the hibernation of hedgehogs. It was Jenner who discovered the extraordinary behaviour of the cuckoo, which deposits its eggs in the nests of other species. He was the first to observe how the oversized young cuckoo ejects the other nestlings and eggs from its adopted nest, using its wings to scoop its prey into a hollow in its back and then lifting it to the lip of the nest, before shrugging it over the edge with a convulsive jerk. Jenner sent this description to Hunter, who passed it on the Royal Society, where its publication caused a flurry of national interest and temporary fame for Jenner, who was honoured with an invitation to become a fellow of the society.

During this period Jenner also made his first original findings in the medical field. Angina pectoris, with is characteristic severe suffocating pain in the chest, had only been diagnosed as a separate ailment in 1772. It was recognized that angina pectoris (literally 'strangulation of the chest') could eventually result in death, but its mechanism and how it caused such pain remained unknown. Jenner vividly describes how he performed an autopsy on a patient who had died of angina pectoris: 'After having examined the more important parts of the heart, without finding anything by the means of which I could account either for his sudden death, or the symptoms preceding it, I was making a transverse section of the heart, pretty near its base, when my knife struck against something so hard and gritty as to notch it. I well remember looking up to the ceiling, which was old and crumbling, conceiving that some plaster had fallen down. But on further scrutiny the real cause appeared: the coronaries were become bony canal's. Later he discovered that 'the coats of the arteries were hard, and a sort of cartilaginous canal was formed within the cavity of each artery and there attached, so, however, as to be separable as easily as the finger from a tight glove.' He concluded that this calcification of the coronary arteries prevented the blood from flowing, causing angina pectoris, which eventually resulted in death.

This discovery caused Jenner some sorrow. He was aware that his dear friend and mentor John Hunter was suffering from angina pectoris, and now realized that one day this would undoubtedly prove fatal. With characteristic selflessness, Jenner decided against publishing his remarkable discovery, not wishing to cause distress to his friend.

Smallpox outbreaks were prevalent in the English countryside, and in Gloucestershire this was one of the main causes of death. Jenner was a firm believer in the comparatively new practice of variolation, but he was well aware that this was a far from perfect preventative measure. The mild outbreak of disease in the variolated patient could on occasion become virulent and result in death. Also, he noticed that the variolated patient could act as a carrier, passing on the full-blown disease to others who had not been variolated.

It was in his youth, while working as an apprentice, that Jenner had first encountered the country belief that cowpox somehow prevented smallpox. The surgeon to whom he was apprenticed was examining a young milkmaid from Sodbury who had developed a rash of pustules on her skin. The milkmaid firmly assured the surgeon that this could not possibly be smallpox, as she had already had cowpox, and after that you never got smallpox. Again and again, Jenner would encounter this story on his rounds. For some 30 years he did nothing about it, though he frequently brought up the subject with his friends, who soon learned to avoid this topic.

Milkmaids would catch cowpox on their hands from the pustulated nipples of infected cows. The disease resulted in unpleasant lesions, but was not otherwise dangerous. Jenner eventually concluded that if cowpox prevented smallpox, then variolating a patient with live material obtained from a cowpox pustule might well prove more effective and less dangerous than variolating with smallpox material. He remembered the words of his mentor Hunter: 'Why think? Why not try the experiment?'

In May 1796 Jenner finally took the plunge when he encountered a young dairymaid called Sarah Nelmes who had fresh lesions of cowpox on her fingers. He took a sample, and on 14 May he inoculated an eight-year-old boy called James Phipps with the living cowpox material. The boy developed a slight fever, and minor lesions, which soon disappeared. On 1 July Jenner inoculated the boy with smallpox. The boy consequently developed no symptoms. The cowpox had worked!

Jenner set to work, writing a short paper for the Royal Society, announcing his sensational claim to have found a cure for one of the worst scourges of humanity. He named the living cowpox material used on the boy a 'vaccine' (from the Latin *vacca*, meaning 'cow') and he referred to the material which caused smallpox as a 'virus' (from the Latin *virus*, meaning 'slimy liquid or poison'), the first medical use of this term in the modern sense. Jenner confidently despatched his paper to the Royal Society. One can but imagine his astonishment when it was refused. His paper was rejected as being too revolutionary; it was considered inconceivable that one disease could prevent another. More pertinently, it was also pointed out that Jenner's finding had insufficient evidence in the form of confirming cases.

Jenner immediately set about confirming the success of his vaccination with several further trials, and wrote up his findings in a 75-page booklet entitled *An Inquiry into the Causes and Effects of Variolae Vaccinae* (Cow Pox). This he published at his own expense in 1798. It achieved an immediate and growing groundswell of effect. By the end of 1799, some 5,000 people had been vaccinated in England. Soon pieces of cloth soaked with cowpox vaccine and sealed in glass vials were being shipped to the United States, where a vial was despatched to President Jefferson, who vaccinated his entire family. It was soon discovered that lymph taken from smallpox pustules could remain active for as long as three months if it was dried and sealed in tubes, and in this way in 1801 smallpox inoculation was transmitted full circle back to Istanbul (from where it was shipped to the Persian Gulf and on to India, where thousands were soon inoculated).

Despite Britain being at war with France, samples of the vaccine were presented to Napoleon in 1804. He ordered a gold medal to be struck in Jenner's honour, and when the Gloucestershire doctor wrote to him on behalf of two friends of his who were imprisoned in France as a result of the war, Napoleon declared, 'Anything Jenner wants shall be granted' – and Jenner's friends were released. A year later Napoleon made vaccination compulsory throughout the entire French army. Meanwhile Sweden made it compulsory throughout the entire country. Such measures demonstrated much more than the success of Jenner's vaccine. They showed how progressive rulers were beginning to recognize that if a modern state was to function effectively, it required healthy citizens. Medicine was increasingly becoming a national concern.

Paradoxically, the vaccine did not prove a great success for Jenner, who selflessly chose to donate his discovery to the world, forswearing any financial gain. Jenner now spent so much of his time and money campaigning on behalf of the vaccine that he neglected his own practice and soon found himself heavily in debt. Fortunately, by this stage he had many sympathizers in high places, who encouraged parliament to vote him the sum of £10,000 in gratitude for his discovery. Others proved less grateful, and saw no reason to emulate Jenner's high-mindedness. A London doctor called George Pearson established the Institute for the Inoculation of the Vaccine-Pox, where patients were charged for inoculation. This was soon making good money for its president, Dr Pearson; though the first Jenner heard of the Institute was when Pearson sent a letter graciously inviting him to become a fellow of it!

Others, such as the Quaker physician Dr William Woodville, leapt on the bandwagon without being fully aware of what vaccination entailed. Woodville inoculated some patients with vaccine contaminated with smallpox, and several of these patients subsequently developed smallpox. Woodville at once blamed Jenner, declaring that his claim regarding his vaccine was false. He then began mounting a campaign against vaccination, which attracted a number of influential supporters of varying credibility.

Among these was Dr Benjamin Moseley, physician to the Royal Medical Hospital at Chelsea, who suggested that after vaccination 'the human character may undergo strange mutations from quadrupedan sympathy' so that these patients might become 'wild, with horns on their heads'. This inspired the artist James Gillray to ridicule vaccination with a cartoon showing people sprouting cows from their arms and other parts of their body. When a number of patients from Dr Pearson's Institute also developed smallpox, almost certainly for the same reason as Woodville's patients, he too joined Woodville's campaign. Jenner was forced to spend much time and energy combating these claims, finally opening an institute of his own, the Royal Jennerian Society, to ensure that his vaccine was properly administered. Unfortunately the Society's resident inoculator embezzled the funds and Jenner was left with further debts. An indication of the size of these debts is seen from the fact that in 1806 parliament was once again forced to come to his rescue, saving him from the prospect of a debtors' jail, this time voting him a grant of £20,000. This represents a colossal sum (a few years later the young surgeon and poet John Keats was able to live and travel on £200 a year). Jenner's biographer Dorothy Fisk notes that taxes 'had eaten up so much of the previous grant', and it seems clear that Jenner was not good at handling money. However, the need for such a vast sum hints at more than simple financial incompetence. Jenner did not live an extravagant lifestyle, and the farming land he owned should have been largely self-supporting, so where did the money go? The need for all this money remains as much a mystery to us, as it doubtless was for Jenner.

Jenner would die in 1823 at the age of 73, by which time he was world famous. At the end of the century the great French chemist Pasteur would suggest that in honour of Jenner vaccination should be adopted as the general term for inoculating modified germs to give immunity from more virulent ones. By the mid-twentieth century smallpox had been eliminated from all developed countries, and only lingered on in certain tropical regions. A few decades later the World Health

Organization would announce that smallpox had been entirely eliminated. This was the first such disease to have been completely eradicated from our planet, all as a direct consequence of Jenner's discovery.

Along with vaccination, a number of familiar features of modern medicine would originate during this period. One of these was the diagnostic method known as percussion – rapping the patient's chest and listening to its resonance – which was introduced by Leopold Auenbrugger, a renowned eighteenth-century Viennese physician. The story goes that Auenbrugger, who was the son of an innkeeper, learned the technique of percussion from rapping on casks of wine to discover how full they were. As early as 1761 he described his technique in a short treatise entitled *Inventum Novum*. By striking the thorax (ribcage) it was possible to determine 'the internal condition of its cavity by the resonance of the sounds it produced . . . The sound thus elicited from the healthy chest resembles the muffled sound of a drum covered with a thick woollen cloth.' A duller, more sonorous sound, or one more high pitched, indicated diseased lungs. However, he was at pains to stress that the main element of this technique was practice, both in tapping and diagnosis. Experience alone enabled the physician to hone his diagnostic abilities with this new method.

Auenbrugger was a sophisticated man of equable temperament and many talents. Among his accomplishments was writing a libretto for an opera called *The Chimney Sweep* by Mozart's great rival Salieri. Auenbrugger does not seem to have been too upset when his medical colleagues dismissed his claims concerning percussion; though he continued to use this method himself, learning to determine the outlines of the heart and lungs. It was not until 1808, the year before Auenbrugger's death, that his *Inventum Novum* was translated into French by Jean-Nicholas Corvisart, Napoleon's personal physican. Corvisart immediately recognized the potential of this diagnostic technique, broadcasting it far and wide.

Ironically, one of the many Viennese colleagues who dismissed Auenbrugger's claims was Anton de Haen, who pioneered the introduction of another revolutionary technique which would become a modern standby: namely, temperature-taking. De Haen was born in the Netherlands, and had been one of the last pupils to study under the legendary Boerhaave, before travelling to Vienna where he later became a professor of medicine in 1756. The Austrian Empire was currently the greatest, and richest, in Europe, extending from the Netherlands to the borders of the Ottoman Empire. Vienna, as capital of this Europe-wide empire, was establishing itself as the leading medical centre of the continent, with its vast hospitals being able to administer to more patients than any yet seen. Such opportunity for extensive medical experience led de Haen to his belief in regular temperature-taking, which enabled the physician to chart the course of any patient's disease in comparatively simple fashion. It was already known that the human body was able to maintain its normal temperature regardless of outside temperature. Normal external human body temperature had been established as 98.6° fahrenheit by Gabriel Fahrenheit himself, the Polish-born Dutch physicist who had in the previous century perfected the mercury thermometer and calibrated the scale which was named after him. (On this scale, 0° was fixed as the freezing point of an ice–salt mixture; 32° was the freezing point of water; and 96° external human body temperature. This latter temperature was adjusted to 98.6°, when he fixed the boiling point of water at 212°, precisely 180° above freezing water.) De Haen favoured the regular use of an invasive thermometer, such as could be placed under the tongue; although these were in practice somewhat crude, having long stems and taking around a quarter of an hour to determine temperature. De Haen understood that the higher the temperature, the higher the fever (the notion of 'high fever' originates from this use of the thermometer). A temperature moving towards normal indicated recovery, a consequent rising temperature indicated relapse. In this way the course of a disease could be charted, and with a temperature chart placed at the foot of a bed it was possible to monitor in simple fashion the condition of large numbers of patients.

De Haen had a deeply contradictory nature in all senses of the word. He was dictatorial in manner and constantly contradicted his colleagues; at the same time, besides being responsible for the efficient scientific advance of regular temperature-taking, he still clung to a firm belief in witchcraft. De Haen was no exception here. Despite medicine's advances as a science, many otherwise accomplished physicians still clung to outmoded historical beliefs. Such was also the case with another pioneer of medical technique, and in this instance it would initially detract from his great innovation. Half a century earlier than de Haen's innovation in the wards, the English physician Sir John Floyer had introduced counting the pulse rate as a diagnostic aid. As we have seen, the first instrument for measuring the pulse rate had in fact been invented a century previously by Sanctorius. This 'pulsilogium' had consisted of a lead weight which swung on an adjustable length of thread, acting as a pendulum. Floyer was to use a special 'pulse watch' which ran for precisely one minute, against which he could count the number of pulses. In practice however, he would place much greater emphasis on the 'feel' of the pulse, resurrecting the ancient Galenic notion that each disease had its own specific quality of pulse. Not until this aberration was dismissed a century later as 'observation going minutely mad; a whole Lilliput of symptoms; an exasperating waste of human intelligence' would pulse-taking in its present form become an accredited part of diagnostic technique. Apart from Floyer's work on the pulse, he was a great advocate of cold bathing in the Roman style, and was also obsessed with prophecy. As a result, alongside his medical milestone *The Physician's Pulse Watch* he would publish such works as *The Ancient Psychrolusia Revived* and *A Vindication of the Sybilline Oracle*.

Another stalwart of diagnostic medicine would be introduced by the French physician Laennec, who invented the stethoscope. This instrument, along with the previously mentioned diagnostic standbys which came into general use around this time, were all attempts to penetrate the inner workings of the human body, to enable the physician to 'see' the living organs which he had known only from post-mortem anatomy. The stethoscope (literally 'an instrument to look into the chest') would prove by far the most effective tool in this sphere until the use of X-rays.

René Hyacinthe Laennec was born in 1781 at Quimper in Brittany in the northwest of France. He had poor health, suffering from asthma, and grew up in the troubled times of the Revolution, which broke out in 1789. From the beginning Laennec was a sensitive youth with a retiring character, who preferred to play the flute and write poetry rather than join in rough and tumble games with his contemporaries. He first studied medicine at Nantes, where he quickly established himself as a brilliant student. After this he studied in Paris under Corvisart, who would remain a major influence. Laennec would eventually succeed Corvisart as Physician at the Hôpital de la Charité; and it was from Corvisart that Laennec learned of percussion, the first major advance in the process of auscultation since the Hippocratic era. Until this time, auscultation had still basically consisted of the physician pressing his ear to the patient's chest or abdomen, and listening for any indication of what might be taking place in the lungs and heart within.

The almost accidental circumstances which led Laennec to invent the stethoscope are on record. A friend of his recalled how 'One day whilst walking in the courtyard of the Louvre [Laennec] saw some children playing. One had his ear pressed to the end of a long piece of wood, which transmitted the sound of a pin, being scratched at the other end.' The story is taken up by Laennec himself: 'In 1816 I was consulted by a young woman presenting general symptoms of heart disease. Owing to her stoutness little information could be gathered by application of the hand and percussion. The patient's age and sex did not permit me to resort to auscultation.' Then he remembered the boys playing by the Louvre, and decided to adapt this acoustic phenomenon to his own purpose. 'Taking a sheet of paper I rolled it into a very tight roll, one end of which I placed on the precordial region, whilst I put my ear to the other. I was both surprised and gratified at being able to hear the beating of the heart with much greater clearness and distinctness than I had ever before by direct application of my ear.'

Laennec realized at once the significance of his discovery. Physicians could now listen in clearly to the sounds of the body at work, the hush of air passing in and out of the lungs, the gurgle of the blood passing to and from the heart. Laennec quickly developed a workable stethoscope in the form of a 30-centimetre-long piece of hollow wood, to which could be screwed an earpiece at one end and a chest piece at the other. Laennec was a patient and observant physician, with an ability to evoke vividly the experience of using his discovery. 'On applying the cylinder . . . to the breast of a healthy person we hear, during inspiration and expiration, a slight but distinct murmur, answering to the entrance of the air into, and its expulsion from, the air cells of the lungs. This murmur may be compared to that produced by a pair of bellows whose valve makes no noise, or, still better, to that emitted by a person in deep and placid sleep, who makes now and then a profound inspiration.' Passing from the healthy lungs, he went on to distinguish between their various ailments. 'The moist crepitus rattle has evidently its site in the substance of the lungs. It resembles the sound produced by the crepitation [light crackling sound] of salts in a vessel exposed to a gentle heat.' Laennec demonstrated how to classify the sounds which indicated crepitation, bronchitis, pneumonia, and consumption (or phthisis). The latter disease, now known as tuberculosis, was becoming a scourge in the urban conglomerations of the new industrializing nations. During the ensuing century it would become the greatest cause of death among all age groups in western countries.

At the same time, Leannec's original stethoscope would undergo various modifications. By the 1850s the wooden tube had been replaced by a rubber tube, and the single earpiece would be replaced by the two-eared instrument we know today. The stethoscope meant that the physician no longer had to rely upon the patient's own description of his or her symptoms, which were liable to be inaccurate or even imaginative. Yet this apparent advantage also had its detrimental effect. The encounter between the physician and the patient lost a certain personal element; the patient was now regarded less as a human being, leading the eminent German physician Robert Volz to remark, 'The sick person has become a thing.'

Laennec's superlative observational and descriptive powers left their mark on that second scourge of Paris, and other urban conglomerations: alcoholism. It was he who first described the yellowish, lumpy, shrunken liver – so characteristic of damage from excessive alcohol – as 'cirrhosis' (from the

Greek *kirrhos* meaning 'tawny-coloured'). Having done so much to advance the study of tuberculosis, ironically Laennec himself would succumb to this disease at the age of 45 in 1826. During the ensuing years the disease would reach pandemic proportions in Europe, becoming known as the 'white plague' or 'consumption' (because it was thought that in the course of this disease the lungs consumed themselves). Just five years before Laennec, the poet and surgeon John Keats had succumbed to 'consumption', which would later become so much a part of everyday life that it would feature in operas from *La Traviata* to *La Bohème*, as well as in the works of playwrights from Chekov to Ibsen.

Other medical techniques developed during this period which remain a feature of medicine today have proved more controversial. Volz's observation that patients were becoming alienated by their doctors had already drawn the sympathetic attention of another German physician Samuel Hahnemann, who would be responsible for the introduction of homoeopathic medicine. Homoeopathy (from the Greek *homoios* meaning 'similar', and *pathos* meaning 'suffering') revived the ancient medieval doctrine of similarities, a variant of the old doctrine of signatures so favoured by Paracelsus. According to the doctrine of similarities an illness could be cured by a substance which produced similar symptoms. For example, the old peasant remedies of treating burns with a hot compress, or treating a cold with onions (because they made the eyes and nose run).

Samuel Hahnemann was born in 1755 at Meissen in Germany. This was a centre of the porcelain industry and his father worked as a porcelain painter until he fell into poverty early in Hahnemann's life. However, the young Hahnemann showed such promise at school that his schoolmasters sponsored his further education and entry into the University of

Leipzig, where he studied medicine, supporting himself by teaching Greek and French. From here he travelled to Vienna, where he was employed as a librarian and personal physician to a local aristocrat, at the same time continuing with his medical education at the university, where he would probably have attended lectures by Auenbrugger. In Vienna Hahnemann joined the semi-secret quasi-religious order of Freemasons, which was becoming increasingly popular among the aspirant professional classes (Mozart would join a few years later). Having saved enough money to support himself, Hahnemann travelled to Erlangen in southern Germany, where he would complete his medical studies in 1779.

For the next few years Hahnemann practised medicine in the small towns of Saxony, becoming increasingly exasperated at the effects of the medicine practised by himself and his colleagues upon their patients. This was hardly surprising, as the medicine practised in the late eighteenth century in provincial Germany (and elsewhere) remained a somewhat haphazard and primitive business. Drugs were prescribed with little regard to precise dosage, patients were regularly bled with leeches, and even among many accredited professionals there remained a distinct tendency to quackery and the promotion of their own 'patented cures'. In the end, despite all the time and effort Hahnemann had invested in qualifying for his profession, he despaired of medicine and abandoned his role as a physician. Instead, he took up pharmacy; and it was while prescribing a treatment for malaria that Hahnemann would make the 'discovery' that would lay the foundations of homoeopathy.

Since ancient times malaria had been a scourge of low-lying marshy areas throughout Europe – even as far north as England, where the whole of East Anglia was notorious for this disease. It was thought to be caused by 'miasmas' (noxious airs) arising from marshes. Galen is known to have treated malaria in second-century Rome, and its prevalence in Italy would cause it to be known there as *mal aria* (bad air). In the rest of Europe it was usually referred to as the 'ague' (a corruption of the Latin for 'acute fever'). Its symptoms began with a headache and violent shivering fever. These recurred at regular intervals, weakening the patient and laying him or her low, to such an extent that in extreme cases this resulted in death. During the late Renaissance, malaria reached such epidemic proportions in Rome that the pope offered a reward for anyone finding a cure. In the seventeenth century Jesuit missionaries in Peru discovered that the bark of the cinchona tree alleviated malarial symptoms. Cinchona (which would later give us the name 'quinine') was brought to Europe in 1640, where its use quickly spread and it became known as Jesuit's Bark. During this period Europe was riven by wars between Catholics and Protestants, with the result that many Protestants were suspicious of the poisonous-tasting Jesuit's Bark, and refused to take it. According to a persistent story, Oliver Cromwell was among these abstainers and his premature death may well have been a consequence of this.

In the course of Hahnemann's pharmaceutical practice, he often came into contact with patients suffering from malaria. On one occasion he observed, or thought he observed, that when an otherwise healthy patient was accidentally given an overdose of quinine, this caused symptoms which were the same as those of malaria. He decided to test this finding on himself, and he too experienced feverish symptoms after taking quinine. This narrow and flimsily based finding led him to a huge generalization. He concluded that disease was cured by drugs which produced similar symptoms to the disease, a revived version of the old medieval 'doctrine of similarities'. By another quirk of logic, this induced Hahnemann to believe

that such drugs should be administered in tiny but very pure
doses, and the smaller the dose the greater the effect. When the
'material' dose was reduced, its 'spiritual' quality increased.
Hahnemann would take this doctrine to extreme limits, directing that a tincture of pure medicine should be diluted with
sugar milk, or alcohol, to one tenth of its strength, which liquid
should then be diluted to a further one tenth of its strength.
This process should be carried out *thirty times*. In the case of
solids, the adulterating substance should be sugar, but otherwise the process should be precisely the same – resulting in a
potency of one part medicine to 10^{30} parts mixing agent. Each
dilution should be accompanied by vigorous shaking, or
pounding for solids, in order to release the 'vital force' of
the medicine. Only then should it be administered to the
patient. Such was the basis of homoeopathy: like was always
treated with like. Thus opium was used for sleepiness, onions
for colds, and so forth.

Hahnemann believed there was no point in seeking a cause
for a disease, the nature of which would always remain open to
different interpretations. The homoeopathic physician should
only be concerned with treating the symptoms. In his controversial *Concept of Diseases* Hahnemnann claimed that
apart from syphilis and 'sycosis' (cauliflower-like veneral
warts), all chronic symptoms were caused by psora (the 'itch').
Such symptoms resulted from the itch being forced deeper into
the body; homoeopathic treatment would bring it to the surface and expel it. This was true of diseases from gout to
hysteria, from cancer to paralysis.

The folk wisdom of treating like with like had proved
effective in the case of smallpox and cowpox, but there were
no scientific grounds for elevating this to a universal principle.
Also, given the apparatus of the period, such copious dilution
of medicines would in fact result in the almost certain elim-

ination of all the original pure medicine. Homoeopathy appeared to be based upon a false premise and non-existent medicine, as many were quick to point out. Despite this drawback Hahnemann persisted, and in 1810 he wrote *Organon der Rationelle Heilkinde* (Handbook of Rational Healing), which was published in Leipzig, where he was now lecturing on pharmacy at the university.

Hahnemann himself was as filled with contradictions as the medical theory he invented. Convinced that his was the only rational approach to healing, he would tolerate no contradiction or discussion of his principles. The only reasoning which could possibly prevail was his reasoning. Nonetheless he found it necessary to spend much of his time vilifying any other approach to medicine. His lectures frequently descended into diatribes against medical orthodoxy, and became a source of great entertainment to his students. The authorities were less amused, and banned him from teaching. Hahnemann replied that, 'He who does not walk along the same path as me is a traitor to medicine.' In the manner of Paracelsus, he saw himself as a Martin Luther of medicine, protesting against a corrupt orthodoxy. Despite the evidence, he insisted that homoeopathy was 'a therapeutic axiom not to be refuted by all the experience in the world'.

Such an approach inevitably required persistent efforts if it was to convince, but Hahnemann proved up to this difficult task, producing a veritable avalanche of publications arguing his case. He would eventually publish over 60 volumes, as well as personally translating several of them into French and English.

This was a period when all manner of unorthodox sects and beliefs were beginning to proliferate throughout Europe. Often these were the creation of charismatic leaders, and the beliefs disappeared with the disappearance of their inventor. The transformations wrought by the new industrialization had left many disillusioned with the old ways. A dispossessed rural population now worked in the 'dark satanic mills' of the Industrial Revolution, which had begun in Britain and was now spreading to Germany and elsewhere. The skies of the new manufacturing cities were permanently overcast with smoke from the belching chimney stacks, leaving filth and squalor in the slums beneath this rain of soot and sulphur. Many who suffered, and others who simply witnessed this suffering, felt that something was going hideously wrong. There was an almost universal nostalgia for a more 'natural' way of life. (Only a few years later, Karl Marx would propose another 'natural' way of life, where the Communist revolution would eventually bring about a glorious semi-rural utopia.) Hahnemann's insistence on pure highly diluted medicines, which 'allowed the body to cure itself', his belief that 'nature should be permitted to take its course', and his advocacy of 'pure living and fresh air', all struck a chord. Likewise his attacks on the 'elitism and vested interests' of orthodox medical treatment, with its 'shot-gun medicine' approach involving harmful drugs, and its unwillingness to accept any alternative, also attracted many. Soon homoeopathic clinics were opening all over Europe and even in America.

In his later years Hahnemann moved to Paris, where his medicine attracted such a following that he was soon earning 200,000 francs a year. Yet despite his inconsistencies and his arrogance, he does not seem to have been a charlatan. He believed in what he preached. Hahnemann would die in 1843, a rich man, by now recognized as the founder of a new worldwide medicine.

Disappointment with the strictures of more orthodox medicine was now manifesting itself in a variety of forms. Homoeopathy was accompanied by such widespread fads as hydropathy, 'the water cure'. Spas all over Europe benefited as fashionable visitors came to 'take the waters' at such spots as Spa, Baden-Baden, Vichy and Bath. The waters at these spas were thought to cleanse the body of its accumulated poisons, and provide a natural cure for the ailments of modern life. The craze for hydropathy gradually began to subside through the nineteenth century, but homoeopathy continued to flourish. By the beginning of the twentienth century an International Congress of Homoeopathic Physicians had been formed, while homoeopathic hospitals had been established all over Europe and in North America. Although the craze for homoeopathy would never threaten the position of orthodox medicine, its various beliefs would persist, such that homoeopathy remains very much alive today as an 'alternative' medicine. Despite the scientific invalidity of its methods, it did little harm from the outset. In the words of the medical historian Ackerknecht: 'At least Hahnemann's system offered a fairly innocuous alternative to the heroic and often fatal orthodox therapeutic methods of the age, which still consisted of extensive bloodletting, purging, large doses of toxic drugs, and induced vomiting.' General medical practice still had a long way to go while doing nothing remained a viable alternative.

10

GIANTS OF PHYSIOLOGY

During the nineteenth century medicine would undergo a transformation. Previously, its researchers had largely been medical practitioners or even amateurs. Now they would become 'pure' scientists, attached to universities. This was aided by the revolution which took place in the leading universities, especially in Germany and France, where physiological research became a standard feature. British medicine, which had contributed so much, would suffer from a series of scandals which plagued anatomical research for many decades. Suffice only to mention the most notorious, the case of Burke and Hare.

The Irish-born William Hare ran a squalid boarding-house in one of the poorest quarters of Edinburgh, where another Irishman William Burke was a lodger. When an elderly lodger died in November 1827, Hare and Burke decided against burying the body legally. Instead they secretly sold it for seven pounds ten shillings to the distinguished surgeon Robert Knox, a larger-than-life character who had been wounded at the Battle of Waterloo and now ran his own anatomy school. Inspired by the success of this scam, it appears that Burke and Hare may now have became body-snatchers, setting out under cover of darkness and robbing graves of recently interred cadavers to sell to Knox. Perhaps finding this too risky, they then certainly turned to the more efficient method of murder. Using their wives as bait, Burke and Hare began enticing strangers into the boarding-house, getting them drunk to the point of unconsciousness, and then suffocating them (a method which ensured that the cadaver showed no sign of any murderous struggle). During the course of the next eleven months Burke and Hare murdered at least fifteen unknown people in this manner, selling on their corpses to Knox for sums between eight and fourteen pounds. Finally the neighbours became suspicious when a local woman disappeared, and the police were called in. At the ensuing trial Hare confessed and turned king's evidence, enabling his eventual release; while the lodger Burke was hanged. Such was the huge public outrage, and ghoulish interest, that after being hanged Burke's body was flayed, his skin tanned, and strips sold as souvenirs. Although the local woman's body had been discovered in a box in the cellar of Knox's anatomy school, at the trial Burke had made it plain that Knox was entirely innocent. Regardless of this an angry mob burnt Knox's house to the ground, and he fled to London, where he eventually died a broken man. Shortly after the hanging of Burke, the police sought to bring charges against Hare for the murder of one of his victims, a character known as Daft Jamie; but it was decided that Hare could not be charged. On his release he also fled the city, and was never seen or heard of again.

As a consequence of this and a number of similar grave-robbing scandals, dissection in Britain remained under something of a cloud. Meanwhile on continental Europe physiological research continued apace. The leading figure of this field in Germany was Johannes Müller, one of the last great physicians, whose expertise spanned the entire spectrum of an increasingly specialized medicine.

Johannes Müller was born in 1801, amidst the German wine-growing region at Koblenz, where his father was a prosperous shoemaker. At school Müller showed exceptional talent and exceptional amibition, the latter in both the theoretical and the practical sense. He appeared to want to know everything, as well as to succeed at everything. He read all that he could lay his hands on, from the ancient Greek philosophers to the poetry of Goethe, and soon became enamoured of the *Naturphilosophie* that was sweeping Germany in the wake of the Romantic movement. Although Müller chose to study medicine, *Naturphilosophie* gave him a mystical belief in the underlying unity of nature which would continue to inform even his most specialized scientific work for the rest of his life. In 1819 he entered the University of Bonn, which had only been founded a year previously and was already established as a centre of *Naturphilosophie*. The school of medicine included believers in 'natural' medicine, quasi-homoeopathists, and even a few who believed in supernatural cures.

Müller qualified at Bonn in 1822, and then travelled to the Prussian capital Berlin, where his medical studies took on a more orthodox scientific tenor. Here Müller found himself studying under the leading anatomist Carl Rudolfi, whose stated aim was to purge medical research of the 'turbid mire of mysticism'. It was Rudolfi who liberated Müller's mind from the futile philosophical speculations which abounded in *Naturphilosophie*. These included arguments about negative and positive 'forces', questions concerning which 'archetypes of nature' various plants and bones derived from, and similar metaphysical enquiries, all in the attempt to see the world in a holistic manner. Although Müller would retain a holistic viewpoint – which would enable him to unite his vast learning – from now on his pursuit of knowledge was carried out in a strictly scientific fashion. Research became a matter for experiment, not speculation.

In 1824 Müller returned to Bonn, where he joined the faculty of medicine and would be appointed professor of physiology at the exceptional age of 24. His large distinguished head, his evident brilliance, and his enthusiasm for his subject gave him a charismatic persona which made him a superb teacher. According to one eyewitness, his presence in the lecture hall 'seemed like that of some warrior of old'. Yet even at this early stage, some could not help remarking on a certain darkness in his character. Such was the man who would prove a formative influence on the ensuing generation of German medical minds. But it is Müller's meticulous, bold and far-reaching research which is best remembered today. It was he who first detected that the blood leaving the embryo was a different colour from that entering it, thus indicating that the embryo respired. His work on glands and their secretions opened up a whole new field of chemical enquiry, as did his examination of tumours. He explained colour sensation in the retina, how sound is propagated by the eardrum, and how the voice originates in the larynx. His wide-ranging scientific knowledge enabled him to advance our understanding of the chemistry which takes place in the human body, and his philosophical inclinations provoked him to psychological discoveries. Though with regard to the latter, he insisted: 'No one can be a psychologist without being a physiologist.'

Unlike many such dominating personalities, Müller did not have the effect of overwhelming his students. His researches opened up so many different fields that he could never have fully developed these all himself. As a result, his students were frequently left aware of further exciting work to be done, possibilities which quickened the minds of his more brilliant students.

By 1832 Rudolfi was a sick man, and the authorities in Berlin needed someone to replace him in his prestigious chair. Never one to underestimate his own abilities, Müller took it upon himself to write to Berlin outlining what precisely was required of a modern professor of physiology, explaining at the same time how he was in fact the only suitable man for the post. After some hesitation, the Prussian authorities were suitably convinced and he got the job. In Berlin, Müller quickly established himself once more as an inspirational teacher, assuring his pupils that he was always willing to entertain original thinking 'so long as we keep to the solid ground of observation and experiment'. Though he no longer regarded *Naturphilosophie* as scientific, he corresponded with Goethe on matters of philosophical and theoretical interest – such as comparative anatomy, and the hunt for the archetypal 'ur-bones' and 'ur-plants' from which all plants and bones were thought to have originated. In the long summer vacations Müller would set off for the North Sea or the Mediterranean in search of palaeontological specimens, and make studies of the comparative anatomy of marine animals.

The Romantic movement had stirred a deep interest in the wonders and varieties of nature, as well as its many unexplained curiosities. This was the era that saw the birth of archaeology, as well as a huge interest in fossils. When Napoleon had invaded Egypt in 1798, he had taken with him scholars of all kinds to study the remains of its ancient civilization, and their findings were at last being published. At the same time the German naturalist and explorer Alexander von Humbolt had undertaken his ground-breaking exploration of the South American jungle, and was now back in Berlin writing up his findings. Müller's far-ranging abilities may have been exceptional, but they were also part of a general awakening of interest in the new discoveries and new knowledge which were sweeping Europe.

In 1840 Müller finally completed the last volume of his masterwork, *The Handbook of Human Physiology*. This superseded the great *Elementa Physiologiae* which had been published by the Swiss anatomist Haller almost a century previously, and it would prove a similar mine of detailed and comprehensive information on human anatomy. It also contained Müller's single most important contribution to medicine, his theory of specific nerve energies – the most radical advance in our understanding of the nervous system since Haller's discovery of 'sensibility'.

By the mid-nineteenth century the importance of the nerves had been understood, but how precisely they functioned had remained obscure, prompting all manner of unfounded speculation. By painstaking dissection Müller managed to show that each nerve, when it is stimulated, can only give rise to one specific sensation. For example, no matter whether the optical nerve is stimulated by heat, electrical or mechanical impulse, it can only transmit the sensation of light. Likewise, by means of a simple experiment with a frog, he was able to show that sensations were relayed from the periphery (e.g. palm of the hand, or other skin surfaces) to the central nervous system by the posterior roots of the spinal nerves. Conversely, the anterior roots transmitted motor impulses outwards (e.g. causing muscles to raise the hand, or withdraw skin surface). This he managed to show by cutting the posterior root to the frog's leg, which left the leg insensible, but not paralysed. When he cut the anterior root, the frog's leg was paralysed but remained sensitive.

The implications of this finding were of the profoundest importance to our existence as human beings. Our philosophical understanding of ourselves, and our psychology, would never be the same again. What Müller had shown was that we in fact had no understanding of any outside world beyond ourselves. The external world, as we knew it, resulted from the perceptions of our particular nerve endings: those in the optic nerve, the skin, and so forth. The human mind did not perceive what was going on in any external world, all it knew was the alterations taking place in its nerve endings.

In any science, including medicine, experimental work will always tend to reductionism. The full richness of reality is reduced to a specfic aspect for the purposes of an experiment. Here was the ultimate reductionism: Müller's theory of specific nerve energies can be seen as the final reduction of the empirical theory first proposed by the philosopher John Locke 150 years previously. If the only utterly reliable truth we can have is from experience, then the only certainty that is available to us is the sensations we experience at our fingertips, on our retina, within our ears, and so forth. We do not experience any outside reality as such.

Needless to say, such implications were of little importance to medicine, though it seems they may have wreaked their effect on the essentially Romantic sensibility of Müller, whose manic-depressive tendency was now becoming more evident. In 1848 Müller was appointed Rector of Berlin University. Unfortunately, this was 'the year of the revolutions', when the people took to the barricades in cities the length and breadth of Europe. Berlin was to be no exception, and the students quickly joined the revolutionaries, demanding social and educational reform. Müller was so deeply immersed in his medicine that he simply could not understand the demands of the students, to whom he had always felt so close. He became terrified that the rioting mob would burn down the university, destroying all its accumulated treasures, not the least of which was its exceptional anatomical collection that he had done so much to build up. When the revolution was finally and savagely suppressed by the Prussian authorities, Müller was plunged into despair. Asking for leave of absence, he set off home to Koblenz with his family. But he was too agitated to settle there, and journeyed on to his old university town of Bonn, which proved no more restful and he set off once more. Finally he reached the end of the road at Ostend, where the winter storms of the North Sea seem to have rekindled his Romantic spirits.

Müller returned to Berlin, but from now on his periodic depressions deepened. After a few years he became gripped by an obsessive fear that medical research was approaching its limits, leaving nothing further to be discovered. Fatigued beyond endurance by his worries, he finally died in his sleep in 1858 at the age of 57, having left strict instructions that there should be no autopsy carried out on his body. This meant that the cause of his death was never discovered, though several of his colleagues were convinced that he had committed suicide by taking an overdose of morphine.

Among Müller's many brilliant students, two are transcendent – Helmholtz and Virchow, both of whom happened to be born in 1821. Hermann von Helmholtz would go on to become the great German physicist of his age, but also made crucial contributions to medicine. Extending the work of Müller, he described how pitch and tone are perceived by the ear, as well as pioneering the measurement of nerve impulses. Müller had found it impossible to detect the passage of electricity in the nerves, and felt sure that such impulses could not be measured. Using frogs, Helmholtz succeeded in measuring the speed of nerve impulses as approximately 20 metres per second, around one tenth of the speed of sound. Much of Helmholtz's research was aided by instruments which he himself invented, and the ophthalmoscope which he developed provided him with 'the great joy of being the first to see a living human retina'.

It was Helmholtz's investigation of the chemical changes in the muscles of frogs which led him to formulate his famous principle of conservation of energy, which would be one of the founding principles of nineteenth-century physics. Helmholtz would also show how vital this principle is to physiology, by demonstrating that energy in the body is obtained from the oxidation of food substances. Like Müller, Helmholtz was also interested in philosophy, publishing a number of papers on the subject. Unfortunately, one of these led to vituperative and impassioned charges of plagiarism from the misanthropic philosopher Schopenhauer. By this stage philosophy in general, and the intellectual influence wielded by German metaphysical philosophers in particular, was becoming something of a nuisance to science. The philosophical implications of Müller's nerve theory could safely be ignored on the grounds of common sense; also Helmholtz had sufficient confidence in his own originality to dismiss Schopenhauer's ravings. Yet when the great mathematician Gauss discovered non-Euclidean geometry during this period, he chose not to publish this finding which would revolutionize both mathematics and science. He simply could not face wasting his time answering the wrath of the likes of Schopenhauer, whose philosophy it fatally undermined. Philosophy, and the 'natural philosophy' to which it had given birth, were now parting company once and for all.

Müller's second great pupil, Virchow, would achieve fame

as the man who transformed pathology. Two centuries previously Morgagni had emphasized the organs in which disease is located, and subsequent pathology had very much concentrated on the appearance of diseases. Virchow's originality was to understand that disease originated in cells. As a result, disease could now be examined afresh on a purely scientific basis.

After studying under Müller, Rudolf Virchow accepted a post at the Charité Hospital in Berlin in 1843 at the age of 22. Here he made such an impression that early in 1848 he was despatched by the Prussian government to Silesia to report on an outbreak of typhus among the Polish mining community. He found that the epidemic was due to the appalling conditions under which the Polish minority were forced to live, and he concluded that this was an 'artificial' disease which could best be cured by 'democracy'. Such a finding would normally have outraged the autocratic Prussian authorities, but they now had other things on their mind with the outbreak of the 1848 revolution in Berlin, which Virchow quickly joined, manning the barricades with his friends. When the authorities finally got round to Virchow's report, and also heard of his activities on the barricades, they were so outraged that Virchow was dismissed from his post and banished from Berlin. Fortunately he managed to obtain a post at the more liberal University of Wurzburg, which was only too pleased to have him as a professor.

Here Virchow studied cell theory. This had originated in botany where it was claimed that plants consisted solely of accumulations of cells – single organizations which were capable of reproducing themselves. Virchow realized that this could also apply to the human body, and formulated his famous principle *omnia cellula e cellula* (every cell comes from a cell). He understood that every cell in the human body is descended from a previous cell. The body itself is originally derived from one previous cell, the fertilized ovum, which in turn is derived from the cells of the parents and by way of them from previous ancestors. Microscopy had long since observed that cells replicated by division of the nucleus. Virchow saw that diseases resulted from abnormal changes in cells, and these abnormal cells then divided and multipled causing the disease to spread.

Müller had undertaken microscopic examinations of malignant tumours, and Virchow was now able to explain these tumours in terms of cellular abnormality. He also recognized that 'pus cells' consisted largely of white blood cells which had leaked from the blood vessels during inflammation. This led him to understand the nature of leukaemia as a mutation taking place in a white cell, which then proliferated by means of uncontrolled divisions, giving rise to a vast excess of white cells in the blood and bone marrow.

The realization that all bodies consisted of cells would transform medicine, and indeed the whole of biology. Here was a blueprint whereby scientific method could be applied to all living substances. The entire scientific endeavour was now entering a new era. It is no accident that around this time chemistry and physics too were discovering a similar scientific foundation, with Dalton's atomic theory which posited that all matter was composed of atoms or combinations of atoms. For Virchow, the atoms of disease were cells.

In 1855 Virchow returned to Berlin where he became professor of medicine, and three years later he published *Cellularpathologie*, which outlined his theory. Despite this great theoretical advance, Virchow always believed: 'Medicine is social.' As a result, he continued with his work in public medicine, which would be responsible for the transformation of the poorer streets of Berlin from 'cauldrons of disease' to more sanitary accommodation. He would always remain politically active, and together with a number of colleagues he formed the Progressive Party. He was soon elected to the Prussian parliament, where his views so outraged the conservatives that Bismarck challenged him to a duel, which he wisely ignored. During his later years Virchow would become one of the founders of the new field of anthropology (literally, 'the study of humanity').

Following the wave of patriotism engendered by the Franco-Prussian war, Germany had become a unified nation in 1871, with Bismarck as its 'Iron Chancellor'. Extreme nationalism now became rife as the new nation began to define itself, asking what it meant to be a German. Anti-slavism (especially against Poles) and anti-Semitism reached epidemic proportions, and many began championing the notion of a 'pure Ayran German race'. In response to this, Virchow conducted an anthropological survey throughout Germany, which discovered that there was in fact no such thing as a pure German race, only a mixture of several different racial types. It is a commonplace that science in itself is ethically neutral, and only the uses to which it is put can be ascribed moral value. Here was a purely scientific finding which appeared to contradict this view. Indeed, the borderline between scientific discovery and moral use has been seen to be increasingly blurred – for instance, in research into nuclear weapons, which may yet result in the destruction of humanity (thus leaving the entire universe morally neutral). On the other hand, the case for a science having a positive moral value in itself would seem most arguable in the instance of medicine.

Virchow would live on into the twentieth century, finally dying in 1902. Although his work was never truly original – even his cellular theory built upon previous botanical and other discoveries – the transformation he wrought in medical thinking has led many to see him as the greatest of all pathologists. Even so, Virchow's cellular theory was far from being the most influential medical idea to appear at this time. With hindsight, it is easy to see behind many of the preceding ideas – Dalton's theory of atoms, Goethe's search for 'ur-bones' and 'ur-plants', Müller's comparative anatomy and study of fossils, and Virchow's understanding of the role of cells – the ghost of one all-embracing unifying idea of nature beginning to emerge. As the nineteenth century progressed, many began to have inklings of evolution, but this idea would only come to full fruition with the advent of Darwin – a botanist and scientific thinker who had no medical training whatsoever, yet whose all-embracing idea would deepen our entire understanding of what medicine is about.

Charles Darwin was born in 1809 at Shrewsbury, amidst the rolling countryside near the Welsh border. Twenty-two years later, by now a somewhat bumbling enthusiast for all things botanical and zoological, he read von Humboldt's account of his travels in South America. Later in the same year he signed on as shipboard naturalist on HMS *Beagle*, which was setting out on a five-year survey that would take it around the globe. Darwin's many archaeological and biological findings along the remote coasts of South America inspired a ferment of ideas, which finally crystallized when the *Beagle* arrived at the tropical Galapagos Islands, in the Pacific Ocean, 700 miles off the coast of Ecuador. Here he found a variety of species, from seawater iguanas to giant tortoises and finches, which had bred for centuries in complete islolation. Most intriguingly, the varieties of finches which lived on the separate islands had each developed differently, their beaks adapting to the requirements of their distinct feeding habits. Those that fed off large seeds had large powerful beaks, those that ate smaller seeds had smaller beaks, and those that fed off insects had fine beaks. Each type of beak appeared suitably adapted. The finches were all different, yet they must all have developed from the same original species.

In 1859 Darwin would publish *The Origin of Species by Means of Natural Selection*, which explained how all plants and all species, every living thing which inhabited the world, had gradually evolved, over millions of years, from the primeval slime, the first primitive life on earth. This process of evolution worked by survival of the fittest: a blind process of adaptation which had resulted in everything from jungles of flora to dinosaurs, from the higher apes to the emergence of *Homo sapiens*. This was certainly the most profound idea which humanity had ever had about the world and our place within the scheme of things. It would affect our entire way of thinking – spiritually, philosophically, and scientifically. In this way, it would also inform medical thought. Our understanding of embryology and anatomy, especially comparative anatomy, would never be the same again. Each limb, each organ, had reinforced, through evolution, that aspect which enabled it better to perform its task. Even the optical and physical complexities of the eye had evolved from the simplicity of particular, light-sensitive cells. Our understanding of life itself would be transformed for ever. Instead of a vast purposeful process, involving a metaphysical guiding hand and an animating spirit somehow beyond our rational understanding, we now realized that we were simply part of a blind and purposeless evolving process that could be studied in entirely scientific terms. And in the words of Roy Porter: 'As with Darwin's vision, the panorama of medicine is an arena of waste, pain, death and imperfect mechanisms – but also remarkable developments.' All further developments in medicine – whether remarkable or wasteful – would take place in the light of Darwin's supreme vision, which remains as true today as it appeared then.

The first comprehensively scientific physiologist of the nine-teenth century was the French experimentalist Claude Bernard. The German physiologist Müller, his only near rival in the field, had still retained a remnant belief in vitalism: ultimately, he believed, there was some kind of 'life force' which animated the human body. Bernard was scornful of such ideas. The human body obeyed the same scientific laws as governed inanimate matter. There was no aspect of living matter which remained beyond such discoverable laws. This view had received a powerful boost in 1828 when the German chemist Friedrich Wöhler conducted an experiment which showed that it was possible to synthesize organic (i.e. living) urea out of ammonium cyanate, a crystalline inorganic (i.e. inanimate) chemical compound. It appeared that 'life' could be created in the laboratory.

Bernard felt certain that the human body could ultimately be explained entirely in terms of physics, chemistry and biology. Yet he was no mere reductionist. It was his genius to under-stand that 'in order to follow step by step and experimentally all of those transformations of materials which the chemists were explaining theoretically [it was necessary] to carry experimentation into the internal environment of the organism.' Bernard was convinced that many of the vital functions which took place within the human body were highly complex. These could not be explained simply by observing its outer perfor-mance, for this would be 'like trying to tell what is taking place inside a house by watching what enters through the door and what leaves by the chimney.' The internal workings of the human body could only be explained by means of experiments on living human beings. Since it was for the most part not possible to experiment on living human beings, it was neces-sary to conduct such experiments upon whichever living animals functioned in a similar way. Bernard was the standard-bearer of systematic scientific vivisection, a topic which was as controversial in his time as it is today, and he would suffer dearly for his advocacy of what he himself readily conceded was an often cruel practice. As he put it: 'The science of life is a superb and dazzling lighted hall which may be reached only by passing through a long and ghastly kitchen.'

Like his German counterpart Müller, Bernard grew up in a wine-growing district, to which he would return in times of distress. He was born in 1813 in the village of Saint-Julien in the midst of the Beaujolais region of eastern France. His father was a vineyard owner who was reduced to poverty during the economic vicissitudes which swept France after the fall of Napoleon, and he was forced to work as a vineyard labourer. During the months when he was not needed in the fields, Bernard's father would educate the local children in his house, and this was how his son Claude received his first schooling. After showing little educational promise, at the age of 18 Claude Bernard was apprenticed to an apothecary in Lyon There is no doubt that Bernard had an interest in chemistry, but his secret ambition was to be a playwright. Two years later, his play *The Rose of the Rhône* was performed in Lyon; after this he set out to seek his fortune in Paris, carrying the rolled up manuscript of his five-act tragedy *Arthur in Brittany* and a letter of introduction to Saint-Marc Girardin, the distinguished Parisian literary critic. Girardin read the manuscript, but advised Bernard to try and obtain some professional qualification in order to support himself. The critic was being kind but realistic; this was a time when the attics of the Left Bank were crammed with penniless artists and poets, a percentage of whom would starve to death during any hard winter.

Having worked as a pharmacist, Bernard decided to study medicine, supporting himself by teaching in a girls' school.

This left him no time for literature, which gradually faded from his life, though he always kept the manuscript of his tragedy. (*Arthur in Brittany* would be published after his death, on the grounds that it showed 'the future qualities of the great investigator'. Despite its occasional purple passages it has its moments of drama, though it must be said that none of its characters reveal any great investigative qualities.)

Once again Bernard proved nothing more than a run-of-the-mill student. It was not until he began serving as an intern at the Hôtel-Dieu, the large historic hospital on the banks of the Seine, that he discovered his second vocation. Here, as part of his duties, he was required to undertake physiological experiments in the hospital laboratories. This not only fired his imagination, but also revealed an unexpected talent for meticulous, ingenious and painstaking research.

Bernard finally graduated as a doctor at the late age of 30, but would never actually practise. He was determined to follow a career in physiological research. This was by no means an easy choice, especially when a year later he failed the exams for a teaching post. On top of this, there was the problem of physiological research itself. Science was now entering a major stage of its development, with physics and chemistry to the fore. The chemistry laboratory had freed itself of tarnishing associations with alchemy a century previously, and was now producing a cornucopia of novelties from original dyeing processes to more efficient explosives. Likewise, physical research was viewed with awed respect following such inventions as the steam engine and the electric generator. Even pharmaceutical and general medical laboratories were viewed with some respect, on account of the new medicines and cures which they produced. However, the physiological research laboratory was another matter altogether. Vivisection was regarded with revulsion, and was widely seen by the public as nothing more than the unnecessary torture of living animals. In Bernard's own words: 'As soon as an experimental physiologist was discovered, he was denounced, became the abomination of the neighbourhood, and was handed over to the police for prosecution.'

In 1844 there was a regrettable incident with a dog, which Bernard had purchased from the stray dog pound and fitted with a small silver tap in order to draw off its pancreatic juices from its stomach. The dog was otherwise in fine condition, and Bernard would let it out into the backyard for exercise. Unfortunately the dog escaped – whereupon all the neighbours' worst suspicions were immediately confirmed, and Bernard was eventually summoned before the outraged local police commissioner. At his side sat the evidence, in the form of the dog, its fitted silver tap protruding from it stomach. When Bernard tried to explain himself the commissioner angrily interrupted him, and it soon became clear to Bernard that owing to a sequence of grotesque mishaps the dog was in fact the commissioner's own missing pet! This was a period in France when people who fell foul of the police could end up rotting on Devil's Island, and in order to defend himself Bernard was forced to resort to all his forsaken dramatic powers. This he did with such eloquence that in the end the commissioner was completely won over to his cause, and assured Bernard of his continuing protection in the name of medical science. (This proved no idle assurance, and during the years to come Bernard made sure that his laboratory always remained within the jurisdiction of his friendly police commissioner.)

However, the initial effect of this incident was to bring Bernard to the brink of despair. He now decided to abandon physiological research and return home to Saint-Julien as a country doctor. When his medical colleagues heard of this, they hatched a scheme to rescue him. The 32-year-old Bernard was persuaded to enter into an arranged marriage with Marie-Françoise Martin, the 26-year-old daughter of a prosperous Parisian physician, who brought with her a dowry of 60,000 francs. Arranged marriages were not unusual during this period in France, and both parties appear to have entered into the arrangement in an amicable fashion, with the result that Bernard soon had two daughters. However, it became clear that each partner had very different expectations of this marriage. Marie-Françoise saw her future as the wife of a distinguished Parisian physician whose practice would bring considerable fortune and social prestige, such as enjoyed by her father. Bernard, on the other hand, finding himself freed from financial restraint, outfitted his laboratory with the finest equipment and threw himself into his physiological researches with renewed vigour. All his waking hours were now devoted to his beloved obsession. Night and day he persisted with his experiments on the animals in his laboratory, and when he returned home he would continue his experiments upon himself. His notebooks from the period record the precise time and details of what he ate, along with the time and acidic or alkaline nature of his excretions.

According to Bernard's biographer J. M. D. Olmsted, Marie-Françoise was of 'narrow intelligence and a limited capacity for sympathy', which left her 'unable to share or understand her husband's intellectual life'. This would appear to be a harsh judgement upon a woman forced to endure a life which was very different from that which she had been led to expect (by her father and his colleagues, if not by Bernard himself). At any rate, Marie-Françoise proved quite capable of her own harsh judgements, and soon became a passionate anti-vivisectionist, making regular charitable contributions to the very people who sought to put her husband out of business. As a result, once again Bernard found himself on the brink of abandoning his career. Yet at the same time he was also on the brink of his most far-reaching discoveries. Fortunately for medicine, he decided to continue with his work, and in consequence our understanding of the human body and its complex mechanisms would be transformed. What had previously been a series of more or less imaginative probings, would now become an informed and comprehensive science.

Arguably the most important of Bernard's countless discoveries was his understanding that the body has its own internal environment. In Bernard's view, physiology was the study of how our organs helped maintain this constant environment, whereas medicine dealt with how this process went wrong. As he put it: 'Medicine is the science of sickness; physiology is the science of life; thus physiology must be the scientific basis of medicine.' Previously, illness had been regarded as a process which tended towards the death of the body. Bernard understood that illness was in fact the body attempting to combat some malfunction, rather than the malfunction itself. Even in everyday healthy life, the body fought to maintain its control over its internal environment in the face of external influences. When the temperature in the external environment rose, the body balanced this by sweating to cool itself, thus maintaining its constant internal temperature. Similarly, when external oxygen was reduced, the respiratory system panted and gasped to draw in more oxygen quickly. Other complex physiological processes were responsible for changing the balance of sugar or salt in the blood.

Until now, the body had been seen as containing a collection of organs, each with its own specific purpose. The nature of this purpose had usually been evident from its position and structure. For example, the liver's position between the heart and the stomach indicated its role in the digestive process. But

Bernard was able to show that certain organs, such as the glands, secreted substances which affected other parts of the body. Some secreted hormones into the blood, thus regulating the behaviour of other organs, whilst yet others secreted sweat onto the surface of the skin to cool it.

Botanists already knew that plants could synthesize complex substances. Yet it was thought that in the case of animals and humans the opposite took place. The digestion of fats, sugars and proteins involved breaking these complex substances down into their more simple constituents. Bernard conducted an experiment which entirely altered this view. When an animal was fed sugar, glucose (a simple form of sugar) could be found in the portal vein leading from the digestive system to the liver, and then in the hepatic vein which carried blood from the liver into the circulatory system. From this it was easy to conclude that the sugar passed through the liver. However, when the animal was fed a sugarless diet, Bernard noticed a vital difference. Naturally, the portal vein into the liver contained no sugar; yet the hepatic vein leading out from the liver did contain sugar. Further investigation revealed that the liver itself contained sugar: the liver was capable of producing sugar, and evidently did so when the body was deprived. Bernard named this and similar gland-ular processes 'internal secretion'.

Further experiments led Bernard to a deeper understanding of digestion. His method of observation and experiment is best revealed in his own words:

One day, rabbits were brought in from the market to my laboratory. They were put upon the table where they urinated, and I happened to observe that their urine was clear and acid. This fact struck me, because rabbits, which are herbivores, generally have turbid and alkaline urine; while on the other hand carnivores have clear and acid urine. These observations of

acid in the rabbits' urine gave me an idea that these animals must
be in the nutritional state of carnivores. I assumed that they had
not eaten for a long time, and that they had been transformed by
fasting into veritable carnivorous animals, living on their own
blood. Nothing was easier than to verify this preconceived idea
or hypothesis by experiment. I gave the rabbits grass to eat; and a
few hours later their urine became turbid and alkaline.

Ensuing experiments led to a deeper understanding of the
entire digestive process, especially that part played by the
pancreas. Two hundred years perviously, the microscopist
Leeuwenhoek's mentor Regnier de Graaf had been the first
to collect pancreatic juice from a living animal. In doing so, he
had discovered that pancreatic juice was acidic, and had
concluded that this acid took part in the chemical process
of digestion, separating the nutritional elements from the
ingested food. Bernard found that this was far from being
the whole story. He conducted a series of experiments on a dog
using a silver tap, such as he had fitted into the stomach of the
police commissioner's dog. By this means he was able to show
that pancreatic juice secreted into the stomach in the course of
gastric digestion acted as an emulsifying agent on the fatty
foods passing through it. These foods were split into fatty acids
and glycerin, and at the same time the pancreatic juice also
converted starch in the food into sugar. But the action of
pancreatic juice was not the entire digestive process, as de
Graaf had supposed; indeed, as Bernard put it: 'Gastric digestion [in the stomach] is only a preparatory act.'

In this case, and many others, Bernard was able to demonstrate that the body and its functions were a great deal more
subtle and complex than had previously been supposed. There
was no possibility that physiology was approaching the end of
its researches into the human body, on the point of a final

understanding of all its workings, as Müller had feared in his paranoid final years. Such fears would intermittently beset several branches of science during the coming years of the nineteenth century, when knowledge was being accumulated at a hitherto unprecedented rate. The most striking example of this recurrent scientific phenomenon would be physics at the end of the century, when it was widely believed that all major discoveries in this field had now been accomplished and only 'mopping up' research needed to be done. Indeed, the young Max Planck would be advised against entering physics because 'there was nothing left to discover'. Several years later his discovery of quantum theory, along with Einstein's theory of relativity, would reveal an entirely new layer of hitherto unsuspected complexity in physics, posing fundamental questions many of which remain unanswered to this day. Bernard's work on 'internal secretion' brought to light an unrealized complexity within the human body, a network of balance and self-control which none had suspected. This would form the basis of an entirely new medical specialization, which would become known as endocrinology (which incorporates the Greek for Bernard's term 'internal secretion').

Bernard was to make other formative discoveries concerning how the body balanced its internal environment. Fundamental amongst these was his understanding of how nerves, controlled by the vasomotor centre in the brain stem, regulate the internal width of the blood vessels to control the flow of the blood. His painstaking experimental work would also detect how the red blood cells transported oxygen through the body. This latter finding was confirmed by his work on the poisonous gas carbon monoxide (CO), which readily absorbs oxygen (O_2) to become carbon dioxide (CO_2).

$$2CO + O_2 = 2CO_2$$

When carbon monoxide entered the blood stream through the lungs it immediately began to strip the red blood cells of their life-giving supply of oxygen.

Bernard's experiments with drugs and poisons would pave the way for pharmacological advances. Previously it had been thought that the effects of drugs permeated the whole body, but Bernard's careful experiments showed that many drugs only affected specific parts of the body. In particular he worked with curare, an alkaline poison used by the South American Indians on the tips of their arrows, which immediately paralysed their prey. Bernard showed that curare managed this by preventing impulses from nerve endings reaching the muscular fibres. He at once saw the value of this, but realized that medical research still had some way to go before such a drug could be used safely and effectively. Curare would in time be used for a variety of medical purposes – such as overcoming the muscular spasms caused by tetanus, and inducing complete muscular relaxation throughout the body during major operations (while breathing is maintained artificially).

In 1860 Bernard suffered a serious nervous breakdown, induced by the pressures of overwork and marital conflict. He retired to a house he had bought back home in Saint-Julien, and sought recovery in the rural peace of the vineyards. His estranged wife, together with the daughters she had alienated from him, stayed behind in Paris. Bernard would remain in Saint-Julien for over two years; yet even here he could not stop working altogether. He began planning a book which would justify his work and reveal to the world the benefits of physiological research. This would eventually be published in 1865 as *An Introduction to the Study of Experimental Medicine*, a work of rare style filled with philosophic insight into medical practice. It is studded with pithy remarks ('Observation shows, experiment teaches', 'Conjectural medicine must necessarily precede exact medicine'), psychological reflections ('Men with excessive faith in their own ideas are ill-prepared for making discoveries'), and justifications ('Without the comparative study of animals, practical medicine can never achieve a scientific character').

Although his work had by now been recognized, and he held prestigous chairs at both the Sorbonne and the Collège de France, he would continually be forced to defend his method of work. Vivisection remained as reviled as ever. At one point even the faculty members of the Collège de France launched a campaign against it. Bernard contemptuously dismissed this as 'Don Quixotery'. Darwin too had initially harboured misgivings, writing of vivisection: 'It is a subject which makes me sick with horror.' Though later he would change his mind: 'Physiology cannot possibly progress except by means of experiments on living animals, and I feel the deepest conviction that he who retards the progress of physiology commits a crime against mankind.'

Bernard's wife Marie-Françoise finally obtained a divorce in 1870, but by then he had spent all of her dowry on his researches. He would be heaped with honours, and his distinguished appearance on the streets of Paris would cause heads to turn. But the years of struggle had taken their toll. A friend from his youth who encountered Bernard found that although he had achieved 'everything which the ambition of the savant could wish for . . . he was weighed down . . . by serious bodily ailments and by the saddest of domestic misfortunes . . . pleasant and kindly, as of old, but grey-haired, with his head inclined on one side.' Bernard died at the age of 65 in 1878. Revered throughout France, he was given the honour of a state funeral – the first to be accorded anyone but statesmen and military leaders.

Another contemporary who suffered for his medical beliefs would not be so fortunate. The Hungarian-born German Ignaz Semmelweis would make just one major discovery, and its effect would eventually transform the hospitals of the world, saving innumerable lives; though his advocacy of this discovery would be the ruin of his career, and almost certaintly cost him his life.

In 1847 Semmelweis was working as a teaching assistant at the maternity clinic in the Vienna General Hospital, which was at the time the largest clinic of its kind in the world. Yet, like such clinics all over Europe it was beset by an appalling mortality rate. Puerperal fever (which attacked women after they had given birth) had reached epidemic proportions, and even some of the finest European clinics occasionally reported mortality rates of over 50 per cent. The fever was accompanied by a puzzling range of symptoms, which could vary from skin eruptions filled with pus to peritonitis (resulting in serious abdominal swelling), from highly malodorous vaginal discharges to pleuritis (damaging the lungs and bringing severe breathing difficulties). It was always extremely painful, and few survived its onslaught for long. Such was the variety of symptoms that some considered 'puerperal fever' to be no more than a blanket term for a number of similar post-natal diseases.

The Vienna General Hospital had two large maternity sections. The first was used for training medical students in obstetrics, while the second was used for training midwives. Semmelweis was surprised to note that whereas the mortality rate in the first section was was 13 per cent (sometimes rising to 30 per cent), the rate in the second section remained at around 2 per cent. There were a number of myths accounting for this discrepancy. The women who came to give birth in the Vienna General were for the most part poor single mothers and prostitutes, who had nowhere else to turn. For such people, death was regarded as a punishment by God. The lower mortality rate in the midwives' section was put down to the fact that the patients felt less humiliated when they were treated by women. Pregnant women entering the clinic would tearfully plead to be allowed into the midwives' section, which even had certain feminine touches such as a few jars containing flowers. It was also kept marginally cleaner than the medical students' section – though cleanliness was not a major concern in the maternity clinic. Vienna was by now a rapidly expanding commercial city, with a proliferation of factory suburbs where the slum districts housing the poor were notoriously filthy, as were the people who inhabited them. It was felt that there was little point in having clean hospitals to tend for such people, who invariably brought in their own dirt.

Semmelweis would conduct autopsies on the puerperal fever victims, and he soon became convinced that this was in fact a single disease despite its varying symptoms. Around this time his colleague Jakob Kolletschka, who was professor of forensics (criminal medical investigation), died after cutting his finger during a post-mortem examination of a cadaver. The consequent autopsy revealed that Kolletschka had what appeared to be the symptoms of puerperal fever. Yet how could this have happened? Kolletschka had no contact whatsoever with the maternity clinic. In Semmelweis's words: 'Day and night the image of Kolletschka's illness pursued me. As we found identical changes in his body and those of the childbed women, it can be concluded that Kolletschka died of the same disease.' Yet Semmelweis remained unable to provide an explanation for this.

Some time later, Semmelweis noticed that the medical students entering their section of the maternity clinic often came directly from their practical anatomy classes, which included post-mortem dissection and the actual handling of diseased organs. When they were finished with their dissection classes, their hands would frequently be wet with blood or pus, yet all they did was douse them under a tap and wipe them on their aprons. Many did not even bother to do that. The cadaver smell on a student's hands was regarded as a mark of distinction. This distinguished the future physicians in the students' maternity section from those who were merely studying obstetrics.

Semmelweis drew a simple conclusion. The students from the anatomy labs came into the maternity clinic bringing 'invisible cadaver particles'. These were what had infected the cut in Kolletschka's finger, and these were what infected the post-natal patients with puerperal fever. Immediately after birth the uterus was in a raw condition similar to an extensive wound, and could easily become infected by any decomposing organic material. A conducive environment for the foetus was transformed into a conducive environment for infection.

Semmelweis issued orders that from now on before entering the maternity clinic all students should wash and scrub their hands in a chlorine solution until the cadaver smell had been entirely eliminated. The results were immediate and spectacular. In the following month the mortality rate in the medical students' section of the maternity clinic fell to just 2 per cent, the same as in the midwives' section.

Yet Semmelweis was hardly prepared for the reaction which followed. The students were indignantly opposed to having to wash their hands. Semmelweis's immediately superior Professor Johann Klein was even more opposed to the measures, which he considered to be an underhand criticism of his running of the maternity clinic. And it soon became clear that the women patients too were opposed to it: they saw such measures as implying that they were dirty. Even Semmelweis himself was far from pleased at what he had discovered. As he wrote dejectedly, 'God only knows the number of women I consigned prematurely to the grave.' He felt himself to be little better than a murderer.

Semmelweis found himself becoming increasingly unpopular at the Vienna General Hospital; and when his post came up for renewal, Klein refused to reappoint him. Several colleagues were sympatheric towards Semmelweis, and obtained work for him elsewehere. In the close-knit professional world of Viennese medicine this was not easy, and in going against the powerful Klein they were jeopardizing their own careers. Suddenly Semmelweis decided that he had put up with enough, and without telling anyone he simply packed up and caught the train home for Budapest. This precipitate action succeeded in alienating him from his few remaining friends.

Back in Budapest Semmelweis eventually obtained a post in the medical department at St Rochus, a large city hospital. This post was unpaid, but he gradually managed to build up a fairly lucrative private practice. He soon implemented his new hygienic methods in the maternity clinic, and here too the high death rate in the wards diminished spectacularly. But even when Semmelweis published a paper on his discovery some years later in a Hungarian medical journal, he continued to be ignored. No one outside Hungary read Hungarian medical journals.

In time, Semmelweis would become professor of obstetrics at the University of Pest (across the Danube from the twin municipality of Buda). Despite such professional recognition in his home country, he was becoming increasingly frustrated by the reception of his great idea abroad. Plagued alternately by his guilt at having earlier been responsible for so many deaths, and by his defiance in the face of international neglect of his ideas, he began to show signs of emotional instability.

Finally he decided to set matters right once and for all by writing a book about his discovery. The first half of the book was devoted to a painstaking elaboration of his discovery, backed by page after page of the supporting statistics which he had gathered over the years. The second half of the book was devoted to a vituperative case by case rebuttal of the many criticisms which had been levelled against him and his discovery. In the course of this, he spared none of his critics. One leading international figure was informed that before writing on medicine he 'should first attend at least one semester in logic'. He even attacked the Society of Obstetricians in Berlin, ridiculing the great Virchow, insisting that medical students in Budapest 'would laugh [him] to scorn if he attempted to lecture them on epidemic puerperal fever'. When Semmelweis published *Etiology, Understanding and Prevention of Childbed Fever* in 1861 it was initially ignored in Vienna. A few reviews appeared in Germany, and most of these were unfavourable. Other senior figures in obstetrics came to the same conclusion as Professor Klein: Semmelweis's so-called 'discovery' was nothing more than an unwarranted attack on the way they ran their hospitals.

The reception of Semmelweis's book all but unhinged him. He began to suffer extreme mood swings, fluctuating between periods of apathetic despair and spasms of dancing rage. He gave vent to his feelings in writing, and the leading medical figures who had criticized his book were soon receiving letters filled with violent abuse: 'your teaching is founded on the dead bodies of women murdered through ignorance'; 'I denounce you before God and the world as an assassin . . . a medical Nero'; 'This murder must cease.' In the middle of 1865 Semmelweis started showing signs of clinical derangement. His wife and a friend managed to persuade him to accompany them to Vienna, where he entered a mental hospital. Two weeks later he was dead, aged just 47. Ironically, his death was said to have been caused by sepsis resulting from a wound in his finger, with the same tell-tale symptoms as his colleague Kolletschka, the professor of forensics. It appeared that he had died from the very infection he had fought so hard to allay.

This canard would remain intact for over a century, until in 1977 the Hungarian physician and writer Georg Sillò-Seidl discovered documents describing the events leading up to Semmelweis's death. These events too should perhaps have involved a professor of forensics. It appears that Semmelweis only left Budapest with his wife and friend because he thought they were taking him to Gräfenberg, a spa in southern Germany where he could recuperate by taking the water treatment. When the train stopped in Vienna he was tricked by his friend into leaving the train. His friend said that he wished to show Semmelweis the hospital where he was working, and drove him to an imposing building. Unbeknown to Semmelweis this was the large public insane asylum on Lazarettgasse, which all agree 'was certainly not among Vienna's best'. As soon as Semmelweis entered the building, he was overpowered and forcibly committed. The document outlining the reasons for his enforced commital was signed by three doctors, not one of whom had psychiatric training (one was a surgeon, another a paediatrician, the third a local internist). Unfortunately Sillò-Seidl rather undercut his claims by turning this material into a book which was 'intended for a popular audience and reads like a spy novel'. He also came to the 'lurid conclusions' that Semmelweis 'was murdered through a conspiracy between his in-laws and several prominent Hungarian physicians'. Not until nearly twenty years later would a more balanced account appear in an article by K. Codell Carter and other American scholars. Its findings would be hardly less sensational. 'The autopsy revealed major injuries that could only have been sustained in beatings to which Semmelweis had been subjected while in the asylum.' They quote an investigator: 'It is obvious that these horrific injuries were the consequence of brutal beating, tying down, trampling underfoot,' and they conclude, 'it seems most likely that Semmelweis was severely beaten by the asylum guards and then left essentially untreated.' K. Codell Carter and his colleagues mention that Semmelweis's funeral was attended by just a handful of former colleagues from the Vienna General Hospital, adding 'Apparently not one family member, not one in-law, not one colleague from the University of Pest was in attendance. Semmelweis's wife later explained her own absence on the grounds that after her husband had been committed she had become so ill that she had been confined to her bed for six weeks.'

After Semmelweis's death, his diagnosis of puerperal fever would soon be overtaken by radical new medical discoveries. Ironically, it was only then that the hygienic precautions he suggested would eventually become accepted by medical authorities throughout the world, thus saving the lives of countless women. At present the major maternity hospital in Vienna is called Semmelweis Klinic, and Budapest has a large prominent public statue in honour of the man who became known posthumously as 'the saviour of mothers'.

11

ELIMINATING THE
SURGEON'S ENEMY

At the same time as Semmelweis was campaigning against needless death, another scourge of hospitals was also being confronted – needless pain. Anaesthetics had been used during operations since ancient times. As early as the fourth century BC Aristotle described how pressing a finger against the carotid artery in the neck caused a patient to become unconscious. This prevented blood from reaching the brain, though Aristotle was probably not aware of this. Around 500 years later the Greek physician Dioscorides, a predecessor of Galen in Rome during the time of Nero, prescribed drugs such as henbane or mandrake root marinated in wine as anaesthetics. Indeed, it was Dioscorides who first used the word anaesthetic – which comes from the Greek meaning 'lack of sensation' – in the medical sense we use it today. Drugs extracted from hemlock, henbane and mandrake root continued to be used well into the medieval era. Various sources confirm that soporific sponges soaked with drugs were employed in the hospital of the celebrated medical school at Salerno in the thirteenth century. However, a recent experiment involving the precise ingredients known to have been used to prepare these sponges has shown that they produced no anaesthetic effect upon animals. It is thus possible that these so-called 'soporific sponges' were in fact an early form of placebo. But this must have been the exception. Truly soporific agents were well known enough for Shakespeare's lovesick Cleopatra to demand,

> Give me to drink mandragora [mandrake] . . .
> That I might sleep out this great gap of time
> My Anthony is away.

Until well into the Enlightenment anaesthesia remained a largely haphazard business, often involving ill-administered opium or over-administered alcohol. This usually had the effect of making the patient easier to restrain, rather than giving any great relief from pain. As a result, the quality of a surgeon was often judged by the speed with which he operated, rather than any notion of finesse. The boast of Napoleon's chief military surgeon Jean Larry was that he could perform any amputation in under a minute. He also claimed that at the Battle of Borodino he amputated 'in the first 24 hours about 200' – a gruesome feat which bespeaks the skill of a lumber-jack more than a surgeon.

Even in civilian hospitals, the operating theatre held a particular horror. When the London Hospital was built in 1791 it became the model for hospitals all over Europe and America; yet its layout was to a large extent dictated by the lack of any dependable anaesthetic method. The operating theatre was placed on the top floor, where the skylight brightly illuminated the operating table. But this was not the main reason for its location. When operations were to be performed, a bell would be rung summoning all the staff to the upper floor of the building. The heavy doors at the top of the stairs would be firmly closed, and the staff would then begin the noisy, violent and exhausting business of restraining the patients being operated upon, relieving each other in teams. The screams of the patients on the top floor would be muffled from the lower floors by the heavy doors. Even so, the abandoned patients on the floors below would be aware of the distant screams, and many would take this opportunity to escape from the hospital, for fear that they would soon be enduring the same terrifying experience.

Surgery was heavily hampered by the lack of any dependable anaesthetic, and each surgeon had his own preference. The greatest French surgeon of the early nineteenth century Guillaume Dupuytrien was said to anaesthetize his upper-class female patients by making a 'brutal remark' which sent them into a faint. Dupuytrien, the son of a peasant from Limousin in central France, developed such exceptional surgical skills that he became a millionaire, with a Parisian practice of some 10,000 patients. His pioneer work included the first excision of a lower jaw, as well as innovations in plastic surgery to replace scars and disfigurements. A character of some eccentricity, he operated wearing a cloth cap and carpet slippers, conducting his operations as consummate high-handed performances with little regard for either the patient or his assistants. He brooked neither competition nor contradiction. This prima donna trait would become more noticeable in surgeons as their status underwent the long and gradual transformation from despised barber-surgeons to revered maestros of the operating theatre. Observing the beginnings of this trend in the surgeons and anatomists of Dupuytrien's time, the contemporary Scottish physician William Hunter perceptively observed that 'the passive submission of dead bodies, their common objects, may render them less able to bear contradiction.'

For patients it was another matter altogether. There was still widespread objection to anaesthetics on religious grounds, especially during childbirth. Pain was a visitation from God, and any interference with this was sacrilege. Operations without anaesthetic were an unimaginable agony, which the novelist Fanny Burney evokes with chilling detail in her description of a mastectomy (breast amputation) she endured without anaesthetic in 1810. The following brief quotation will suffice:

> I saw the glitter of polished steel – I closed my eyes . . . when the dreadful steel was plunged into the breast – cutting through veins – arteries – flesh – nerves – I needed no injunctions not to restrain my cries. I began a scream that lasted unintermittingly [sic] during the whole time of the incision . . . so excruciating was the agony . . . the air that suddenly rushed into those delicate parts felt like a mass of minute but sharp & forked poniards [daggers], that were tearing the edges of the wound, – but when again I felt the instrument – describing a curve – cutting against the grain, if I may so say, while the flesh resisted in a manner so forcible as to oppose & tire the hand of the operator, who was forced to change from the right to the left – then, indeed, I thought I must have expired . . .

The discovery of a viable anaesthetic reads like a tale out of Edgar Allen Poe. Perhaps it is no coincidence that Poe himself lived out his tragic life at the same time on the same eastern seaboard of America as the flawed characters who emerged from the fringes of medicine to live out their own tale of mystery and imagination. Yet their fated quest for immortality would result in one of medicine's most significant achievements.

During the early decades of the ninteenth century various European poets and bohemians began experimenting with nitrous oxide, giving it the name 'laughing gas' on account of the feelings of hilarity it provoked. This eventually spread across the Atlantic, where a craze for 'laughing gas parties' soon caught on in America. Early in 1842 a physician called Crawford Long, who lived in the remote small town of Jefferson in Georgia, was approached by a group of young landowners' sons, who asked if he would prepare them some nitrous oxide for a laughing gas party. An indication of the contemporary attitude towards laughing gas, and its prevalence, can be seen in the fact that Long found nothing exceptional in this request.

Crawford Long had been born in 1815, the son of a well-off Georgia merchant who owned an extensive amount of property. He appears to have been an exceptional pupil in an exceptional class at Franklin College in Athens, Georgia. He graduated at the age of 14 from a class which included no less than two future Confederate generals, one state governor, two senators, a secretary of the treasury and three celebrated scientists (of which Long would be one). He then gained his medical degree at the Poetically named Transylvania University in Virginia, and later undertook some ground-breaking research at the University of Pennsylvania. This might have received wider attention, but for the fact that his professor was a stickler for detail, insisting upon the need for extensive back-up research before any original paper could be submitted for publication. For him, rushing into print was a vainglorious pursuit fraught with danger, and in medicine this could well cost lives. Long absorbed this lesson, before leaving to take up general practice in Jefferson, a town of just 400 population amidst the southern countryside some 40 miles northeast of Atlanta. Although Long's family owned land near Jefferson, and Long himself was naturally modest, it remains a mystery why such a highly talented man should choose to bury himself in the depths of Georgia. Even so, he soon established a thriving practice, and was much in demand throughout surrounding districts.

When the local landowners' sons approached the 26-year-old Long, asking him to prepare some laughing gas for a party, Long replied that they would be better off trying ether instead, because it had much better effects. Evidently Long's days as a medical student had not all been devoted to arduous study. Long's friends gladly accepted ether instead of nitrous oxide, and Long himself even participated in a few of their 'ether frolics'. Taking the ether was simple: the drug was poured onto a handkerchief, which was held under the nose and inhaled – until the taker fell back unconscious, his hand falling away at the same time, thus ensuring that he received no overdose. Usually Long found that this produced a blissful stupor, but occasionally he would thresh about under the influence of the drug, to such an extent that he often suffered considerable bruising next day. It was then that Long came to a profound realization. Whilst he was inflicting these bruises upon himself he had experienced no sensation of pain.

Some time later Long found himself dealing with a troublesome young patient named James N. Venables, who kept making appointments for the removal of two cysts from his neck, and then not turning up because he was afraid of the pain this operation would involve. Long recalled the numbing effect of ether, and finally persuaded Venables to let him try a new painless method of operating. On 30 March 1842 Venables inhaled deeply over an ether-soaked towel, became unconscious, and Long removed the two cysts. Venables experienced nothing. When he woke up, he was so oblivious to what had happened that Long needed to show him the two cysts he had removed in order to convince him that the operation had taken place!

In keeping with the views of his professor, Long decided not to rush into print with his findings. Instead, he continued using this method sparingly over the next few years, extending its use to amputations and then obstetrics. Each time his original finding was confirmed: the patient experienced no pain during the operation. Long had discovered modern surgical anaesthesia; he had found a method for both overcoming pain and at the same time rendering the patient unconscious, so that a surgeon could operate unhindered. The trouble was, this discovery remained unknown outside the remote Georgia region of his practice.

Meanwhile the laughing gas craze continued in America. An enterprising huckster named Gardner Colton even began demonstrating its properties at fairs. 'Professor' Colton, a self-proclaimed 'travelling lecturer in chemistry', would invite a volunteer on to the stage and ask him to breathe in some nitrous oxide. The crowd would then laugh and jeer as the hapless volunteer reeled drunkenly about the stage, laughing uproariously as he banged into things. In 1844 'Professor' Colton's act reached Hartford, Connecticut, where it made a deep impression upon Horace Wells, a local dentist. Wells was a handsome 29-year-old farmer's son who had previously been a schoolteacher; but his hypersensitive temperament had ill-equipped him for this task and he had resigned his post with the intention of becoming a church minister. Then, on the spur of the moment, he decided instead to become a dentist. He attended the Harvard School of Dentistry and graduated with honours, becoming a lecturer and writing learned articles on dentistry. Highly impressionable and unstable in temperament, he soon abandoned his academic career to pursue various short-lived ventures. For a while he bought art works in France for sale in America, and when this failed he set up as a manufacturer of portable baths. After the failure of this, and several other ambitious schemes, he ended up as a dentist in Hartford, where he was viewed as a somewhat volatile character prone to rash decisions.

Inspired by the fairground performance of 'Professor' Colton, Wells decided to try out nitrous oxide for himself. He had Colton render him unconscious with nitrous oxide, while a colleague extracted one of his teeth. The operation was a painless success, and on coming round Wells exclaimed that the world was about to embark upon 'a new era of tooth-pulling'. He soon moved to Boston and went into partnership with a friend called William Green Morton, who had in fact been one of his students at Harvard. Wells assembled a 'laughing gas apparatus' consisting of a bellows and a tube with a wooden mouthpiece, which was placed in the patient's mouth. Convinced that his apparatus would be perceived as a major breakthrough, he arranged for a public demonstration before the assembled doctors and students in the surgical amphitheatre at the Massachusetts General Hospital. A highly suspicious and frightened young patient was led into the amphitheatre, and anaesthetized with nitrous oxide; then a resident dentist proceeded to extract a tooth. Unfortunately, the supply of nitrous oxide proved insufficient, the young boy awoke, and immediately began shrieking with terror. The assembled doctors and students were outraged, and Wells was dismissed in ignominy.

This incident proved traumatic for Wells, whose sensitive temperament never fully recovered from his public humiliation. However, to begin with this was not fully apparent. Wells dissolved his partnership with Morton, and left Boston under a cloud. He then set up practice in New York, still using his laughing gas apparatus. This time he learned from experience, and increased the supply of nitrous oxide, performing scores of successful operations. Each patient readily agreed to give Wells a signed testimonial confirming the success of his operation, but by now the damage had been done. No one in the medical or dental profession was willing to believe Wells' claims. Showing increasing signs of manic depression, Wells began taking nitrous oxide to console himself. He was soon exhibiting symptoms of hopeless addiction.

When Wells had left Boston, his partner William Green Morton had decided to return to Harvard and study for a full medical degree. During the course of his studies, Morton married and soon had a son. This reduced him to poverty, whereupon he was forced to abandon his medical studies without a degree and return to dentistry. Fortunately his professor at Harvard, the eccentric and brilliant Charles T. Jackson, took pity on him and allowed Morton and his family to stay in his house. It was now that Morton conceived of the idea of making a fortune from nitrous oxide. He had learned of its properties from Wells, and like Wells he still believed in its efficacy. But he regarded Wells as a bungler, who had missed his chance for ever by antagonizing the medical profession. Morton set about conceiving his own plan for achieving lasting fame with nitrous oxide, which he confided to Jackson, his benefactor, who listened with interest.

Jackson was another oddity, in this cast of odd characters. A multifaceted and intensely competitive man with a somewhat paranoid temperament, he appears with some justification to have regarded himself as a genius who had been thwarted in his several bids for world recognition. By this stage Jackson had already achieved a measure of renown, and notoriety, in several fields. On a trip across the Atlantic in 1832 he had become involved in a smoking room discussion about electricity. One of his fellow passengers asked him whether a small pulse of electricity would transmit along a wire for any great distance, and Jackson assured him that it would. This passenger was Samuel Morse, who then went on to develop this idea and invent the electric telegraph, which he patented. When Jackson heard of this, he immediately claimed the invention was his idea. In the ensuing court case, it was agreed that Morse had used Jackson's idea, but that Jackson had no claim because he did not develop his idea and 'had failed to realize its commercial value'.

Two years later Jackson's competitive nature landed him in further trouble, when he learned of a unique patient who had been placed in the charge of a local military doctor by the surgeon general. The patient was a 19-year-old Canadian trapper who had suffered a serious gunshot wound in the stomach. This had healed leaving a fistula, a permanent hole into his stomach wide enough to admit a finger. The hole had to be plugged with a wad of lint to prevent food spilling out, but it provided a unique opportunity to study the human digestive process first-hand. Jackson realized that if he could somehow gain possession of this patient he could make discoveries about the human disgestive process which would earn him a place in medical history. Secretly taking matters into his own hands, Jackson hid the Canadian trapper, and then sent a petition to Congress asking for him to be removed from the care of a mere military doctor and placed under his own sole jurisdiction. This petition evidently came to the notice of the surgeon general, who was so enraged that Congress threw out the petition forthwith.

Such was the man to whom William Green Morton confided his belief that he had discovered the first modern anaesthetic in the form of nitrous oxide. After listening to the excited ideas of his impecunious lodger Morton, Jackson suggested a modification: instead of nitrous oxide, he should try ether. Astonishingly, there is evidence that four years previously, in 1842, Jackson had travelled through Jefferson, Georgia, and had heard about Crawford Long's pioneer anaesthetic method. Much like his knowledge of electric pulses passing along a wire, Jackson had not realized the significance of Long's discovery.

Morton decided to proceed with caution, and tested Jackson's ether suggestion – first on his son's goldfish, then on a hen, and finally on his pet spaniel. All proved successful, and in September 1846 he anaesthetized a patient with ether and extracted a tooth. After several further successful operations, and some fine-tuning of his anaesthetic equipment, Morton approached the Massachusetts General Hospital and was given an opportunity to demonstrate his new discovery. Mindful of Wells' earlier debacle, he assured the medical authorities: 'Gentlemen, this is no humbug.' In the course of the demonstration a patient had a tumour removed from his neck, and next day a woman had a tumour successfully removed from her arm under anaesthetic. The surgeons of the Massachusetts General Hospital concluded that Morton's demonstration had been an unmitigated success, and endorsed his claim to have discovered an effective modern anaesthetic, which both rendered the patient unconscious and insensible to pain.

Morton now found himself faced with a problem. Having endorsed his anaesthetic, the Massachusetts surgeons demanded to know the secret of his method. If he told them that it was just ether, then everyone would soon be using it, and he would reap no benefit. Morton consulted Jackson, who suggested mixing the ether with some aromatic oils to disguise its smell, and naming it Letheon (after the legendary ancient

Greek river Lethe, through which the dead passed on their way to the underworld, whose waters erased all memory of their earthly life). Morton then applied for a patent on Letheon. But this was the opportunity which Jackson had been waiting for, and he immediately contested Morton's application, claiming that he was the co-inventor of Letheon. On legal advice, Morton was reluctantly forced to include Jackson as his co-inventor.

News of this great discovery soon swept around the world. Surgery would be revolutionized, and all manner of daring new operations would now be possible. In recognition of the gift to humanity of Letheon, the French Academy awarded a prize of 5,000 francs to its joint discoverers. But Morton refused to accept his share, still convinced that he was the sole discoverer and as such should be awarded the entire prize.

It was now that Morton's erstwhile partner, the disgraced Wells, emerged from his obscurity in New York, to launch a claim of his own, insisting that *he* was in fact the discoverer of the first anaesthetic. There followed an unseemly uproar of litigation and counter-litigation, which even ended up before the Senate, where it became known as the 'Gas War'. While Wells, Jackson and Morton continued their bitter dispute over priority, the original discoverer of the first modern anaesthetic refused to join in the fray. Crawford Long continued going about his general practice amidst the Georgia countryside, administering his anaesthetic when necessary, and carefully recording its effect.

All three of the protagonists in the Gas War would come to a bitter end. In the tradition of Poe, it was as if each claim placed a curse upon the claimant. While pressing the courts for recognition of his priority, the nitrous oxide addicted Wells continued as a dental anaesthetist in New York, exhibiting increasingly severe symptoms of manic depression. From taking nitrous oxide, he moved on to taking chloroform, becoming more addicted and more erratic in his behaviour. In 1848, just two years after lodging his initial claim, he attacked two prostitutes with sulphuric acid and was jailed. From his cell he wrote, 'I feel I am fast becoming a deranged man.' He then inhaled a large dose of chloroform and slashed himself to death with a razor.

Morton would fare little better. Although the secret of Letheon was quickly exposed, Morton persisted in his legal battle to establish his priority as the inventor of the first anaesthetic, and with it a generous grant which had been promised by the government in recognition of this feat. The expense of Morton's legal battles soon plunged him into debt. Beset by increasing monetary and emotional problems, he retired to a smallholding in the country, where he descended into abject misery. In the end some supporters took pity on him, and began raising a testimonial subscription for 'the founder of anaesthesia'. When Jackson got wind of this, he immediately contested Morton's claim to the title, threatening to scupper the entire subscription. Meanwhile, Morton travelled to New York. He first read of Jackson's threat in a newspaper while travelling through Central Park in a carriage. Whereupon he became so enraged that he suffered a fit of apoplexy, from which he died.

Jackson's life too would be cursed. The continuing litigation in which he had involved himself had only served to increase his tendency to paranoia. This had become evident as early as 1846, when he had first contested Morton's sole claim to the patent. In that same year the German chemist Christian Schönbein announced his invention of gun cotton, an early form of explosive. When Jackson heard of this, he immediately claimed that he had invented gun cotton several years earlier – another claim which was not upheld by the courts.

In 1852 Crawford Long was finally persuaded to publish a paper describing the use of ether as an anaesthetic, and many now recognized that he was the true claimant to priority. Eventually the Senate became so tired of the Gas War that its members suggested Jackson should visit Long, and they should settle the matter between themselves. In 1854 Jackson duly travelled south to Georgia to meet Long in Athens, where he now resided. According to all reports this meeting passed without incident. Long behaved like a southern gentleman, duly deferring to the older and more forceful Jackson. However, it soon became apparent that amidst all this courteous hospitality nothing had actually been resolved.

Despite this, Jackson returned from his meeting with Long convinced that victory was his. Yet by now all these trials and tribulations had begun to render Jackson's mental state increasingly unstable. For years he alternated between fits of paranoia and long bouts of deceptively calm depression. Eventually in 1873, exhausted and deranged, Jackson was confined to a lunatic asylum in Somerville, Massachusetts, where he died seven years later.

After the secret of Letheon had been exposed, ether had quickly begun to be used as an anaesthetic in hospitals throughout Europe and the Americas. In England, a newspaper headline announced: 'Hail Happy Hour! We Have Conquered Pain!' Even so, anaesthesia still encountered widespread opposition on religious grounds. Popular feeling remained largely unconvinced, especially concerning the use of anaesthetics during childbirth. According to the Bible, God had decreed that our entry into this life must be accompanied by pain. More serious objections arose from medical opponents of ether. It was found that this could damage the lungs, and occasionally caused vomiting, which during an operation could have fatal consequences.

In 1847, while searching for an alternative anaesthetic, the Scottish professor of surgery Sir James Simpson inadvertently discovered a substitute in the form of chloroform, which proved both safer and more powerful. He reported his findings to his colleague John Snow, one of the physicians to Queen Victoria. In 1853 Snow successfully administered chloroform to the Queen during the birth of Prince Leopold. When it was reported in *The Times* that Queen Victoria had received chlorofom, public opinion immediately began turning in favour of anaesthetics.

The age of anaesthesia had arrived. Yet even today the administering of anaesthetics remains at best a quasi-scientific enterprise. It is still not fully understood how anaesthetics work, which is why the patient's heartbeat, breathing and so forth, are carefully monitored throughout any operation.

12

THE PIONEER WOMEN

During the same decade, another major transformation in medicine would also be initiated by a remarkable woman, this time one of Queen Victoria's subjects. The woman was Florence Nightingale, who was a prime mover in the establishment of modern nursing. Prior to the nineteenth century nursing had not been a profession, and its practitioners had largely been female members of Catholic religious orders or ill-educated helpers who looked after hospital wards. The latter were often of dubious moral character and frequently drunk – hardly a surprise, when one considers the state of the wards. Prior to its rebuilding in the late eighteenth century, the wards of the Hôtel-Dieu in Paris were described as having: 'six unhappy patients heaped in a bed, annoying and frightening one another, infecting one another, and one throwing himself about and shrieking when the others had need of repose.' Only when the wards opened for the day would the dead be removed from the beds, or from the floor if they had been ejected. Even as late as the 1850s such conditions were not exceptional.

The first school for nurses was established at Kaiserswerth on the River Rhine in Germany in 1836. It was run by the local Protestant pastor Theodore Fliedner and his wife Frederike. Here local young women were trained as 'deaconesses'. They were given lessons by a physician, instructed in pharmacy, and unlike Catholic nuns they were allowed to marry. This was the school which was attended in 1850 by the 30-year-old Florence Nightingale, when she had finally managed to break away from the stifling influence of her upper-class Victorian family. Nightingale found that the school was run with 'no luxury, but cleanliness' and contained 'only peasants – none were gentlewomen'. The latter was not intended as a disparaging remark: in the years to come it would inform her choice of 'those best suited to nursing'. Despite being so favourably impressed by Kaiserswerth, Nightingale only lasted there two months, largely because she found herself unable to submit to the discipline enforced in the school.

Far from being the selfless heroine of popular legend, Nightingale was a psychologically complex woman: a conflicting mixture of egoism and compassion, wilfulness and vulnerability. She was an early exemplar for female emancipation, and she had the foresight to recognize this, often alluding to 'the deep feeling I have for the miserable position of educated women in England (or rather half-educated)'. Nightingale was born in 1820, while her family were on the grand tour in Florence (hence her first name). She was educated at home by her father, an intelligent but otherwise idle man who had inherited a fortune. In the course of this intense but suffocating education she learned five languages, as well as philosophy, the scriptures, mathematics and history. Despite this, she quickly recognized that no matter how much she learned, like other women in her class she remained not educated but 'rather half-educated'. She was beset by a powerful but inarticulate feeling of unfulfilment; she wanted to do something, to live a life of her own. At the age of 17 she had a religious experience in which God informed her that she had a mission. The precise nature of this mission remained obscure, but she continued to chafe: 'There is so much misery in the world which we ought to be curing instead of living in luxury.' In the course of her continuing studies, she came across the contemporary Belgian mathematician Adolphe Quetelet, whose work was revolutionizing statistics and probability theory. According to Quetelet, statistics was the key to understanding society: the causes and effects of public behaviour, including health, could not only be monitored but also predicted by this method. Then at the age of 30 Nightingale finally managed to break away from her family and register at Kaiserswerth for a course in nursing. On her return she secured, through social connections, an appointment as live-in superintendent at the Institute for the Care of Sick Gentlewomen in London.

Her great opportunity arose in 1854 with the outbreak of the Crimean War, in which British, French and Turkish armies confronted the Russians on the northern Black Sea coast. The British expeditionary force was accompanied by the first accredited war correspondent, William Russell of *The Times*, who would sit on his shooting stick on a hillside above the battle, peering down through his opera glasses as he took notes – it was from this vantage point that he would coin the phrase 'the thin red line' to describe the British army formation in battle. Russell was outraged to discover the appalling muddle and chaos behind the lines, reporting: 'It is with feelings of surprise and anger that the public will learn that no sufficient preparations have been made for the care of the wounded. Not only are there not sufficient surgeons . . . not only are there no dressers and nurses . . . there is not even linen to make bandages.' Russell's reports provoked an outrage in Britain, and Nightingale immediately petitioned her social connections: she wanted to take out a party of nurses to tend the wounded. Many in the military were implacably opposed to such an unprecendented move, but Nightingale's principal contact happened to be the Secretary for War, and on 21 October 1854 she and her 38 nurses set sail. Two weeks later she disembarked at Scutari on the Asiatic shore of the Bosphoros in Turkey.

The conditions which greeted Nightingale and her nurses at the military hospital in Scutari were horrific. Almost 2,000 soldiers lay wounded, sick and dying amidst stinking rat-infested wards. The very day after her arrival, the Battle of Inkerman was fought in a thick freezing mist, resulting in such anarchy and slaughter that no one knew what was happening. Many of those who survived recounted tales of their glorious and fantastic exploits, confident that no one could contradict them – the reason why in Britain there there are pubs ironically named 'The Hero of Inkerman'. Those less fortunate were shipped on the 400-mile sea journey south across the Black Sea to the hospital at Scutari, which was soon overflowing. According to Nightingale's biographer Hugh Small, drawing on centemporary descriptions of these survivors: 'Many of them were starved and frost-bitten, so that it seemed a miracle that they were alive at all. Their limbs were blackened and mortified; some had lost their hands and feet to frostbite and their bones protruded from their disintegrating extremities. Long-untended wounds were infested with maggots.' Nightingale and her 38 nurses did their best, though she had to start from scratch. As she wrote, in a letter back to England: 'I am a kind of general dealer in socks, shirts, knives and forks, wooden spoons, tin baths, tables and forms, cabbages and carrots, operating tables, towels and soup.' In the midst of all this, she found herself pestered by government commissioners, who told her that her first priority should be to clear the clogged foul-smelling sewer-drains beneath the building, scrub out the filthy wards and get the place properly ventilated. Nightingale dismissed these commissioners as interfering busybodies: there were far more important things than sanitation. Men were dying, at an alarming rate.

During the first winter, Nightingale and her nurses had to deal with 12,000 soldiers, of whom 5,000 died. So many arrived at Scutari beyond hope of recovery that many considered it surprising the figures were not worse. Not until the following summer did the government commisioners manage to convert Nightingale to the cause of sanitation, whereupon she and her team set to work with a will. A few months later the death rate in the wards at Scutari was reduced from 40 per cent to 2 per cent. Meanwhile, Nightingale continued to rule her team with a firm hand. Except in emergencies, no nurses were permitted in the wards after dark – to avoid any temptation or even hint of impropriety. Nightingale alone would tour the wards with her lamp, comforting and giving succour to the suffering. It was these men who gave her the name 'The Lady of the Lamp'.

But soon Nightingale was travelling further afield to the Crimea itself, busying herself with the welfare of the British soldiers, transferring nurses to the hospitals behind the front lines, becoming ill herself with 'Crimean Fever'. Not all welcomed her efforts, but by now reports were beginning to reach England about the 'The Lady of the Lamp'.

When Nightingale returned to England in 1856, she was acclaimed as a national hero. She had a private meeting with

Queen Victoria, and assisted with a Royal Commission which was appointed to look into the performance of the British Army's medical services in the Crimean War. But all was not as it seemed with Florence Nightingale. In the midst of this, she suffered a serious nervous breakdown – from which she would never fully recover. This was certainly in part due to the illness and exhaustion of her Crimean experience; but it seems that the largest contributory factor was guilt. This was due to her belated realization that far from being a saviour she had in fact been the opposite. Her obstinacy in opposing the hygiene suggestions of the government commissioners had been responsible for the deaths of many thousands of soldiers during the winter of 1854. The facts uncovered by the Royal Commission spoke for themselves. Death rates had been high in all hospitals; but they had been much higher at Scutari. The arriving soldiers had been in such a pitiful condition that no one had expected any of them to survive – as a result the appalling death rate had been accepted as inevitable.

The Royal Commission would recommend the establishment of the Royal Army Medical Corps, but its other findings were buried in a typical government cover-up. The public remained unaware of the facts, and The Lady of the Lamp's reputation remained unscathed – except in her own eyes. In 1857 Nightingale took to her bed, where she stayed for the remaining 53 years of her life. Her frail physical condition appears to have been largely psychosomatic. Yet incredibly, her mind remained as alert, forceful and manipulative as ever. Using her invalid status to her own advantage, she sought interviews with the highest in the land. Ministers, and even the prime minister, came humbly to her bedside to listen to her proposals.

At the height of her fame, after her return from the Crimea, a Nightingale Fund had been established. This had attracted huge popular support. The celebrated opera singer Jenny Lind – 'the Swedish Nightingale' – had given a charity performance, with all takings donated to the Nightingale Fund; and Queen Victoria had gone so far as to donate one of her royal jewels. In the end the fund had attracted a massive £45,000, which Nightingale now used to found the Nightingale School of Nursing at St Thomas's Hospital in London. This was the first nursing school attached to a general hospital, and would be the model for future nursing schools. Nightingale also produced *Notes for Nursing*, which would become a standard text for the teaching of nurses. Nightingale insisted that nursing was more than just 'the administration of medicines and the application of poultices'; she placed great emphasis upon the 'proper use of fresh air, light, warmth, cleanliness, quiet and the proper selection and administration of diet'. Among her great achievements was to have learned from her own horrendous mistakes. Another of her achievements was the introduction of statistics into nursing. Even in the Crimea, Nightingale had found time to put into practice the statistical ideas she had learnt from Quetelet. She had gathered statistics concerning her patients, thus enabling her to follow the fluctuations of disease and recovery. During the course of this work she had even gone so far as to invent the pie chart. Despite such pioneering achievements, she would in later life be denied a professorship at Oxford. Nightingale did not always get her own way, and many wished to limit her achievements to the more acceptable female field of nursing.

One of the first tasks of Nightingale's school for nurses was to produce 'training matrons', who could run teams of nurses. Ever the independent woman, Nightingale astutely understood that trained female nurses in a hospital should remain under the control of a female matron, rather than the male medical staff – a control structure which remains largely in position to this day. As a result of Nightingale's efforts, hospital nursing in Britain became transformed from a degraded occupation for slatterns and social unfortunates into an honourable vocation aspired to by a wide social class of women. Nightingale's training matrons were soon spreading the word, as nursing schools were established throughout Britain and the British Empire. By the 1870s there were also nursing schools in Sweden, Denmark and the United States – though in Catholic countries the profession remained in the hands of the religious orders. The spread of the nursing profession would also play a leading role in the proliferation of the Red Cross, which Durrant had founded in 1864.

However, no history of modern nursing could be complete without the larger-than-life figure of Mary Seacole, whose legend even came to rival that of Florence Nightingale. Mary Seacole was born Mary Grant in 1805 at Kingston in Jamaica, the daughter of a Scottish soldier. Her mother Jane was of mixed race, ran a boarding house for visiting British army officers and their families, and was also an 'admirable doctress', specializing in Caribbean herbal remedies. Such alternative medicine was in some demand amongst the white colonial community, which was liable to be in the care of a young visiting doctor who had no previous experience of tropical disease. Not surprisingly, local remedies passed on by word-of-mouth were sometimes more efficacious than the leeches and powders prescribed by more orthodox medicine. Mary's mother Jane achieved more than a little respect as a 'doctress' amongst the white colonial community, and much of her knowledge she would pass on to her daughter.

Little is known of Mary's early life, though she seems to have visited England twice. At the age of 31 she married Edwin Horatio Seacole, a godson of Lord Nelson. Nine years later she had what she described as her 'first great trouble' when Seacole died. She now travelled to Panama, where she ran a boarding house with her brother. In such a climate, running a boarding house often involved looking after guests suffering from cholera or yellow fever, and Mary Seacole gained considerable nursing experience in this way. But she also gained a reputation as 'Aunty Seacole', a convivial host dressed in extravagant and colourful clothing who served excellent champagne at 12 shillings a bottle in her hotel bar. Despite this, she maintained strict order on her premises: drunkenness was not tolerated, and offenders were liable to be sharply dismissed. Of her character, her biographer Jane Robinson writes: 'her greatest qualities were her warmth and spontaneity, and her most precious possession was her own idiosyncrasy. All her life people responded to her instinctively, and rarely analysed her motivation or her rationale . . . Mary was a true eccentric, relying entirely on herself to make the decisions that shaped her life.'

In 1849 many Americans began passing through Panama on their way to the California Gold Rush, and at one stage Mary Seacole considered joining them. But she was soon put off this idea. Because of her coloured face, Americans regarded her as a slave. Mary had not encountered such naked prejudice in Jamaica, or in Panama, where the local blacks were free to hold municipal office the same as anyone else.

When the Crimean War broke out in 1854, Mary Seacole embarked for England, where she volunteered to join Florence Nightingale's group of nurses, but was turned down. Seacole was now 51, but she refused to be put off, and travelled at her own expense to the Crimea. Here she joined forces with a distant relative of her husband, and opened the 'British Hotel'. This acted as a rest home for officers from the front, and also housed an officers' club which served good meals as well as being well stocked with whisky and champagne. Always independent, Mary Seacole now began travelling on her own initiative the few miles up the road to the front. On her regular missions she would take two mules, one bringing much-needed medical supplies, the other carrying food and wine. Her activities at the front were similarly even-handed. She tended casualties, nursing the sick and diseased as best she could. On the other hand, on the day following the Battle of Chernaya she organized 'a capital lunch' for an inter-regimental cricket match. At the British Hotel she had a bet with some officers that she would be the first woman into Sebastopol when it fell, and duly won her bet, leading a mule train into the burning city just hours after it had fallen. This and similar exploits gained the dark-skinned indefatigable figure of 'Aunty Seacole' legendary status amongst the troops. Her actual nursing is said to have been as effective as possible under the circumstances, despite retaining its unorthodox herbal elements.

Back in Scutari, some 300 miles from the front, Florence Nightingale was not amused by reports of her rival. Jealousy certainly played a part here, but there was concern too at Seacole's unorthodox methods. The prim Nighingale was also suspicious of the fact that Seacole ran a hotel rather than a hospital, and indeed supected that Seacole's establishment might be offering something more than empty beds. Despite the rumours, this was not the case: beneath her eccentric mannerisms Seacole is said to have retained a Victorian attitude to morality.

Seacole was in many ways all that Nightingale was not. By now stout and middle-aged, she was a raucous character who dressed herself 'like a gypsy at a fair'. She was also undeniably part black, though she herself preferred to ignore this – and expected others to follow suit. Despite her idiosyncratic command of English, she was not above a certain snobbery. This appears to have been her way of forestalling both sexual and colour prejudice.

In 1856 Mary Seacole returned to England, left penniless by officers who had run up bills at her hotel. Sympathetic friends encouraged her to write her memoirs. When these were published, under the title *Wonderful Adventures of Mrs Seacole*, they quickly became a huge success, and Mary toured the country giving talks. Friends in high places organized a Seacole Fund, with the Prince of Wales as its patron, and Seacole gained the status of a national treasure. She survived in some style until the age of 76, when she died of 'apoplexy'. Seacole's achievement, as a woman and as a black, was in being a pioneer. Unlike the well-connected Nightingale, she left no permanent nursing legacy; but as we shall see, those who came after her would often begin in the Seacole manner. She had shown that it was possible to do something as an individual, despite all manner of prejudice. Pioneer nursing would owe a great deal to such individuals.

By now, modern nursing was becoming established further afield. Even before Nightingale's disciples crossed the Atlantic, local nursing traditions were being established in America. Two remarkable women would play leading roles here. Of these, the most influential was Dorothea Dix, who is today best remembered for her campaigning on behalf of better treatment for the insane. Dorothea Dix was born in 1802 at the pioneer settlement of Hampden in Massachusetts. Her family were poor and fanatically religious; in her own words, 'I never knew childhood.' By the age of 14 she was teaching. Just over a decade later she had risen to become headmistress of a girls' school in Boston. She also had literary aspirations, writing sentimental poems, hymns and children's stories. At the age of 32 she suffered a nervous and physical collapse – a consequence of ill-health and weak physique, as well as thwarted and repressed aspirations.

In 1841 Dix visited a jail to teach Sunday school. Some of

the women prisoners complained about the treatment of the insane inmates, whereupon Dix discovered to her horror that they were kept in squalid cells in an underground cellar. This stirred her to action, and she was soon uncovering even worse conditions. Near Providence, Rhode Island, she discovered an insane man locked in a cell 'six to eight feet square, built entirely of stone and entered through two iron doors, excluding both light and fresh air . . . The internal surface of the walls was covered with a thick frost . . . the only bed was a small sacking stuffed with straw [its] outside covering was completely saturated with drippings from the walls and stiffly frozen.' Elsewhere insane prisoners were frequently kept in chains, in permanent darkness, goaded by foul-mouthed warders, even used as grotesque entertainment. Worse still, some of the confined women were sane, committed to asylums by jealous husbands or authoritarian families.

Dix now devoted all her considerable energies to campaign for the establishment of proper insane asylums, completely separate from prisons. This took her to England where her message so inspired Queen Victoria that she ordered a Royal Commission on the matter. Dix then toured Europe, even travelling as far as Constantinople (modern Istanbul). As a result of her campaigning, there would be an 'era of awakening' with regard to the incarceration of the insane – in Europe as well as in America. One direct result of her work was that no less than 32 new asylums for the insane would be founded in America.

Dix was now a public figure, and at the outbreak of the American Civil War in 1861 she was appointed Superintendent of War Nurses. She immediately set about establishing a nursing corps for the treatment of the wounded. This proved no simple task, as female family members of the fighting men, and other less worthy female volunteers, frequently offering their services, infiltrated the front, to the extent that many military commanders banned all women from the war zones. Dix used her persuasive powers, and began recruiting nurses with precise qualifications 'very plain-looking women . . . no curls, no jewelry, and no hoop skirts'. Although later, as the demand increased, she reluctantly allowed good-looking women to train as nurses.

The American Civil War would also produce its own Florence Nightingale, in the form of Clara Barton, 'The Angel of the Battlefield'. Her war exploits would become the stuff of legends, though they were in fact very real accomplishments with no mythical exaggeration. A slight figure, only five feet tall, with a head of thick brown hair and blazing brown eyes, Barton was an exceptional combination of extreme courage and extreme sensitivity. Incapable of taking orders, she was also often incapable of ordering her own existence. She would frequently drive herself beyond endurance, both physical and mental, as if she did not know how to stop until she collapsed. These traits would both make her and break her.

Born in 1802 in Oxford, Massachusetts, Clara Barton was the only daughter of a local politician and his fiery-tempered wife 13 years his junior. Home life was volatile, but Clara would remember for ever her father's stories of life in the army. He had fought in the Indian Wars under the command of General 'Mad' Anthony Wayne, and delighted in passing on to her all the survival skills he had learned. As a result, when she finally arrived in the war she said that she found herself more at home than most of the combatants.

But all this lay in the future. Barton took practically the only way out for a woman of the time, and became a schoolteacher. Overwork brought on the first of the nervous breakdowns which would continue to dog her throughout her life. After recuperating in Washington, she obtained a clerical post in the government. One of only a few female government employees, she suffered from extreme chauvinist harassment. This came to an end when the new Democrat administration took office in 1857 – whereupon all female government employees were dismissed. When the Republicans came to power in 1861, she was reinstated.

On the outbreak of the Civil War, Barton was determined to take an active part. She quickly saw her opportunity. Noting the appalling lack of supplies, she obtained passes which enabled her to travel along the main military routes encouraging civilian contributions to the passing forces. In between times she spent the ensuing years of the conflict 'anywhere between the bullet and the hospital' as she so graphically put it. She would see action at many major conflicts, including Antietam, Fredericksburg and Fort Wagner. In the course of these battles, she assisted army surgeons under appalling conditions during makeshift operations, on one occasion even improvizing dressings with corn leaves when the bandages ran out. After battles she would be found moving among the wounded, her long dresses hitched up, her face blotched blue with gunpowder, doling out soup, cutting bullets from their flesh (as her father had taught her), holding the hands of the fatally wounded as they groaned and cried their last. On one occasion she almost drowned crossing a river, when her blood-soaked dress became waterlogged, its sheer weight dragging her slight figure downstream. Such were her exploits that the chief surgeon himself dubbed her 'the angel of the battlefield', rating her contribution even greater than that of General McClellan.

Throughout the war Barton operated as an independent; she avoided joining Dix's nursing corps. Temperamentally averse to receiving commands, military or otherwise, she relied upon personal contacts. Never at any time did she receive any payment nor was she given any official post. As a result, when the war was over she was left penniless. In order to earn money, she was persuaded to embark upon a lecture tour, telling dramatic tales of her exploits. The strain of this tour, which she had embarked upon reluctantly, brought on another nervous collapse. But by this stage she had earned so much that she would remain without financial worries for the remaining 47 years of her life.

As soon as Barton heard about the founding of the Red Cross, she travelled to Switzerland to join the organization, taking an active role in its work in Europe. During this period she also made contact with Florence Nightingale. On her return home to the United States, Barton finally managed in 1881 to establish an American branch of the Red Cross – despite considerable opposition. At the time, the US was against getting involved in such international European organizations, for fear of becoming dragged into conflicts which it felt were none of its concern. In 1884 Barton was responsible for the famous 'American Amendment' to the Geneva Convention, which permitted the Red Cross to operate outside wartime in undeclared conflicts, as well as in all kinds of emergencies and humanitarian disasters.

Based in Washington, Barton also worked strongly for the Woman's Suffrage movement and campaigned on behalf of disenfranchised blacks. Unfortunately, her involvement with the Red Cross came to a sad end. Her unwillingness to delegate her authority meant that by the end of the century the American branch of the Red Cross was descending into administrative and financial chaos. In 1904, at the age of 83, she was finally forced to resign. Typically, she at once made plans for a trip to Mexico City, with the intention of reorganizing the Mexican Red Cross, only being dissuaded from this when her bags were already packed. She spent her last years at Glen

Echo outside Washington, where she died at the age of 91 in 1912.

By now the first women were also beginning to penetrate the all-male preserve of the medical profession itself. The obstacles placed in their way were formidable, and the male logic used to buttress these defied all argument. Women who concentrated on intellectual pursuits deprived their womb of energy, leading to hysteria and fainting fits. Young women were not psychologically adapted to thinking, which rendered them sterile. Unlike men, their capacity for rational thought was limited, being dominated by their ovaries, and so on . . .

The first woman to become a doctor in the modern era was the Prussian doctor's daughter Dorothea Erxleben-Leporin, who qualified in 1754. Not surprisingly, she was a remarkable woman. Her father, a firm believer in educational reform and the spread of the Enlightenment, began passing on his medical skills to his daughter when she was still a teenager. In 1740, at the age of 25, she sent a petition to the Prussian king Frederick the Great, asking to be allowed to attend the medical course at the University of Halle. This was granted, but she eventually gave up her studies to marry a local clergyman, who already had four children from a previous marriage. She then had five children of her own. Even so, she still found time to write a book called *Rational Thoughts on Education of the Female Sex*, which was published in 1849. With the outbreak of the Prussian–Silesian War, her father left the country and she took over his practice. Other doctors in the neighbourhood began to regard this as a threat, and caused her to be charged with quackery, a serious offence at the time. To overcome this, she submitted her doctoral thesis and was examined by the university authorities at Halle, who granted her a medical degree at the age of 39.

Another exceptional forerunner was the Italian Maria Dalle

Donne, who obtained a medical degree at the age of 23 in 1799. Three years later she came to the notice of Napoleon, who appointed her professor of obstetrics at the University of Bologna. She taught midwifery in her own home, thus allowing her also to reach students who could not afford the university fees. In this way she ensured that a network of qualified midwives was established in the local villages.

But these were the exceptions who proved the rule. They had no immediate followers. Even more exceptional, in many senses of the word, was the woman who was probably born Miranda Stuart in 1795. Her childhood remains a secret which she carried with her to the grave, though she may well have been of Scottish aristocratic lineage. Adopting the enveloping name of James Miranda Stuart Barry, she disguised herself as a man and joined the army as a hospital assistant at the age of 18, qualifying as an assistant surgeon two years later. In 1816 she was posted to the Cape of Good Hope colony, at the tip of southern Africa, which was then something of a wild, frontier settlement on the fringes of the empire. Here her independent and wilful manner soon attracted attention; but this attitude was tempered by a genuine compassion for her patients, and her exceptionally humane treatment of the most unfortunate among them – which included prostitutes, sailors with venereal disease and black slaves. Yet it was undoubtedly her appearance which attracted most attention. A contemporary report remembered her as

> the most skilful of physicians and the most wayward of men; in appearance a beardless lad, with an unmistakably Scotch type of countenance, reddish hair and high cheek-bones. There was a certain effeminacy in his manner which he was always striving to overcome. His style of conversation was greatly superior to that one usually heard at a mess-table in those days.

Barry went to great lengths to establish her manliness, becoming a skilled marksman and convivial raconteur. On one occasion she is said to have made love to a fellow officer's Dutch girl-friend. As a result, Barry was challenged to a duel, in which she contrived to receive a superficial wound, thus satisfying her fellow officer's honour. She later confessed that she had not really loved the girl.

However, her feelings for the governor of the Cape colony, Lord Charles Somerset, were another matter. Somerset was an attractive and distinguished aristocrat, a contradictory character who exhibited both the assured superiority of his class and determinedly enlightened ideals, especially towards the colony's black slaves whose emancipation he sought. One of Dr Barry's duties was to act as personal physician to the governor, which entitled her to an apartment in the governor's residence. In an early demonstration of her medical acumen, Barry managed to save the governor's life, when he appeared to be dying of cholera. Contradicting the opinion of her superiors, who had already sent to England for the governor's replacement, she used all her considerable medical skills in nursing him back to health.

It was probably during this episode that Barry fell in love with Somerset. Disregarding his wife, it seems that Somerset also fell in love with Barry, and was probably the only person during her lifetime to have had certain knowledge of her secret (though there would be a few who suspected it). All the indications are that James Miranda Barry and Lord Charles Somerset embarked upon an intense love affair. Somerset even gave Barry a small dog called 'Psyche'. (In Greek mythology, Psyche is the beloved of Eros, or Cupid (love), and also means 'soul' – the name was almost certainly a private joke between the two lovers.) Lady Elizabeth Somerset was aghast, and gossip about the governor's suspected homosexual entanglement with his personal physician quickly spread through the colony, and thence to London. A bishop presented a petition to parliament on the matter, and a royal commission was set up to look into this scandalous state of affairs. The commission travelled out to the Cape, and eventually exonerated Barry; yet by now Somerset had returned to England.

The rest of Dr Barry's career was a story of success and promotion, punctuated by occasional incidents of flamboyant insubordination which never quite sabotaged her rise. She served in many parts of the British Empire, including the West Indies, Canada and the Mediterranean. In all these postings she demonstrated great surgical skill and instituted a range of medical reforms. Her insistence upon the highest standards of cleanliness in the hospitals under her command certainly saved countless lives. For the first time, colonial military hospitals were no longer places where you were taken simply to die (especially in the tropics). Her treatment of incurable tropical diseases and leprosy was seen as both humane and understanding. Pioneers of medicine have often been such unsung heroes, especially in the public sphere. One instance of Barry's far-reaching, but unacknowledged influence will have to suffice.

By the outbreak of the Crimean War, Barry had risen to the rank of Inspector-General. She immediately volunteered her services, but was ordered to remain at her post in charge of the hospital at the Greek island of Corfu (then under British rule). War casualties were soon being shipped from the Black Sea, around the Peloponnese to Corfu. Despite this voyage of well over a thousand miles, the recovery rate of the soldiers treated by Barry and her team speaks volumes for her abilities. Out of the initial 462 sick and wounded who arrived, only 17 died. When Barry got wind of the appalling death rate at Scutari, where Florence Nightingale had taken over, she characteris-

tically flouted orders. Going on 'leave', she boarded a ship for
Scutari, where she saw for herself the atrocious and unhygienic
conditions of Nightingale's hospital. This resulted in a decisive
encounter between Nightingale and Barry, when Barry rode
into Nightingale's hospital. During their meeting, Barry remained on his high horse (in every sense). Standing beneath
Barry, Nightingale was forced to endure what she always
remembered as the worst 'scolding' she received in her life.
It is more than likely that this 'scolding' by Barry played a
decisive role in helping to change her mind on the fundamental
need for hygiene.

When Barry eventually retired she returned to England,
where she lived a bachelor existence, attended by her West
Indian manservant 'Black John' and her dog Psyche (the last of
a long line to be given this name). By now she was the senior
Inspector-General on the British Army List. Only when she
died at the age of 70 in 1865 was her secret revealed by the
autopsy. Even 'Black John' had not known the truth. The
revelation caused huge public interest in prudish Victorian
society, to such an extent that Charles Dickens published an
account of her life in his popular journal *All the Year Round.*

In her own way, Barry too inevitably proved an isolated
case. But by now the all-male preserve had been breached. The
first woman to establish a genuine tradition of women in the
medical profession was Elizabeth Blackwell, who graduated in
America in 1859. Blackwell had been born at Bristol in
England in 1821. Her father, a prosperous sugar refiner
and believer in reform, would prove a decisive influence.
Yet when Elizabeth was just eleven her father was ruined after
his business was destroyed by fire, and the family emigrated to
the United States.

Upon leaving school Elizabeth Blackwell became a teacher
in Charleston, North Carolina, studying medicine privately in

her spare time. This was a curious choice, for Blackwell claimed that she had despised everything to do with the body since she had been a child. So why did she choose medicine? Apparently to dissuade a persistent suitor, and also to register her outrage over the unequal treatment of women. She certainly encountered the latter, for her persistent efforts to gain entry into a medical school were turned down again and again (at one stage she was turned down by all four schools in Philadelphia). Blackwell began casting her net further afield, applying to the Geneva Medical School in upstate New York, which finally decided to accept her – though ironically this decision did not reflect well on any involved in it. The authorities had fallen out with the students, and in a gesture to heal the breach they delegated the decision concerning Blackwell's entry to the students. With the intention of getting back at the authorities, the all-male student body voted for Blackwell's acceptance 'as a practical joke'. Fortunately, Blackwell took it seriously – but she had to pay for this. Shunned within the school community (and particularly by the doctors' wives), she was also ostracized socially in town, where it was reckoned that she must be either 'mad or bad'. Blackwell's views on the human body must have mellowed somewhat, for she was now spurred on by the belief that women were more suited to be doctors than men, on account of their 'superior healing powers'. At any rate, she finished top of her class.

After this, Blackwell returned briefly to England for further training. She wanted to be a surgeon; but when she contracted ophthalmia, which led to blindness in one eye, she was forced to abandon this idea. She now returned to America and set up practice in New York, but met with little success. During this period she met Marie Zakerzewska (pronounced Zak-shef-ska), a recent immigrant from Germany. Zakerzewska's father was descended from Polish minor aristocracy and her mother from a distinguished medical family of gypsy origin. She had qualified in midwifery at Berlin in 1851 at the age of 22, and a few years later she was appointed professor of midwifery – but this was blocked on account of her age, her sex, and academic jealousy. In disgust, she emigrated to the United States, where she was fortunate to encounter Blackwell. As a result of Blackwell's encouragement and peristence Zakerzewska was accepted to study medicine at the Western Reserve College in Cleveland, where she graduated in 1856. She then joined Blackwell, and together they established, in a tenement district, the New York Infirmary for Women and Children, the first ever hospital run entirely for women by women. The first few women doctors were now beginning to qualify in the United States, though the battle was by no means won. Harvard continued to stand by its declaration that it would admit 'no women or Negroes' to avoid devaluing its degrees. Not until after World War II would Harvard and Yale medical schools open their doors to women.

In 1869 Blackwell crossed the Atlantic back to England, where six years later she established the London School of Medicine for Women. The first British woman to qualify as a doctor in Britain had begun the long and devious journey to full recognition just a decade previously. This was the woman now remembered as Elizabeth Garrett Anderson, who had been born in 1836 in Whitechapel, one of the poorest districts of London's East End. Her father was a pawnbroker, whose business flourished to such an extent that young Elizabeth was sent to a private 'boarding school for ladies' across the Thames in salubrious Blackheath. On leaving, Anderson became interested in the women's movement, which was then in its infancy. She now encountered the newly qualified Dr Elizabeth Blackwell, during her first short return journey to England. Inspired by Blackwell, she decided to become a doctor. This led to trouble at home, where her father was outraged at this 'disgusting' idea, and her mother wept at the family 'disgrace'. Undeterred, Anderson began her determined and ingenious struggle to overcome all obstacles. In 1865 she obtained a diploma from the Society of Apothecaries, which technically allowed her to enrol on the medical register, even though she was not qualified as a doctor. She then took a medical degree at the University of Paris in 1870 – thus becoming both a doctor and a member of the medical register. She then enrolled at the British Medical Association, allowing her to set up in practice. The BMA would later claim that her enrolment was due to 'a bureaucratic error', because it did not officially admit women, but nothing could now be done about this.

In Europe, the University of Paris had opened its doors to women medical students in 1865. It was followed by the University of Zurich in Switzerland, which soon began attracting women students from all over Europe, especially Russia. However, this remained something of an anomaly within Switzerland itself, where women would not even receive the vote until *over a hundred years later* in 1971. By the end of the twentieth century, over half the students in British medical schools were women, most of whom appeared not to be suffering unduly from sterility, hysteria, fainting fits or even the de-energized wombs which male logic had so confidently predicted during the previous century.

13
PRIDE AND PREJUDICE

Few physicians have had their names immortalized in everyday speech, though not all of these deserved it, or even wished this upon themselves. One who inadvertently won this accolade was Dr Samuel A. Mudd, who gave rise to the saying, 'Your name is Mudd' (as it was originally spelt). After John Wilkes Booth assassinated President Lincoln in 1865 he fled the scene badly wounded, and later called in on Dr Mudd. True to his Hippocratic oath, Dr Mudd treated Booth for an injured back and put his broken leg in a splint, before allowing him to go on his way. Although the doctor had nothing to do with the assassination plot, he was arrested for assisting Booth. His name was Mudd. At his trial he was sentenced to hard labour for life, to be served at Fort Jefferson on the notorious Dry Tortugas, a cluster of reefs 100 miles west of the Florida mainland in the Gulf of Mexico.

In 1867 there was an outbreak of yellow fever on the Dry

Tortugas and over half the prisoners and garrison, including the governor and the doctor, died from the disease. Dr Mudd had treated yellow fever several years beforehand during an outbreak in Baltimore, and understood that it was highly contagious, suspecting that it was carried by mosquitoes. He was permitted to take over and was instrumental in saving many lives, before he himself fell ill. Fortunately he recovered, only to be clapped in irons once more by the new governor, and returned to hard labour. Two years later Mudd received a presidential pardon and returned to his small Maryland to-bacco farm, where he eked out a living, frequently acting as unpaid doctor to the poor locals, many of whom were impoverished released slaves. While Mudd lived out his days in obscurity, gaining a good name for himself, his bad name travelled by word of mouth around the world, gaining infamy and immortality in the famous saying.

A contemporary medical figure whose name was more deservedly immortalized was the Frenchman Louis Pasteur, who gave his name to pasteurization. Even more importantly, he would also be responsible for showing why Semmelweis was correct in his diagnosis of puerperal fever. Pasteur's understanding that infectious disease, as well as putrefaction and fermentation, are all caused by microbes, would be the founding insight of contemporary medicine. Unlike almost all others in the history of medicine so far, Pasteur was not a medical man. His French predecessor Bernard had qualified as a doctor, but had never practised; Pasteur would not even qualify. He remained strictly a chemist – a further indication of the ever-increasing scientific specialization of medical research.

Louis Pasteur was born in 1822 in the rural Jura region of eastern France. His father was a tanner who had been a sergeant major in the Napoleonic army, a proud Bonapartist who would instil in his son the republican patriotism of 'Liberty, Equality and Fraternity' – even though France had now restored the monarchy. His mother appears to have been a passionate but devout woman from whom young Louis would inherit a fervent religious faith. His earliest memories were of his father's small tannery business in the little provincial town of Arbois: the house above the river, the tannery yard, and the pits smelling of chemicals where the animal hides were converted into marketable leather. Young Louis's earliest talent was for art, and the succession of portraits which he executed of friends and family during his teenage years show that this was no ordinary talent. However, his academic prowess proved even greater, and after studying both literature and science at the provincial capital Besançon, in 1843 he won a coveted place at the elite École Normale Supérieure in Paris. Here he quickly showed an exceptional aptitude for chemistry, which developed into an obsession that would last a lifetime. Louis Pasteur was an intense and highly ambitious young man, confidently aware of his exceptional scientific abilities.

Such self-confidence was not misplaced. Aided by the luck that would follow him throughout his career, Pasteur soon made a fundamental scientific discovery which would open up an entirely new field of chemistry. Some years previously, it had been found that there existed two forms of tartaric acid, both of which consisted of the same atoms arranged in the same way, yet bafflingly they had different properties. By investigating crystallized salts of the two forms of tartaric acid, Pasteur was able to show that these different properties arose because their atomic structures were in fact asymmetrical. In other words, although they appeared the same they in fact mirrored each other like left- and right-hand gloves. Furthermore, he was able to show that whereas one form of the acid could be absorbed by living micro-organisms as a nutrient, the other could not. This was the beginning of stereochemistry, which would investigate asymmetry in the huge range of organic chemicals. And Pasteur's luck? The particular tartaric salt whose crystals he chose to investigate is now known to have been the only one out of all the tartaric salts which would have enabled him to make his discovery! But as Pasteur was later to remark: 'Chance favours the prepared mind.'

As a result of this sensational discovery, Pasteur achieved fame in scientific circles. He was appointed a professor at the University of Strasbourg at the exceptionally young age of 25; a year later he married the daughter of the university Rector; and four years after this he was given charge of the new science faculty at the University of Lille, the main industrial city in northeastern France. Pasteur was a young man in a hurry, but the rewards of 'pure' academic science were not for him. His family background inclined him towards the commercial uses of science, and he soon began involving his department in the factories and manufacturing processes of Lille. As a result, Pasteur was approached by an industrialist who was experiencing certain difficulties in manufacturing industrial alcohol from beetroot. Pasteur began investigating the fermentation process, and soon discovered that French winemakers were experiencing similar difficulties. During fermentation some wines 'soured', rendering them unpalatable.

Winemakers had been fermenting grape juice since prehistoric times, though without understanding what precisely was taking place in the process. It was simply accepted that during fermentation a few batches of grape juice were liable to go vinegary. But now that wine had become an important part of the French economy, and was being produced in industrial quantities, fermentation that went wrong was proving a costly business.

Fermentation, and similar biological processes, were at this stage thought to consist solely of chemical reactions. This view had been suggested by German chemists such as Wöhler, whose synthesis of organic urea had led him to believe that he had created 'life' in a test tube. The main advocate of this chemical supremacy was Wöhler's friend and colleague Justus von Liebig, the giant of German chemistry who was professor at Munich. Liebig's purely chemical investigations had already resulted in several important medical discoveries. He had also dismissed the so-called 'biological' process of digestion, insisting that this too could be explained in purely chemical terms. There was no need to go into any minute investigation of 'disgestive processes'; all that was required was a study of the input into the bodily system in the form of foods, gases and water, and a study of the output of this system, in the form of acids, salts, urea, and so forth. This approach had already led Liebig to analyse the fundamental elements of human nutrition as carbohydrates, proteins and fats – a major advance in our understanding of the human body.

Pasteur had various reasons for opposing Liebig's views on the supremacy of chemical processes. Firstly, his passionate religious faith remained unaffected by his equally passionate pursuit of scientific truth, and as a result he refused to believe that life could be manufactured in a test tube. In his view, life was the gift of God. Despite all his scientific discoveries, Pasteur would remain throughout his life a vitalist: matter was animated by some 'life force' that remained beyond the reach of science. Liebig's reductionist materialist approach also struck at the very heart of the French biological tradition, as exemplified by such men as Claude Bernard. Was all French biology to be reduced to nothing more than German chemistry? Pasteur's heartfelt patriotism, instilled by his military father, tended to see things in this simplistic way, and he rebelled at the thought of such a French defeat. As would often be the case with Pasteur, his inspiration came from beyond the realms of science – he knew what he wanted to find, well before he started looking for it.

The fact was, fermentation had not yet been investigated in any experimental fashion. Ever the meticulous and thorough investigator, Pasteur soon showed that fermentation was produced by living micro-organisms in yeast. He was also able to show that when successful fermentation took place the wine contained spherical globules of yeast cells, yet when the wine went sour it also contained yeast cells which were elongated. The round cells produced alcohol, whereas the elongated cells produced lactic acid which soured the wine. Fermentation was not a simple chemical reaction, it clearly resulted from the activity of these tiny organisms. He also managed to show that paradoxically fermentation did not require oxygen, despite the fact that it involved living micro-organisms (though it could be speeded up by the presence of oxygen).

In 1860 Pasteur finally published his conclusive evidence that fermentation involved living organisms, but Liebig refused to believe it. Over the years, Pasteur became so incensed at this that he eventually visited Munich and confronted Liebig in his laboratory. The silver-haired chemist in his distinguished long frock coat politely greeted Pasteur, but refused to discuss science with him on the grounds that he was now old and ill. As the great German physicist Max Planck would later wryly observe: 'A new scientific truth does not triumph by convincing its opponents and making them see the light, but rather because its opponents eventually die, and a new generation grows up that is familiar with it.'

Pasteur had demonstrated that if the yeast cells which produced lactic acid remained in the wine, they would eventually sour it. But how to avoid this? Pasteur invented an ingenious method of forestalling this process. After the good yeast had produced alcohol, the wine should be heated to around 55°C. This would kill off all the yeast, good and bad. The producers of the great vintage wines were horrified at the prospect of heating up their lovingly and carefully produced wines, but they quickly discovered that Pasteur's method worked, without affecting the taste of the wine. This was the process which became known as pasteurization, and it would eventually be adapted for the semi-sterilization of a wide range of products, especially milk.

Pasteur now embarked upon a further investigation of micro-organisms. Despite Leeuwenhoek's discovery some two centuries previously that 'animalcules' reproduced and had life cycles like other insects, many still believed in 'spontaneous generation'. Ironically, this view was reinforced by the latest scientific thinking in the light of Wöhler's creation of 'life' in a test tube. Many now considered that the spontaneous generation of the tiniest microbes from inorganic chemicals was much the same process. Here again this eliminated any reason for divine intervention.

Once more Pasteur entered the fray with his own agenda, determined to protect the world against atheists, materialists and Germans. Yet although his motives may have been scientifically suspect, his science was sound. Pasteur had noticed that although fermentation did not require oxygen, it could still be speeded up by exposure to air. This appeared to imply that the air itself contained microbes. To test his conjecture, Pasteur set up an experiment in which air was passed through gun cotton. He then dissolved the cotton, and found that it contained microbes similar to those in fermenting liquids. It appeared that even the most microscopic dust in the air was filled with invisible spores of living organisms.

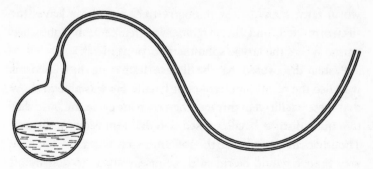

Figure 7. Pasteur's flask for collecting dust particles in air

Pasteur now set up a further experiment to confirm his findings. He boiled some meat extract in a flask, and this was then exposed to the air by means of a long thin tube with a U-bend in it. Under normal circumstances, the beef extract exposed to the air would soon have begun to putrefy, but this time it did not. As the air passed through the long slender tube, the dust particles were deposited on the lower U-bend of the tube and only air passed on up the tube and into the flask, so that no living organism reached the meat extract. Pasteur concluded that microbes in the air were also responsible for the putrefaction of exposed meat, previously thought to have been a process involving the spontaneous generation of maggots. He now concluded that fermentation and putrefaction were evidently the same process, both caused by micro-organisms.

In 1865 Pasteur was called in by the French government to investigate a disease which was devastating the silkworm industry, one of the mainstays of the economy in southern France. Pasteur now had his laboratory at the École Normale Supérieur in Paris, but decided that the only practical way to investigate this disease was in the field. Together with his family, he moved to Alès, 30 miles outside Nîmes in the south of France, in the heart of the sericulture region. Here he took up residence on a silkworm farm – amidst the mulberry trees on whose leaves the silkworms fed, and the *magnaneries* (temperature-controlled barns) where the larvae spun their cocoons of silk.

Pasteur discovered that the disease destroying the silkworms was also the result of microbes or bacilli. He was able to show that these bacilli went through their own life cycle, and also that two quite distinct bacilli caused two different types of disease. The advice he passed on to the government was drastic. The only way France would be rid of these diseases was to destroy all infected worms, and then start again with worms that were indisputably healthy. Pasteur's advice was hardly welcome, but he would eventually be lauded as the saviour of the French silk industry. As a result, he now became a national hero – the first time that a scientist had ever occupied such a role.

The importance of science was beginning to be recognized throughout society: medicine too would benefit from this transformation. Even the necessity for vivisection was reluctantly recognized. These were the years when Claude Bernard was transformed from pariah into widely respected scientist, acclaimed for his physiological discoveries. When Pasteur returned to Paris, he happened to attend some lectures by Bernard, whose scientific work he had long appreciated. Bernard was championing the work of Semmelweis, who had suspected that puerperal fever might be spread by 'invisible cadaver particles'. Instead, Pasteur was beginning to understand that such diseases were caused by living particles, airborne micro-organisms.

The ideas accumulated over 20 years of investigation were now beginning to fall into place in Pasteur's mind. By a stroke of luck, he had been asked to investigate the silkworm disease. This had led him to understand that fermentation, putrefaction *and* infection were all part of the same process, all caused by microbes or bacilli, with different bacilli seemingly causing different diseases. Such ideas flew in the face of medical orthodoxy. How was it possible that such insignificant micro-organisms could affect the workings of any large, powerful and complex animal body? And how could every single disease be caused by an entirely different microbe, when so many diseases responded to the same treatment? Medicine was complicated enough without some ignorant chemist trying to impose his abstruse theories on things which in practice he knew nothing about.

Despite such plausible opposition, the first fundamental principles of germ theory, which would transform medicine, were beginning to form in Pasteur's mind. Though ironically, Pasteur's ideas had orginated in his attempt to show that there was still room for divine intervention in the world – an attempt in which he was convinced he had succeeded. (For this reason, Pasteur would also remain a convinced anti-Darwinist all his life: evolution left no room for God.)

In 1868 Pasteur suffered a cerebral haemorrhage, depriving him of movement in the left side of his body. This had been brought on by overwork and the continuing stress of his angry polemical battles against anyone who disagreed with him – from the atheists to the Germans, and now the medical authorities. Fortunately his mind was unaffected by the stroke; and although the effects would gradually lessen over the years, he would always retain a noticeable limp and a semi-paralysed left hand which considerably hampered him in his experiments.

Even so, by July 1870 Pasteur was well enough to embark upon his celebrated trip to Munich to confront Liebig in his laboratory. Pasteur was not alone in his patriotic anti-German feeling at this time, and in the same month of 1870 the ill-will between France and Germany spilled over into war. Pasteur was lucky to make it back onto French territory in time.

Despite his semi-invalid state, Pasteur was keen to volunteer, but was fortunately dissuaded by his colleagues, who quickly found themselves the only ones left among the deserted court-yards of the École Normale Supérieur. All the students had volunteered for the army. Despite such enthusiastic support, the French military campaign quickly turned into a debacle, when faced with the efficient Prussian war machine, which had long been preparing for this war.

As the Prussians advanced on Paris, Pasteur and his family were persuaded to return to the family home at Arbois in the Jura. By September the Prussians were besieging Paris, and elsewhere the French armies were retreating in disarray. With the coming of winter, Pasteur received some devastating news. As the fleeing local regiment passed through the snow-clogged streets of Arbois, there was no news of what had become of Pasteur's son. Distraught with worry, Pasteur together with his wife and daughter set out in the old family carriage to see if they could find him. They drove on into the night through the snow-covered pine woods. Next day, they arrived at the small town of Chaffois, where the streets were filled with ragged soldiery. Some were camped about makeshift fires, others begging pitifully for food, yet others lying in the gutter frozen dead beside their horses. The news spread through the town that their commander, General Bourbaki, had attempted to blow his brains out. But in the midst of all the misery and despair Pasteur suddenly caught sight of his son, huddled in his greatcoat, in the back of a passing cart. After a rapturous reunion, the Pasteurs all returned home in the rickety family carriage.

In January a starving Paris capitulated; the war was over. After the victorious Germans marched off home, there was a revolution in Paris and a Commune was established – regarded by many as the first communist revolution. The balance of power in Europe was now transformed. The victorious Prussians established a united Germany, which became the first German Reich, displacing France which for centuries had been the largest and most powerful nation in Europe. In France, the Paris Commune was savagely put down, the ineffectual monarchy was deposed, and the Third Republic established.

Pasteur's patriotic answer to this national disgrace was to investigate the problems of fermentation in French beer, determined to make it better than German beer. Using the knowledge gained during his study of fermentation in wine, he soon devised improved fermentation methods for beer, which ensured that it was not liable to spoil. He even visited England, passing on this knowledge to London brewers. In consequence, they began to brew a new pale ale, which was capable of being shipped all the way around the Cape of Good Hope to India without going off – the origin of India Pale Ale. Pasteur could have patented his methods and made a fortune, but instead he believed in the free interchange of scientific knowledge (except to Germany). By now Pasteur was convinced that his germ theory of disease was correct, and this would soon be put to the supreme test.

As if the devastation of war was not enough, French agriculture now began to be ravaged by a succession of diseases. Sheep, poultry and cattle throughout the land were succumbing to widespread virulent and contagious diseases. Most medical experts still believed that livestock diseases were spread by 'miasmas': noxious and pestilential emanations which spread through the air. Miasma theory had originated in ancient times, but had recently undergone a revival in the sphere of public health, where disease was thought to arise from locations with noxious smells, such as cesspools, rubbish dumps and even graveyards. Eliminating these sources of 'miasma' had often proved highly effective. In the countryside, marshes and boggy low-lying pastures were often seen as a source of miasma. Pasteur was determined to show that his germ theory not only accounted for disease, but also explained the occasional 'successes' of miasma theory.

In 1877 Pasteur began a study of cholera in farm animals, and once again his researches were aided by a lucky chance. Pasteur and his staff began injecting healthy chickens with fresh disease culture. After a series of experiments they ran short of fresh culture, and two chickens in the batch had to be injected with culture that was two weeks old and somewhat attenuated (less concentrated). Normally, all injected chickens died within 24 hours, but this time two survived. Pasteur ordered them to be added to the next batch, which were all injected with fresh cholera culture. Once again, the two chickens survived. Pasteur immediately remembered Jenner and how his cowpox vaccine had immunized against small-pox.

Pasteur could hardly believe his luck. It looked as if he had found a vaccine against chicken cholera. But this time the vaccination came from the disease itself. If this was the case, it seemed likely that chicken cholera could be used as a vaccine against *other* diseases as well. Perhaps he had discovered a universal immunizing agent, which protected against all germs. Always ambitious, Pasteur saw this as the fulfilment of his dreams. He set to work with a number of experiments, but all of them proved a disappointment. It seemed that attenuated chicken cholera bacilli only provided immunization against chicken cholera. Unlike cowpox and smallpox there was no crossover. But what if attenuated germs of any disease could provide immunization against that same disease?

Pasteur now turned his attention to anthrax, a violent and fatal contagious disease which attacked the lungs and spleen of sheep and cattle. Stricken animals developed symptoms with such rapidity that often their shaking limbs and exhalations of blood were not noticed among the herd until they died, within hours of being infected. A sheep carcass quickly became distended, any rupture of the skin giving rise to a flow of dark, viscous blood. (The name anthrax comes from the Greek for 'charcoal' or 'ruby'.) By 1877 anthrax was killing 20 per cent of sheep in many regions of France, and in some regions as many as 50 per cent. Worse still, even after the diseased herds had been cleared from the land where they had grazed, the land remained infected and passed on the disease to new herds. The disease was also liable to attack woolcombers and shepherds who had looked after the infected sheep.

Such evidence seemed to support miasma theory, but Pasteur knew otherwise. A year previously anthrax bacilli had been identified by the German physician Robert Koch, and Pasteur's microscopic investigations confirmed the existence in diseased sheep of the characteristic tell-tale anthrax microorganism, consisting of a string of minute beads (now called streptococci, from the Greek words for 'chain' and 'berries'). Pasteur also discovered that these germs occasionally existed as spores which could remain alive in the ground, thus accounting for the diseased pastures.

Pasteur knew that if he had in fact discovered the secret of vaccination for all diseases, the injection of attenuated anthrax bacilli should provide immunization. The trouble was, anthrax proved so virulent that it seemed all but impossible to produce a suitably attentuated version of the bacilli. Using the ageing process either resulted in bacilli that were still so strong they infected and killed the host, or bacilli that were too weak to provide immunization. However, by means of painstaking experiments Pasteur discovered that if the bacilli subjected to the ageing process were heated to a very precise temperature (42–43°C) this produced a suitably attenuated virus. Even so, when this was innoculated it still produced the occasional 'misfires'.

Hearing of Pasteur's latest unsatisfactory experiments, the medical establishment now began to ridicule Pasteur and his germ theory, referring to it as 'microbal madness' and even 'fetishism'. Meanwhile, the German physician Robert Koch had established the important fact that anthrax bacilli were the cause of anthrax, rather than just tell-tale evidence of the disease. Pasteur had long suspected this, but to his chagrin the German had been the first to prove it.

Stung by the persistent rejection of his germ theory, and fearful of the possibility that a German might scoop him in his moment of triumph, Pasteur announced a public demonstration of his cure for anthrax. This would be held on the farm of Pouilly-le-Fort near Melun, which was conveniently on the main railway line, just 25 miles south of Paris. On 5 May 1881, Pasteur prepared to supervise his faithful long-term assistant Emile Roux as he innoculated 24 out of a group of 48 sheep with attenuated anthrax virus. By now Pasteur had developed a new, and apparently more succesful way of attenuating the bacilli by treating them with potassium bichromate. However, he had not yet had time to test this fully to see if it invariably eliminated all 'misfires'. Despite this, Pasteur decided to go ahead and inject the sheep with the attenuated bacilli obtained by his new method – even though his public announcement had specifically mentioned that he was using vaccine obtained by the initial ageing process. Pasteur was not only perpetrating a deception, he was also taking a huge risk.

Just under four weeks later, on 31 May, all 48 sheep were injected with fresh anthrax bacilli. Given the virulence of anthrax, the results of Pasteur's inoculations would be evident within two days. By this stage, the experiment at Pouilly-le-Fort had begun attracting huge publicity – in the press, among the medical and scientific establishments, as well as among the public at large. It also attracted great controversy. Bernard had died three years previously, and the anti-vivisectionist movement had now focused its attention on Pasteur and his experiments involving animals.

Everything depended upon the results of the inoculation, which were to be demonstrated before the assembled crowds of spectators at Pouilly-le-Fort on 2 June. On 1 June news reached Pasteur in Paris that two of his inoculated sheep were showing signs of becoming ill. Already stressed to the limit by the pressure of publicity (which was largely of his own making) Pasteur exploded with rage and began bawling out his assistant Roux. This was all his fault: he had obviously been careless when administering the inoculations. Pasteur was soon screaming at his assistant in an uncontrollable fury. He refused to go to Pouilly-le-Fort next morning and face a public humiliation – which would be the ruin of his reputation, of his career, of the good name of France – all because of the incompetence of his assistant. Yet both Roux and Pasteur were well aware of the truth. It looked as if Pasteur's gamble had failed – the new attenuated vaccine had evidently 'misfired'.

Only later that evening did Pasteur receive another telegram informing him that the two apparently ailing sheep had now fully recovered. Next morning Pasteur set out for Pouilly-le-Fort to review the results of his experiment. Of the 48 sheep which had been injected with fresh anthrax bacilli, it could be seen in the field that just 24 had survived. All of these were sheep which had been inoculated with Pasteur's attenuated anthrax virus. Pasteur received the adulation of the crowd, who cheered and threw their hats in the air when the results were publicly announced. Even the medical establishment appeared convinced by this overwhelming public demonstration. Once again, luck had been on Pasteur's side.

Only his German rival Koch remained unimpressed. When Pasteur had published his earlier researches into anthrax, he had 'forgotten' to mention the German's previous seminal identification of the anthrax streptococcus bacillus, glossing over this as if it was his own discovery. Koch now responded by criticizing Pasteur's methods at Pouilly-le-Fort, insisting that he had not fully solved the problem of how to manufacture a foolproof attenuated vaccine. This evidently hit the mark. At the International Congress of Hygiene which was held in Switzerland in 1882 Pasteur launched into an attack on Koch, who was in the audience. Koch declined the invitation to reply to this attack, remarking sarcastically that he had still learned nothing new about the attenuation of anthrax virus. Later, he would publish a paper severely critcizing Pasteur's methods: 'Such goings-on are perhaps suitable for the advertising industry, but science should reject them vigorously.' German and French science remained at war.

With hindsight, there seems to be an inevitability about the direction of Pasteur's career. To begin with, his work extended chemistry (with the discovery of stereochemistry); this then led to his proof that fermentation was more than chemical (involving microbes). As if by logic he then went on to demonstrate the origin of microbes (dispelling the notion of spontaneous generation). He was thus able to show that the role of microbes was the same in fermentation and disease (silkworm project), finally demonstrating that such microbe-induced disease could be cured by inoculation (in chickens, and then even larger animals such as sheep and cattle). Only now, after over 20 years of research, did his work lead him on the seemingly inevitable step to the study of human disease.

But this was only one progression. With every step, Pasteur's career had become increasingly spectacular, attracting ever greater public notice until he had become a national hero. His next step would bring him to even wider public attention throughout the world. And in a similar progression, he would also take even greater risks, which put his reputation in even greater peril, and would require even greater luck to see him through.

Having dealt with anthrax, Pasteur now turned in 1882 to one of the most horrific of all diseases transmitted from animals to human beings – rabies. This disease had been known since ancient times, its name being derived from the Latin *rabere* meaning 'to rage' (in French, it is even known as *la rage*). When a person was bitten by a rabid animal, most frequently a dog or a wolf, there would be no immediate affect. But between ten days and several months later the appalling symptoms would emerge. The affected victim would suffer variously from delirium and convulsions, foaming at the mouth and paralysis, experiencing extreme dehydration yet unable to drink because of painful spasms of the throat muscles. Death was inevitable and would result in a few days.

Pasteur's initial investigations threatened to overturn his entire germ theory. Despite autopsies on numerous rabid dogs, and microscopic examination of their tissues, he could discover no bacilli for rabies. With characteristic aplomb, he declared that the rabies bacilli were too small to detect with a microscope. (His hunch would not be confirmed until a century later, with the advent of the electron microscope.) Pasteur's subsequent hypotheses reveal his brilliance. Symptoms such as spasms and delirium indicated that the infection attacked the spinal cord and the brain. Pasteur surmised that the infecting micro-organism must enter the body through the bite wound, and then gradually proceed by way of the peripheral nerves into the spinal cord and the brain – thus accounting for the often lengthy interval between the initial bite and the onset of symptoms.

Having been unable to find evidence of bacilli, Pasteur was forced to work with infected tissue from the spinal cord and brain. Once again, he sought a method to attenuate the diseased tissue in order to produce an inoculating agent – or vaccine, as it was now becoming known. Just a year previously, at the Fourth International Medical Congress in 1881, Pasteur had charitably suggested that Jenner's word vaccine should now be used to describe inoculations against all kinds of contagious diease. Pasteur may have been egotistical and ambitious, but he was also capable of self-effacing generosity of spirit.

Searching for a rabies vaccine would involve Pasteur and his assistants in much distressing and highly dangerous work with animals. To begin with, the only way to infect another dog with rabies was to put it in a cage with an infected dog, and then wait for the rabid dog to undergo one of its inevitable fits. In the course of this, the rabid dog would savage the healthy dog, biting it again and again in its frenzy. Even hardened experimenters such as Pasteur and Roux found themselves distressed by the results. As with so many vivisectionists (who, contrary to popular prejudice, are far from being cold-hearted sadists) they frequently had to remind themselves that the aim of their work was to save human beings from the terrible scourge they were investigating.

Eventually Pasteur's experiments began to yield results. Having obtained infectious spinal cord tissue from a rabid rabbit, he was able to attenuate this by allowing it to age for several days. This was usually done by exposing the tissue to air, though in some cases he discovered that the process could be speeded up by introducing pure oxygen, much as he had done in the fermentation process. This attenuated tissue was then injected into some healthy dogs. First, 14-day-old rabbit tissue was injected. Next day, slightly stronger 13-day-old tissue, and so on, for a fortnight. Following a series of experiments, Pasteur found that by the fourteenth day the dog was able to receive full strength rabid tissue from the spinal cord of a rabbit. This would normally have infected the dog with rabies, but now had no ill effects. The course of gradually strengthening tissue appeared to give immunity. But this was not all. Years of experimental work with vaccines led Pasteur to suspect that even if the course of injections was begun after the dog had been infected, but before it began showing symptoms, it might still manage to prevent the disease. It was just possible that he had found both a vaccine for rabies and cure for it.

Pasteur had proceeded with extreme caution, and it had taken him three years to develop this vaccine. He had been determined that there should be no repeat of the anthrax near-disaster. Yet once again Pasteur would succumb to his apparently insatiable desire for sensational publicity. Word had got out that Pasteur was working on a vaccine for rabies, and this soon had the inevitable effect. In July 1885 a distraught baker's wife travelled the 250 miles from Alsace to Paris to see Pasteur, bringing her nine-year-old son Joseph Meister. Two days previously Joseph had been savagely bitten 14 times on the arms, legs and thighs by a rabid dog. She begged Pasteur to save her son's life by giving him the vaccine she had heard about.

The prototype vaccine which Pasteur had just developed had so far been used solely on dogs. Despite this, Pasteur decided to take the risk. As he was not a qualified doctor, he was not permitted to administer the injections to a human being himself, so he asked his assistant Roux, who had recently qualified as a physician, to administer them. Roux had taken part in all the initial 14-day vaccine tests, and was the only other person who was privy to Pasteur's laboratory notes recording the successes, and failures, of these tests. On this evidence, Roux refused point-blank to take part in what he regarded as nothing more or less than a risky experiment using a human being as a guinea pig. So what exactly was this evidence which made Roux so vehemently against this 'human experimentation'? We now know from Pasteur's laboratory notebooks that he had completed the 14-day process on a set of 50 dogs 'without a single failure'. On the other hand, not a single one of these dogs had been given the 14-day course of injections *after* having been infected with rabies, which was the situation with young Joseph Meister.

Undaunted, Pasteur approached two other doctors (who had not seen the contents of his laboratory notebook) and persuaded them to perform the series of injections. At eight o'clock in the evening on 6 July 1885, just 60 hours after Joseph Meister had been attacked by the rabid dog, he received his first injection of Pasteur's rabies vaccine. For the next 13 days Meister was given increasingly potent injections of infected spinal cord tissue. On the last day he was injected with a dose which would have been lethal on the first day of treatment. Joseph Meister survived, and later developed no symptoms of rabies.

With a characteristic blend of recklessness and daring, Pasteur had triumphed. The news that a vaccine for rabies had been discovered quickly spread throughout Europe and its colonies, across the Atlantic and through the Americas. Pasteur's name was now recognized throughout the world, and soon people from around the globe would be making their way to Paris for treatment. In December 1885 four American boys, the sons of port workers at Newark, New Jersey, who had been bitten by a rabid dog, were shipped across the Atlantic to Pasteur. Their daily progress and eventual cure were telegraphed back to America, where they made headline news. Three months later, the Czar of Russia sent 19 peasants from Smolensk who had been savaged by a rabid wolf. Sixteen of these were saved, and the Czar sent Pasteur a cross studded with diamonds, as well as 100,000 francs to enable him to establish a Pasteur Institute for the treatment of rabies. In the years to come, Joseph Meister would be employed as doorman of this institute.

In 1895, at the age of 72, Pasteur died holding a crucifix in one hand and his wife's hand in the other. After a state funeral with high mass at Notre Dame, attended by the President of France and members of European royalty, he would be buried in a specially constructed crypt at the Pasteur Institute. Joseph Meister swore to guard this with his life, and would prove as good as his word. In 1940 Pasteur's hated Germans would once again conquer France. When the Nazis arrived at the gates of the Pasteur Institute, and ordered Meister to open up Pasteur's tomb, he refused. Rather than submit his saviour to this national humiliation, the little white-haired Meister retired to his small appartment in the institute and commited suicide.

Pasteur would prove big enough to survive both the fulsome admiration and the controversy surrounding his name. Both seem part and parcel of his achievement. His self-publicizing and theatrically contrived triumphs would have a transforming effect on public opinion. Here medicine had its first world-famous hero. This would prove a watershed in the public perception of medicine. From now on the persistent mists of quackery enveloping the profession would gradually be dispelled, and it would increasingly be seen for what it had become – a saving grace of humanity.

14

MEDICINE FOR THE WORLD

Semmelweis had recognized that infection could be transmitted, Pasteur's germ theory showed how it could be transmitted, Lister would show how such infection could be eliminated. For this reason, the English physician Lister is generally regarded as the founder of antiseptic and preventive medicine.

Joseph Lister was born in 1827 at Upton Park in West Ham, which in those days was several miles east of London in the Essex countryside. His father was a Quaker wine merchant who became a highly skilled microscopist in his spare time. Lister senior was responsible for inventing the achromatic lens, which eliminated colour distortion in microscopic images, and for this was elected a Fellow of the Royal Society.

Young Joseph Lister grew up in a close family, and was encouraged by his father to follow scientific interests. He developed a particular, and practical, interest in animal skeletons. In a typical letter, the 14-year-old Lister describes how 'when Mamma was out I was by myself and had nothing to do but draw skeletons . . . and in the evening, with [his brother] John's help I managed to put up a whole skeleton, that of a frog, and it looks just as if it was going to take a leap.' A mere two years later, he was ready to enter university. The two leading universities in England, Oxford and Cambridge, still denied entry to Quakers (as well as any others who would not take the oath of allegiance to the Church of England). Instead, Lister attended the recently founded University College, London, which opened its doors to all religions (thus earning it the popular nickname 'the godless college'). Here Lister studied arts subjects as well as anatomy. His ultimate aim was to become a surgeon, and in 1846 he witnessed the first operation in England to be carried out under an ether anaesthetic. This event seems to have inspired him, but two years later he suffered from a nervous breakdown. This was brought about by a combination of overwork and an undermining religious fervour. His intense spiritual feelings persuaded him that medicine was not a sufficiently fulfilling subject in which to immerse his soul, yet his strong and prevailing ambition had always been to enter this profession. Accepting the hospitable offer of a wealthy Quaker friend of the family, he went to Ireland, where several months of rural travels aided his recovery. He then returned to University College, fully reconciled to devoting his life to medicine. In 1852 he achieved high honours in his medical degree, and three years later at the age of 28 he accepted a post as a surgeon at the Edinburgh Royal Infirmary. He was to remain in Scotland for the next 20 years.

By the age of 32 young Lister had risen to become professor of medicine at Glasgow University and surgeon of the Glasgow Royal Infirmary, where he was in charge of the wards and operating theatres. The mortality rate for operations in these theatres (and all contemporary operating theatres) was alarmingly high. This was also the case even for such simple operations as setting bone fractures. What struck Lister most of all was the discrepancy between simple fractures and compound or multiple fractures. The latter, where the bone frequently became exposed to the air, were highly prone to develop gangrene. Mortality rates often rose as high as 60 per cent in such cases. Lister conducted a series of operations on frogs' legs and confirmed that gangrene was in fact a process of rotting. He was unwilling to accept the usual explanation, which was that 'miasma' or 'foul air' was the cause of this. Instead, he began to wonder if perhaps the cause was something in the air, such as dust. These ideas all came together when he read the results of Pasteur's latest researches into putrefaction, which showed that it was a form of fermentation caused by bacteria in the air. Lister's suspicions had been confirmed: it was not the air which caused the disease, but what was in it. (Pasteur's great insight had been that these airborne particles contained living micro-organsims.)

At the time, carbolic acid (phenol) was used to cleanse sewers and disperse their foul smells. Lister found that this was the best agent for killing the airborne bacteria which caused disease. In August 1865 a boy who had been run over by a cart was brought in to Glasgow Royal Infirmary suffering from multiple fracture of the tibia (shin bone). Lister set the bone and dressed the wound with lint soaked in carbolic acid, which he left for four days. The wound suffered no infection, and six weeks later the boy was able to walk home. Lister used this process in several similar cases, and then in a series of amputations. The results were heartening: the mortality rate for amputations in his operating theatre fell from 46 per cent to 15 per cent. He published his results in 1867 in a historic article entitled 'On the Antiseptic Principle in the Practice of

Surgery' (septic stems from the Greek word *sepsis* meaning 'putrefaction').

This article would ultimately save more lives than any other medical paper ever written. Yet as ever, such innovation was greeted with derision in more conservative circles. Some simply refused to believe that bacteria existed, demanding 'Have you ever seen them?' Medical training still did not necessarily involve microscopy; such things were for specialists and research. Others were quicker to welcome this life-saving 'principle of antisepsis', and it soon gained adherents in Britain and Germany – though ironically, not in France, where germ theory had originated. When the Franco-Prussian War broke out in 1870, German surgeons pressed for antiseptic measures to be installed in military hospitals, but with only marginal success. The situation on the French side was observed by Lister's cousin, who volunteered for an international ambulance unit. He wrote back that antiseptic surgery in French military hospitals was 'unknown'. Bottles of carbolic acid sent to field stations at the front were sent back unopened. One French surgeon who had visited Lister in Glasgow was even forbidden to use antiseptic methods. As a result the French war statistics make pitiful reading. Over 13,000 men had limbs amputated; of these, 10,000 died of gangrene or fever.

Meanwhile Lister developed his antiseptic methods, advocating their use in all surgical operations. Wounds, surgical instruments, and surgeons' hands were all to be treated with carbolic acid. A special donkey-engine pump was invented which emitted a fine spray of carbolic acid to purify the atmosphere. Soon the antiseptic principle was being applied in every branch of surgery. (Apart from the military, that is. As late as the turn of the century the commander-in-chief of the British Army during the Boer War, Lord Wolseley, would arrogantly assert: 'Medical advice is a very good thing – when it is asked for.' Despite this pronouncement, the British forces during the 1899–1902 Boer War in South Africa were the first to be equipped 'with all the requisites for antiseptic surgery' – seemingly without their London-based commander's knowledge. When the low mortality figures came to light, these were attributed by the top brass to 'short battles, low British casualties, and the dry fresh air of the open Veldt'. Medicine evidently had nothing to do with it.)

In most civilian hospitals, on the other hand, the *raison d'être* for Lister's antiseptic measures was quickly grasped. In 1875 Lister was invited to Germany and France to instruct in his methods, and a year later he travelled to America. He would receive many honours, being made President of the Royal Society in 1885 and a lord two years later. In 1898 he was given the freedom of the City of London for his services to medicine, coincidentally on the very same day as Lord Wolsley was given the same honour, for whatever reason. A truly modest man, Lord Lister made it known that he had no wish to be buried in Westminster Abbey, one of the greatest honours that Britain can bestow, preferring instead to be buried beside his wife.

As a result of Lister's antisepsis, surgery would undergo a revolution. Previously, surgeons had not dared to invade such vulnerable parts as the abdomen, the vertebrae or the head. The first great surgeon to take advantage of antiseptic surgery was the German-born Theodor Billroth, who reigned supreme in Vienna from the late 1860s until his death in 1894. A man of typical Viennese culture, he was a close friend of Brahms and even wrote a book on musical taste. As early as 1872 he resected an oesophagus (removed a gullet), later performing similar operations on the pylorus (exit from the stomach) and the thyroid gland. The dissection of cadavers had taught surgeons their anatomy, but entering the living body was venturing into the unknown. Billroth's methods were daring and experimental, with the result that his patients sometimes paid the ultimate price.

This was the 'heroic' age of surgery, which threw up such charismatic figures as the pioneer Irish-born surgeon William Arbuthnot Lane, who operated with great panache and regarded the workings of the intestines as largely a matter of plumbing. His operations were drastic and effective: none more so than his pioneer cure for constipation, which simply involved removing a length of the lower intestine to enable more speedy passage. Such colectomy remains part of the surgeon's repertoire; similarly, many of Billroth's operational methods have remained standard practice. During this period such everyday operations as appendectomy (removal of appendix) and kidney removal were also pioneered. The first men to perform these operations certainly risked the lives of their patients, but their discoveries saved many more. The morality of all this remains debatable, though some modern ethical philosophers argue that an act can in fact become moral (or immoral) in the light of what good (or evil) it ultimately brings about.

Along with improved surgical techniques there were further concrete improvements, such as the artery clamp (invented as early as 1862) and the gradual introduction of rubber gloves. Even so, operations were still for the most part conducted in dimly lit rooms by surgeons 'correctly' dressed in frock coats, which were used in operation after operation, and tended to become gruesomely encrusted with blood over time. Only gradually through the 1880s and 1890s would face masks, caps and white coats begin to appear. The modern operating theatre, with gleaming instruments and spotless surgeons attended by starched nurses, was slowly beginning to evolve.

As we have seen, modern medicine as we know it was

founded with Pasteur's discovery during the 1870s that each contagious disease was caused by its own signature bacteria. This was the start of bacteriology, and there would be spectacular advances in this field during the following decade – as even a partial list of the major discoveries makes clear:

1875	amoebic dysentery (bacteria identified by Loesch)
1879	gonorrhoea (Neisser)
1880	typhoid (Eberth)
	leprosy (Hansen)
	malaria (Laveran)
1882	tuberculosis (Koch)
	glanders (Loeffler)
1883	cholera (Koch)
1884	diphtheria (Loeffler)
	tetanus (Kitasato)
	pneumonia (Fraenkel)

As can be seen, Pasteur's great German rival Koch would play a major role in this field – a position overwhelmingly reinforced by the fact that Loeffler was one of his assistants, and that the Japanese Kitasato (who would later go on to isolate the plague bacillus) also worked at the Koch Institute.

Koch has been unfortunate in being overshadowed by Pasteur. His career may have been less spectacular than that of his great French adversary, but it would prove no less controversial. Robert Koch was born in 1843, almost 20 years later than Pasteur. He was one of 13 children born into the family of a mining engineer in the small town of Clausthal in the Harz Mountains of central Germany. In contrast to Pasteur, Koch qualified as a doctor; yet he certainly showed no signs of early brilliance, practising in a number of small provincial towns.

Koch's interest in research is said to have been sparked by a microscope which was given to him for Christmas by his young wife Emmy. He soon became so absorbed in his investigations that he transformed part of his consulting room into a makeshift laboratory. During this period he developed a new way for staining bacteria, making them more visible and easier to identify under the microscope. In 1876, in the course of his investigations, he identified the anthrax virus. At the time, German scientists were finding it impossible to obtain pure cultures of particular bacteria. This had led some of them to propose the theory of polymorphism, which suggested that bacteria were capable of transforming themselves from one type to another. By 1879, Koch was able to prove that this was not the case. He was able to show that bacteria were the cause of disease, rather than its product; and he was able to prove that particular bacteria caused particular diseases. It was these breakthroughs which provided the theoretical foundation to Pasteur's famous anthrax experiment with the sheep at Pouilly-le-Fort in 1881 (whose findings would make no mention of Koch's work).

Koch's profound discoveries now came to the notice of the authorities in Berlin, and he was summoned from his provincial obscurity to work at the Imperial Health Office. Here he had access to the latest equipment and soon made further advances. By using set gelatin, he managed to perfect a technique for obtaining pure cultures of particular bacteria uncontaminated by bacteria from the air. In 1882 he also formulated his famous 'postulates', four requirements necessary to prove that a particular organism was the cause of a particular disease. These insisted that the organism had to be detected at *every* instance of the disease; it must then be cultured for a number of further generations; these later generations must then be capable of causing the disease in a healthy animal; and finally the infected animal must have the same organisms as found in the original victim.

The year 1882 would also witness Koch's greatest triumph. By now the disease we know as tuberculosis – then called consumption, or phthisis – was reaching epidemic proportions, being responsible for 1 in 7 deaths in Europe. Using his new techniques, Koch managed to isolate the tubercule bacillus *Mycobacterium tuberculosis*. The scourge had been identified and named. At last, the development of a cure for this disease seemed only a matter of time. But before Koch could work on this, he was drafted on to a German government commission to Egypt. There had been a serious outbreak of cholera in Alexandria, and it seemed only a matter of time before this spread to Europe. An impending catastrophe loomed, and something had to be done about it.

As ever, Germany and France seemed incapable of cooperation, even in the face of such a serious threat. By the time Koch disembarked in Egypt, a French team under the leadership of Pasteur's trusted chief assistant Roux had already arrived and begun work, though with little success. Using Pasteur's tried and tested technique of trying to reproduce the disease in animals, Roux's team had so far only drawn a blank. Unbeknown to them, cholera is a disease that does not affect animals, only humans. Koch chose to use his own methods, directly investigating the victims themselves. In this way, he succeeded in isolating and identifying the *Vibrio cholerae* (comma-shaped bacillus), demonstrating that it was transmitted mainly through polluted water and lodged in the human intestine. Koch had capped his tuberculosis triumph with a victory over the French by becoming the first to isolate the cholera bacillus.

On his return, Koch was greeted as a national hero. He duly advised the government to carry out regular checks on the water supply, and established courses to enable doctors to recognize cholera. These measures would prove effective in stemming the disease when it duly arrived in the port of Hamburg some years later. Though not everyone was so impressed. Many resented the 'upstart' Koch, a mere country doctor; although jealousy was not the only cause of opposition. The distinguished Munich professor of hygiene Max von Pettenkofer adamantly refused to believe that bacteria were the sole cause of disease: *Vibrio cholerae* could not possibly cause cholera. He demanded that Koch send him a flask of vibrios so that he could check for himself. Upon receiving a flask, he wrote back to Koch thanking him 'for the flask containing the so-called cholera vibrios. Herr Doktor Pettenkofer has now drunk the entire contents and is happy to be able to inform Herr Doktor Professor Koch that he remains in his usual good health.' And so he would remain for the next 18 years, until at the age of 83 he decided upon a more reliable method of suicide and shot himself.

By now Koch had been appointed director of the Institute of Hygiene. A few years later he would become director of a newly founded Institute of Infectious Diseases, which would become known as the Koch Institute, Berlin's answer to the Pasteur Institute in Paris. In 1884 Koch's institute was the scene of yet another triumph, when his assistant Loeffler isolated the bacillus which caused diphtheria, a severe and painful infection of the throat, where the growth of false membranes gradually suffocates the patient. Often the only method of saving the patient was to perform a tracheotomy – cutting open the windpipe to introduce a breathing tube – though even such drastic measures failed if further choking membranes formed. This disease, which principally affected children, was also reaching epidemic proportions, both in Europe and America. By the 1880s in New York, diphtheria rates of 4,000 children per year were being reported, with anything up to 50 per cent of cases proving fatal. Besides identifying the rod-like bacillus, the researchers at Koch's institute also noticed its presence in healthy children, thus leading to the crucial understanding that there can be an unaffected 'carrier' of a contagious disease (a concept which had largely been overlooked since it was first noticed by Jenner). However, these important findings were undermined a few years later by Roux at the Pasteur Institute, who was able to show that diphtheria was not in fact caused directly by the rod-like diphtheria bacteria, but by a toxin (poison) released by this bacteria which passed into the blood-stream. This meant that the efforts of Koch's team to develop a vaccine were unnecessary: the disease could be attacked by the injection of a more simple antitoxin. Undeterred, Koch's team immediately raced to become the first to develop an antitoxin, which was initially used by Koch himself in the dramatic rescue of a child in Berlin on Christmas Day. Not even Pasteur himself could have staged such a coup! Franco–German rivalry remained as fierce as ever.

Koch pressed on, keenly conscious that great discoveries were now being made almost annually at the Pasteur Institute. In January 1891 he dramatically announced his greatest breakthrough. He had discovered a substance which halted the growth of the tuberculosis bacillus. This he called 'tuberculin': Germany had finally triumphed with a cure for tuberculosis. Koch was once again a national hero. The Kaiser personally pinned a medal on his chest, and he was also awarded the freedom of the city of Berlin. In a bid to retain German supremacy, Koch was quietly permitted to keep the secret of 'tuberculin' to himself, which would normally have been against the law. This new cure would be manufactured solely at the Koch Institute. Soon thousands of patients were being treated with tuberculin.

Unfortunately, Koch's announcement proved to be premature. Sufficient tests had not been carried out on tuberculin, and it soon became clear that this wonder cure was only effective during the early stages of a particular type of the disease. In cases of pulmonary tuberculosis, the most prevalent form which attacked the lungs, tuberculin was wholly ineffective and sometimes even worsened the condition. From being a national hero, Koch fell to becoming a national disgrace. Word spread that he had even sold the secret of tuberculin to a drug company for a million marks – which the 47-year-old Koch was using to pay for his divorce from his wife Emmy and his remarriage to an 18-year-old artist called Hedwig.

Just a year after the announcement of its discovery, tuberculin was revealed to be simply a glycerin extract of tuberculosis bacteria. Koch and his new young bride fled to Egypt to escape the furore. Throughout the ensuing years Koch would obstinately maintain that one day an improved form of tuberculin would eventually provide a cure. This hope proved false. On the other hand, it was soon discovered that tuberculin did have its uses as a diagnostic agent for latent tuberculosis. In an effort to publicize this, Koch even injected himself (and his new young wife Hedwig, who insisted upon joining her husband). The result of Koch's test proved positive – like a large percentage of the population, he too had now become infected with a weak latent form of the disease.

Koch would spend his last years leading expeditions to combat disease in Asia and Africa. In India he was able to demonstrate that the plague was spread by rats (although without identifying the rat flea as the actual source of infection), in South Africa he cured cattle plague, but it was East Africa which would see his most sensational late success. Here he virtually eliminated sleeping sickness from the Sese Islands in Lake Victoria. Before Koch's arrival no less than 20,000 of the 35,000 islanders had succumbed to this fatal disease. Koch discovered that it was spread by the tsetse fly, and took measures to destroy the natural habitat of the fly along the shoreline, thus reducing the death rate by 90 per cent. In 1905 he was awarded the Nobel Prize for Physiology or Medicine.

Koch was far from being alone in his fight against tropical diseases. By the end of the nineteenth century, the European powers and America had extended their influence around the globe, in the process encountering many virulent and widespread diseases which they fought to eliminate. The main instrument in this battle was the new science of bacteriology which had been developed by Pasteur and Koch; the way forward now lay through the microscope. Here, the next major insight came from a medical graduate of Aberdeen University, Patrick Manson, who entered the Imperial Chinese Maritime Customs Service in 1866. Manson was an energetic man, who self-effacingly described himself as 'a good carpenter, but an indifferent surgeon'. In reality he was an exceptional surgeon, inventing several surgical techniques which still bear his name. One of these was a method for removing the tumours which are a feature of elephantiasis, a disease which he had first encountered at the Chinese port of Amoy. Elephantiasis causes hideous swelling of the limbs and genitalia, whose skin becomes coarse like the hide of an elephant. Occasionally, the victims's limbs become so heavy and swollen that they are anchored to the ground, unable to move. Manson embarked upon a study of this humiliating disease, discovering that it was caused by a threadworm (*filaria*) which entered the bloodstream by way of a mosquito bite. Here was the breakthrough: Manson was the first to show that mosquitoes acted as a vector (from the Latin *vehere*, 'to carry') for disease, rather than being the direct cause of the disease. While on leave in London in 1894, Manson gave a talk at the prestigious

Linnean Society to announce his findings, but this was greeted with disbelief and even laughter. Fortunately, he struck up a friendship with Ronald Ross, a 37-year-old doctor who was on leave from India.

Ronald Ross had been born in India, the son of a British Army officer. He had studied medicine in England before returning to serve as a doctor in the Indian Army Medical Service (which had been established as a result of the Royal Commission prompted by Florence Nightingale). Ross was a man of many exceptional talents, who despite this had reached middle age without really succeeding in anything. His first love had been mathematics, in which he had produced original work on rational integral algebraic equations. At the same time he had also achieved a reputation as a minor poet, as well as writing two novels and even some plays. Later he had shown talent as an artist, and had also composed a number of original works for the piano. All this he had pursued while practising as a military doctor, where he had developed a particular interest in malaria. But it was not until he met Manson while on leave in London that he discovered his true vocation. Manson managed to convince Ross that the mosquito was a vector for tropical disease. One day, while they were walking together down Oxford Street, Manson had a flash of inspiration. Placing his hand on Ross's shoulder, he exclaimed: 'Do you know, Ross, I have formed the theory that mosquitoes carry malaria, just as they carry my *filaria.*' *Ross was intrigued, and when he returned to India he decided to embark upon an intensive study of malaria.*

Malaria was by now recognized as the most serious epidemic disease operating throughout the world. Its characteristic hot and cold fevers often resulted in death, but even in non-fatal cases the victim was liable to suffer from recurrent debilitating bouts of the fever for the rest of his life. Quinine could alleviate some of these symptoms, but this could not eliminate the disease. The malaria-causing parasite *Plasmodium* had been identified as early as 1880 in Algeria by the French military doctor Alphonse Laveran, who had been influenced by Pasteur. But prevention of malaria remained impossible until it was known how the disease was transmitted.

Meanwhile the situation continued to deteriorate. Widespread figures are not available, but one of the worst instances is well recorded. In 1881 a French project was launched to dig a canal across the isthmus of Panama, linking the Atlantic Ocean to the Pacific. This was led by Ferdinand de Lesseps, who had recently completed the Suez Canal; and one of his collaborators was Gustav Eiffel, constructor of the Eiffel Tower, who was brought in to design the massive locks required. Eight years later the project was abandoned in disarray – the finances had collapsed and over 20,000 workers, most of whom were black West Indian labourers, had died of malaria and other tropical diseases. Panama was now dubbed 'the White Man's grave', an epithet which was also applied to malaria-infested parts of colonial Africa and Asia. Malaria was threatening to render large parts of the globe practically uninhabitable.

Ross's initial investigations of malaria, after his London encounter with Manson and his return to India, met with little success. August 1897 found him still searching for evidence of the parasite *Plasmodium* in the stomachs of mosquitoes which had bitten malaria sufferers, and were therefore thought to be infected. This was a long and laborious business, and he appeared to be getting nowhere. After working at his microscope for several hours continuously in the heat of an Indian summer's day, he found himself despairing:

I was tired, and what was the use? I must have examined the stomachs of a thousand mosquitoes by this time. But the Angel of Fate fortunately laid his hand on my head; and I had scarcely commenced the search again when I saw a clear and almost perfectly circular outline before me of about 12 microns in diameter. The outline was much too sharp, the cell too small to be an ordinary stomach-cell of a mosquito. I looked a little further. Here was another, and another exactly similar cell.

The afternoon was very hot and overcast; and I remember opening the diaphragm of the sub-stage condenser of the microscope to admit more light and then changing the focus. *In each of these cells there was a cluster of small granules, black as jet* and exactly like the black pigments of the *Plasmodium* crescents.

Ross had discovered the secret. He would go on to show that the mosquito acquired the malaria parasite *Plasmodium* through sucking the blood of an infected victim. In the stomach of the mosquito, the malaria parasite bred, and within ten days its offspring had spread into the salivary glands of the mosquito. From this time on the mosquito was infectious, and when biting it passed on droplets of saliva containing malaria parasites. Manson's insight, followed by Ross's discovery, would revolutionize our understanding of tropical diseases.

Just three years beforehand, Koch's Japanese colleague Kitasato had finally succeeded in isolating the plague bacillus *Yersina pestis*. Koch had shown that the disease was somehow caused by rats. In the light of Ross's discovery, another Japanese bacteriologist who had studied under Koch in Germany, Masaki Ogata, was able to show that the plague bacillus was in fact transmitted in a similar fashion to the malaria parasite. This time the vector was a flea which lived on the plague-ridden rat.

By 1904 the Americans had begun a further attempt to dig a canal across the Panama isthmus. Malaria had been only one of the fevers which had led to the collapse of the French project; at one stage yellow fever had been accounting for over 500 workers a month. Despite the French debacle, the American governor of the Panama Canal Zone, General George W. Davis, did not consider disease a problem. He declared that 'spending a dollar a day on sanitation is as good as throwing it in the bay'. The American military doctor appointed to the project was a genial white-haired southern gentleman called William C. Gorgas, whose benign exterior concealed a ruthlessness he had inherited from his Confederate general father. During his previous posting in Havana he had initiated dramatic measures to eliminate mosquitoes, which thanks to Ross and others were now known to be the vector of both malaria and yellow fever. Gorgas had ordered all barrels for the collection of rainwater throughout Havana to be destroyed, and protective screens were erected over all water tanks and wells. At the same time ditches and pools were drained, while kerosene was spread over the surface of larger ponds to exterminate mosquito larvae. As a result, the mosquitoes which carried yellow fever were eliminated, and Havana was cleared of a disease which had been the bane of the city for 150 years.

Gorgas now proceeded to apply similarly ruthless measures in the Panama Canal Zone. With a robust disregard for the local ecology, swamps were drained, the jungle undergrowth was subjected to a scorched earth policy, rivers were liberally doused with kerosene, vast 'mosquito-traps' were set up, and any remnant mosquitoes were mercilessly hunted down by teams of exterminators. When despite this campaign yellow fever flared up again in 1905, Gorgas mobilized every able-bodied man in Panama City to hunt down the culprits with the aid of brushes, ladders and buckets. Those who caught the disease were strictly quarantined, their beds placed within portable isolation cages of sealed mosquito netting. Every room in every house was fumigated, regardless of protest by those who wished to protect their furniture, heirlooms, pets or aged relatives, and the disease was duly eliminated. By the time the Panama Canal was completed in 1916, the Canal Zone had become one of the most disease-free places on earth, far exceeding that of any eastern seaboard city of the United States. Gorgas was now regarded as the leading sanitation expert in the world, travelling to South America and Africa to pass on his expertise. In 1920 he was in London on his way to West Africa when he fell ill. It soon became clear that the 75-year-old Gorgas was dying, whereupon he was visited by King George V, who knighted him for his services to humanity.

15

THE START OF
THE MODERN ERA

On 8 November 1895 the German physicist Wilhelm Röntgen
was in his laboratory at the University of Wurzburg studying
the luminescence which cathode rays cause in various materials. In order to improve the experiment he had darkened the
room and shielded the cathode ray tube with black cardboard.
As he turned on the cathode ray tube, he noticed out of the
corner of his eye a gleam of luminescence on a bench a yard or
so away from where he was working. He found that this was a
sheet of paper coated with barium platinocyanide – one of the
luminescent chemicals he had been testing. When he turned off
the cathode ray tube, the distant luminescence faded. What
was happening? In Röntgen's own words:

No light could come from the tube, because the shield which
covered it was impervious to any light known ... [Yet] I
assumed the effect must have come from the tube, since its

character indicated that it could come from nowehere else . . . I tried it successfully at greater and greater distances . . . It seemed at first a new kind of invisible light. It was clearly something new, something unrecorded . . . Having discovered the existence of a new kind of rays, I of course began to investigate what they would do. It soon appeared from the tests that the rays had penetrative power to a degree hitherto unknown.

Over the next few days, Röntgen conducted a series of further experiments and found that the rays did not reflect off surfaces, like some kinds of invisible light. He remained baffled as to the nature of these mysterious rays, so he gave them the mathematical symbol for an unknown quantity – calling them X-rays.

By now Röntgen was beginning to realize the sensational nature of his discovery. The X-rays could actually see *through* things – not even the scientific fantasies of the great Jules Verne contained anything like this! Röntgen knew that several other scientists were working on luminescence, and realized it would not be long before someone else discovered these rays. Eager to claim priority for his discovery, he set to work on a series of rapid but exhaustive investigations into the properties of his X-rays. He discovered that they could pass through paper, wood and even thin sheets of metal. They may have been invisible, but he found that they did affect photographic plates, which meant that you could record photographic evidence of their passing. Unable to keep the secret any longer, Röntgen brought his wife into the laboratory and took an 'X-ray photograph' of her hand. This clearly revealed the bones and joints of her fingers, as well as the wedding ring on her penultimate finger. Later, Röntgen would confess that only when he saw his X-rays recorded on a photographic plate was he finally convinced that they were not some kind of delusion.

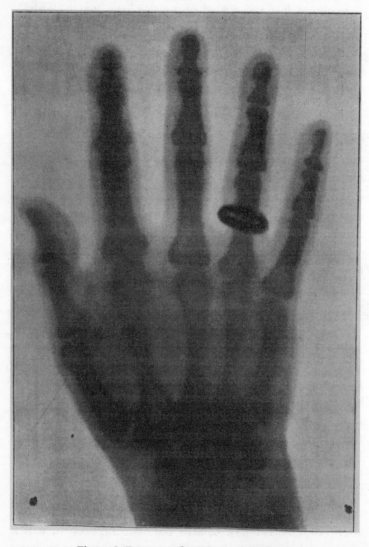

Figure 8. Röntgen's first X-ray photograph
of his wife's hand with a ring on her finger

Within just three weeks Röntgen had prepared a paper on X-rays. News of his discovery spread through the scientific community, and then a newspaper in Vienna obtained the X-ray photograph of the hand of Röntgen's wife. Röntgen's X-rays immediately caught the public imagination, causing an even greater sensation than Pasteur's experiments. X-rays were so simple to produce that in no time they were being put to practical use. Within just four days of Röntgen's discovery reaching America, X-rays had revealed the position of a bullet in a patient's leg. All kinds of dramatic stories began appearing about the properties of the amazing invisible rays. When it became clear that they could see through women's clothing, the state of New Jersey began considering a law banning the use of X-rays in opera glasses in order to protect the virtue of women attending the theatre. Unfortunately, no one else thought of protecting the public from X-rays – it would be several years before it was discovered that prolonged exposure to X-rays caused leukaemia.

Röntgen's almost accidental discovery of X-rays would transform science. It would lead directly to Marie Curie's discovery of radioactive decay and the beginning of nuclear physics. Its effect on medicine would also be immense. Not since the microscope had transformed pathology would an instrument play such a decisive role. Now it was surgery's turn to undergo a similar transformation, and diagnostic medicine too. Previously the physician had relied upon his senses to make a diagnosis – using sight, touch, taste, smell and hearing. Now he had a sixth sense, an entirely new form of vision which enabled his eyes to penetrate the inner space of the patient.

Important developments would soon follow. In 1904 it was discovered that if a patient consumed barium salts the entire digestive tract from the oesophagus through the stomach to the intestines and the rectum could be revealed by radio waves on a fluorescent screen. Likewise, iodine solution injected into the ureter revealed the bladder and the kidneys. And by the 1920s mass X-ray chest screening was being used to detect tuberculosis.

Röntgen had been 50 at the time of his momentous discovery. A good experimentalist, though never a great one, he remained a modest man. He received the many honours, medals and honorary degrees that came his way with genuine gratitude. Though he drew the line at being elevated to the nobility, involving the addition of 'von' to his name. In 1901 he became the first scientist to receive the Nobel Prize for Physics.

Röntgen steadfastly refused to patent his discovery, thus passing up the chance to earn a fortune. He believed that scientific discoveries should be for the benefit of humanity, not their discoverers. At the turn of the twentieth century he was appointed to a prestigious professorship at Munich, a post which he held until 1920 when he was 75. His wife had died the year previously, and the last three years of his life were lived in loneliness and increasing poverty. His savings and pension simply evaporated during the years of the notorious German hyperinflation when the Mark became virtually worthless.

The next major discovery in medicine involved a further advance in our ability to see the inner workings of the human body. This was the ability to grow living cells outside the body from which they came – enabling medical science to experiment for cures to all manner diseases. A century after it was discovered, tissue culture (the artificial cultivation of living matter composed of particular cells) is at the heart of some of medicine's most vital endeavours, such as the search for cures to cancer and AIDS. Unlike X-rays, however, this discovery would not be clear-cut, and would involve three very disparate characters.

The American embryologist Franklin P. Mall grew up during the 1860s on an isolated farm amidst the plains of Iowa. His father had fled Germany during the year of revolution in 1848; his mother, who was also German, died when he was ten. His father soon remarried, but young Franklin's new stepmother felt no love whatsoever for him, and he was soon sent away to a boarding school. Here, perhaps predictably, he buried himself in learning – though not in an expected fashion. Far from burying himself in books, he insisted upon investigating things for himself. This trait would persist through his life (later making him an ardent reformer of medical education). Mall gained his medical degree at the University of Michigan in 1883. Like a number of exceptional American medical students of the period, he then crossed the Atlantic to finish his education in Germany. Mull studied at Leipzig, where he developed a deep interest in the study of the development of the human embryo (embryology). The return home of Mall, and his American contemporaries who had studied in Germany, would mark the beginning of a new era of American medicine, which would soon be on a par with that of Europe.

Mall returned to the United States in 1874, where he ended up taking a position at Johns Hopkins University in Baltimore, at the time the leading medical school in the country. It was here that he published *A Study of Human Monsters* which dealt with the pathology of human embryos. Since earliest times this had been a subject of deep-rooted superstitious fears. Even scientific opinions were deeply divided: was this a matter of heredity, or the environment in the womb? Such so-called human monsters came in a distressing variety of forms, which were studied in aborted foetuses. These included the macerated (wasted, or weakened in some fashion), the compressed or stunted, and the cyclopia (those with a single eye). Experiments carried out on fish eggs had shown that exposing them to anaesthetics at certain critical stages during development could result in deformations such as cyclopia. Mall discovered that pathological human embryos suffered from similar disturbed development, which he called 'dissociation'. The growth of the various tissues and organs in the embryo was controlled by hormones, and Mall found that pathological defects arose when the embryos eluded the control of these hormones, becoming 'dissociated' and allowing the tissues and organs to grow independently, as happens in tissue culture.

Mall would eventually become professor of anatomy at Johns Hopkins. He was a retiring, somewhat dreamy character, but he attracted sharp minds around him who thrived on his original ideas. Early in 1907 he suggested to his colleague Harrison that their work on 'dissociation' might be greatly helped if Harrison could develop a way of artificially cultivating live tissue.

Ross Harrison was a somewhat colourless character, who had also lost his mother at an early age. His father was an engineer who spent most of his time in Russia constructing the St Petersburg to Moscow railway, so that young Ross was brought up by an aunt. He too turned out to be a brilliant and dedicated student, but was always something of a cold fish. Like Mall, he too completed his education in Germany, studying at the University of Bonn, where he finished his medical degree and absorbed a lasting interest in medical biology. At the same time he married a German woman, whom he brought back to Johns Hopkins when he returned to work with Mall.

In 1907 the 47-year-old Harrison was appointed professor of comparative anatomy at Yale. It was in his first year here that he successfully followed up the project which earlier in the year had been suggested to him by Mall – the attempt to grow tissue *in vitro* (literally in glass, as in a test tube or between glass slides under a microscope). The idea may have been

Mall's, but the brilliant technique involved in accomplishing this task was all Harrison's. Using the embryo of a frog (tadpole) Harrison removed the nerve tube and excised nerve cells which had not yet developed fibres. These cells were then viewed through a microscope in a hanging drop of frog lymph containing nourishing protein. As Harrison drily observed of his breakthrough: 'When reasonable aseptic precautions are taken, tissues live under these conditions for a week, and in some cases specimens have been kept alive for nearly four weeks.' Using this 'hanging drop' method, Harrison was able to observe nerve fibres emerge 25 microns from the nerve cells in a period of 25 minutes. This was the first time such 'outgrowth' of nerve fibres had been observed. Not only had Harrison succeeded in growing tissue *in vitro*, but he had also settled the vital question of how nerve fibres are formed. In fact, Harrison was so elated at having discovered how nerve fibres emerge from the nerve cell that he rather overlooked the importance of his discovery that tissue can be grown artifically, independent of the body from which it originated.

The sensational potential of this method for preserving and even creating 'artificial life' would only be exploited some years later by a very different character from the dry, reticent Harrison. After his discovery of 'outgrowth', Harrison gave a series of talks on the subject, during which he would mention how he had developed a method for cultivating live tissue. In 1908 one of these talks was attended by the Frenchman Alexis Carrel, who was working at the newly founded Rockefeller Institute for Medical Research in New York. Carrel immediately realized the importance of tissue culture, and despatched one of his assistants to work with Harrison and discover all he could about the process.

Carrel was a volatile mixture of genuine brilliance, self-promotion and outright charlatanry – along with several less appealing ingredients which would only gradually emerge. He was born Alexis Carrel-Billiard in 1873 on the outskirts of Lyon, the centre of the French textile industry in south-central France. His family were solidly bourgeois and strict Catholics. At school he was bright, but impatient of textbook learning. He quickly displayed an exceptional dexterity and became a medical student with the aim of qualifying as a surgeon. In 1894 the French President Carnot was shot by an anarchist during a visit to Lyon, and the surgeons were unable to save his life owing to their inability to suture (stitch closed) his ruptured artery. This inspired Carrel, who was still a student, to seek a way of overcoming such difficulty. By 1902 he had perfected a method of turning back the ends of severed arteries like cuffs, and sewing them together with fine silk thread in an ingenious manner he had learned from a local lacemaker. This ensured that the only surface exposed to the circulating blood was the wall of the vessel itself, thus avoiding clotting of the blood, which tends to adhere to uneven surfaces in the blood vessel.

Despite this brilliant coup, Carrel did not achieve the promotion that he felt was his due at the University of Lyon. He was an aloof but outspoken character, and also had unscientific views which his colleagues found anathema. Carrel was a devout Catholic, and on his regular pilgrimages to Lourdes, the Catholic holy shrine, he became convinced that he had witnessed a number of miracles. In consequence, he argued that science should broaden its thinking to include the influence of the spirit world. In 1904 he resigned his post at Lyon in a fit of pique; whereupon he left for Canada, saying he was going to work as a cowboy. But this aberration soon passed, and he ended up as a visiting experimentalist at the University of Chicago. Here he brilliantly extended his work on suturing blood vessels by transplanting the kidneys, ovaries and even legs of dogs. He also discovered that animals grafted with organs which were not from their own species invariably died, as a result of rejecting the alien organ. In a matter of a few years, Carrel had laid the foundations for modern transplant surgery, even discovering the concept of 'rejection'.

As intended, these sensational operations brought Carrel to public notice, and in 1906 he accepted a post at the Rockefeller Institute for Medical Research in New York. Here his superior, slightly ridiculous manner made him few friends. He insisted upon wearing his white surgeon's cap at lunch in the staff dining room, where he spoke to no one but important visitors. Yet it was here in New York that he excelled himself. No sooner had he learned Harrison's method of tissue culture than he began using it to spectacular effect. He succeeded in cultivating a wide range of tissues *in vitro*, including human tissue. He also managed to preserve some tissue from a chicken's heart in clotted chicken plasma (blood) for 120 days. Carrel had quickly understood the methods of the American press, and made sure that his scientific feat was widely publicized. The resultant headlines were sensational, if not strictly accurate: 'Scientist Keeps Heart Alive in Test Tube'. He then went one step further, dividing cultured chicken tissue and placing it in further plasma, where it grew. This process was repeated every few days, thus keeping the tissue alive indefinitely. The papers were soon running headlines about the scientist who had managed to create an immortal chicken's heart. This heart would be kept alive for over 30 years, providing a constant source of publicity for Carrel. Each year on New Year's Day, the *New York Times* would carry an announcement that Carrel's chicken heart was still alive.

In 1912 Carrel was awarded the Nobel Prize. This caused a furore in the American medical community, which protested that it should have gone to Harrison. In fact, this outrage was unwarranted: Carrel had been given the prize for his research into organ transplants and repairing blood vessels. Even so, Harrison would never receive the Nobel Prize for his discovery of how to 'grow' tissue – which undoubtedly represented an even greater breakthrough than Carrel's work.

In later years, Carrel's thirst for fame would know no bounds, not even medical ones. He began cultivating famous figures in American society. In 1927 Lindberg flew the first solo flight across the Atlantic and became the most famous man in America. Soon after this Carrel joined up with Lindberg and began using a sterilizable glass pump, designed by Lindberg, to keep his transplant organs alive. In 1935 Carrel published *Man, the Unknown*, which contained 300 pages of his profound thoughts on the future of humanity and the state of history. In the course of this he praised Mussolini, placing him among the 'men of genius', adding for good measure that 'great leaders of nations grow beyond human stature.' He also opined that 'the weak should not be artificially maintained in wealth and power . . . social classes should be synonymous with biological classes.' Carrel may have understood the machinations of the American publicity machine, but he had misunderstood American democracy.

In 1939 at the outbreak of the war in Europe he returned to France. When the Nazis overran France and Petain set up a collaborationist government in Vichy, Carrel was offered the post of Minister of Health. But by now he had even more important things to do. He had set up his Institute for the Study of Human Progress, which began preparing his plans for the future of France after the war (which he expected Hitler to win). Carrel's Institute also launched into what were intended to be literally world-shattering studies of the spirit world, telepathy and other paranormal phenomena.

After the liberation of France by the Allies in 1944 Carrel

was due to be arrested, but died of a heart attack before he could be charged with treason. It would take another 20 years before his 'immortal chicken heart' was revealed to have been a fake. No one had ever managed to duplicate his feat, and it now became clear why. Research showed that chicken heart cells invariably died after they had been subdivided a few dozen times: to retain their appearance of immortality, his original chicken cells must have been surreptitiously mixed with additional live cells at regular intervals. Despite this, Carrel's genuine contributions remain outstanding. Among these, his method of suturing blood vessels (anastomosis) was an astonishing feat of intricate and ingenious surgery. And his pioneer work in organ transplants was truly revolutionary. The less said about the rest, including the man himself, the better.

As the twentieth century progressed, the important advances in medicine came so thick and fast that it would be impossible to describe them all. However, there still remained some outstanding discoveries which transformed both the practice and the understanding of medicine. One of these was the discovery of vitamins. In the mid-eighteenth century James Lind had overcome scurvy by prescribing citrus juice for British sailors. Although he himself did not understand that scurvy was due to a deficiency, others soon began to suspect that this was the case. Yet with no understanding of proper dietary requirements, or how the body absorbed and made use of particular foodstuffs, any advance in the field remained blocked.

The first advance came in 1897, when the Dutch colonial doctor Christiaan Eijkman was part of a team investigating beri-beri in Java (now part of Indonesia). Beri-beri comes from the Sinhalese word *beri* meaning 'weakness', its repetition intended as emphasis. The disease attacks the peripheral nerves, resulting in lack of sensation, especially in the legs, loss of muscle power and general weakness. Its weakening of the cardiac muscles leads to heart failure and death. Similar symptoms were first noted by western physicians as early as 24 BC among Roman sailors travelling down the coast of the Red Sea. By the end of the nineteenth century beri-beri had become the scourge of Southeast Asia, and was so prevalent throughout the Far East that it was known as 'the natural disease of Japan'. In the light of Pasteur's discoveries it was thought that the disease must be caused by a particular bacteria. As the disease also affected animals, the Dutch colonial authorities in Java began a series of trials with chickens. Groups of chickens with beri-beri were studied, together with isolated control groups of healthy chickens. It was Eijkman who first noticed that a number of the isolated chickens also succumbed to the disease. Further tests led him to suspect that perhaps the disease had something to do with diet. He then discovered that some of the chickens had been fed surplus polished white rice from the stores, rather than their usual rough unpolished rice which still retained the husks. The disease only seemed to affect the chickens which had been fed polished rice. Beri-beri was far too dangerous to carry out tests on human beings, but Eijkman knew that it was prevalent in the prisons of Java. He then carried out a survey of all the 84 prisons on the island of Java, sending out a questionnaire to the governors, asking them to list relative conditions, crowd-ing, ventilation, as well as details of diet. Eijkman discovered that in prisons which used white polished rice, 71 per cent were affected by beri-beri; whereas those which fed the prisoners rough unpolished rice only had a 3 per cent incidence of beri-beri. Eijkman concluded that this was due to a toxin in the white rice, whose natural antidote was produced by the husks of the unpolished rice. But before he could make any further tests, he himself fell ill and was forced to return to Europe on sick leave.

The next advance came in 1906 from the British researcher Frederick Hopkins at Cambridge. Hopkins, a relative of the Jesuit poet Gerard Manley Hopkins, had at the age of 37 been appointed the first lecturer in chemical physiology at Cambridge University. The post was ill-paid and he was forced to take on extra tutoring to support his wife and young family. On top of this, he was determined to continue with research he had begun into the constituents of human diet. He experimented with rats, feeding them on cheese, lard, sugar, starch and salt – all the generally recognized constituents of a healthy diet. Yet he found that these rats soon began to languish. He then fed some of them with a supplement of fresh milk, and they immediately began to thrive. He found that 'astonishingly small amounts' of milk were required to bring about such transformation. This led him to develop the idea of 'accessory food factors', which were somehow required to enable the body to benefit from normally required foodstuffs.

As a result of overwork, Hopkins' health broke down in 1910 and he was unable to continue with his research. He would recover, but later in life illness left him blind. However, in 1929 he and Eijkman were jointly awarded the Nobel Prize for their work. This was in recognition of their pioneer research which led directly to a major discovery in 1912 by the Polish chemist Casimir Funk, working at the Lister Institute in London.

Funk had been born in Warsaw in 1884, but owing to Russian restrictions on the education of Poles was forced to finish his education at Bern in Switzerland (at the very same time as Einstein was working there at the patent office, thinking out his special theory of relativity). Funk then did research work in Germany. Unfortunately he produced results which contradicted those of his superior, who wrongly dismissed his work as faulty. Partly on account of this, Funk ended up in London. Here he decided to investigate Eijkman's findings about polished and unpolished rice and its effect on beri-beri. Using pigeons, he managed to confirm Eijkman's findings, but he then discovered that a supplement of yeast to the pigeons' diet also cured beri-beri. This indicated that the cause of the disease was not some toxin contained in polished rice, but a lack of the 'accessory food factors' suggested by Hopkins. Funk speculated that these factors were amines, so he called these dietary supplements 'vitamines' (vital amines). Funk surmised that these vitamines somehow helped the body to use the foodstuffs of its normal diet, and provided it with energy for renewal and growth.

Having linked beri-beri with vitamine deficiency, Funk now felt sure that lack of vitamines was also the cause of scurvy, as well as pellogra (a skin disease) and possibly rickets, all of which appeared to result from a deficiency rather than bacteria. However, such opinions were largely disregarded at the time, mainly because the medical profession remained in the thrall of Pasteur's persuasive bacteria theory.

It soon became clear to Funk that there were probably several different types of amine, which were vital for different processes. Unfortunately, circumstances were to prevent him from playing an immediate role in the development of the vitamine idea. When World War I broke out in 1914, London was overcome by patriotic hysteria, and as a German-speaking Pole Funk had several unpleasant experiences. In 1916 he accepted a post at the Harriman Research Laboratory in New York, and crossed the Atlantic with his new Belgian bride. He arrived to find that the laboratory had no equipment and no funds. In desperation, he was forced to find work as an industrial chemist in New Jersey. After a breakdown brought on by the strain of his situation, Funk finally found work at the more prestigous Metz Company of New York, though still as an industrial chemist. The U-boat war in the Atlantic had cut off the supply of Salvarsan, the new drug used to treat syphilis, but Funk was able to synthesize this and thus ensure limited supplies. In 1920 he became a United States citizen, but later returned to work in Warsaw and then Paris before settling permanently in America where he worked for the US Vitamin Corporation.

The first vitamines were isolated soon after Funk's initial discovery. In 1913 Thomas B. Osborne of the Connecticut Agricultural Experimental Station in New Haven detected in butter a substance which promoted growth. This soon became known as fat-soluble vitamine A (its precise chemical constituents would be discovered in 1933, and it would first be synthesized in 1947). In 1916 Osborne isolated another vitamine which was present in milk, rice polishings and yeast. This became known as vitamine B (chemical constituents discovered in 1926, synthesized 1936).

Other developments in the vitamine field followed much as Funk had suspected they would. For many years the smog-shrouded slums of the industrial cities of Europe and America, as well as poverty-stricken remote rural areas such as the west of Ireland, had suffered from rickets, which causes defective bone growth. In 1900 it was discovered that as many as 80 per cent of the children under two in the city of Boston were suffering from this disease, which Funk hypothesized was due to a vitamine deficiency. In 1919 the British researcher Edward Mellanby managed to induce rickets in puppies which had been maintained on a diet lacking in certain animal fats. When some of the puppies were dosed with cod liver oil this cured the rickets, and Mellanby concluded that rickets was due to a deficiency of fat-soluble vitamin A. In 1922 it was discovered that vitamine A in fact consisted of two vitamines, only one of which was responsible for curing rickets. This became known as vitamine D. This vitamine was then introduced into milk supplies in the United States and proved highly effective in the elimination of rickets. When it was realized that not all vitamines were amines, these substances became known as vitamins.

The way forward lay in deeper understanding of the chemistry of the human body, and the most significant advance in this field came from Germany, where the legacy of Koch still prevailed. The man responsible for this progress would be a biological chemist who for many years worked closely, though not always comfortably, with Koch and his colleagues. This was Paul Ehrlich – whose many achievements included founding haematology (the study of the blood and its diseases), a major breakthrough in immunology, but most of all the founding of chemotherapy (the treatment of infection by drugs).

Ehrlich was born in 1854 in the small country town of Strehlen, in a region of southern Poland that was then part of the Austro-Hungarian Empire. His family was Jewish and his father was an eccentric character who ran a number of local businesses including a distillery and a lottery. Ehrlich would inherit a mild version of this quirkiness, but developed a genius that was all his own. He was only moderately bright at school, his full talents unexpectedly emerging when he went to study medicine at the University of Leipzig. Here he became enthralled by the study of biochemistry, to such an extent that he was making major discoveries even before he received his medical degree and passed on to the Charité Hospital at Berlin.

Ehrlich's major advance was in the technique of staining different cells so that they could be easily identified, and their behaviour observed, under the microscope. Previously white blood cells had proved resistant to ordinary aqueous dyes, but Ehrlich found a way of staining them with aniline dye. This enabled him to discover a new variety of white cells called 'mast' cells, and also to distinguish various blood disorders. This laid the foundation of haematology. He also succeeded in staining the bacilli of tuberculosis, which Koch had only recently identified; Ehrlich's breakthrough facilitated the microscopic diagnosis of the disease. In the course of this work he became infected with tuberculosis himself, and was forced to leave Berlin in 1886 with his new wife and spend two years in the warm dry climate of Egypt. This improved his condition, and on his return to Berlin he underwent Koch's controversial tuberculin treatment. Despite tuberculin's dubious powers, all this must have had a beneficial effect, for Ehrlich remained free of tuberculosis throughout the rest of his life.

After working for a time in a makeshift laboratory of his own, which he set up in a rented apartment, Ehrlich was invited to join Koch's institute. The antitoxin agent which cured diphtheria had recently been isolated here, but the precise method by which bacteria caused disease remained unknown, as did the method by which antitoxins actually worked. Ehrlich's experiments led him to develop his 'side chain' theory, which arose directly from his study of dyes and his study of the blood. If cells had 'receptors' that accepted the dye, thus staining them, Ehrlich reasoned that cells must also have receptors that accepted drugs. His study of the protoplasmic molecule (protein) led him to discover that it had trailing 'side chains' which could absorb foodstuffs and neutralize toxins. When the latter process happened, preventing its normal function, it manufactured extra side chains which were matched to this particular toxin. These 'antibodies' were then shed and passed into the bloodstream, where they served to neutralize the toxin.

Ehrlich found that by injecting horses with diphtheria toxin, and then removing the blood serum containing the antibodies, he could use this as an immunizing agent for injecting into human beings. Measuring the necessary strength of the serum was evidently essential, and Ehrlich managed to develop a standard for gauging the effectiveness of the serum that was adopted throughout the world.

Althought the anti-diphtheria serum proved successful, it soon became clear that serum treatment would not be effective for all diseases, especially those caused not by bacteria but by protozoa (the smallest and simplest of all living creatures). This led Ehrlich to a turning point. Instead of serums, he would seek to discover chemicals that attacked the toxins. In his own words, he would create materials 'in the chemist's retort [that would] be able to exert their full action exclusively on the parasite harboured within the organism and would represent, so to speak, magic bullets which seek their target of their own accord'. This was the beginning of chemotherapy: the treatment of infections by drugs (artificial antibodies) that neutralize, or poison, the infecting agent without harming the patient.

Partly as a result of his success with diphtheria, in 1899 Ehrlich left Berlin and was placed in charge of his own institute in Frankfurt. Another reason for this move appears to have been his inability to get on with Koch's assistants. Ehrlich was not an easy man to work with. Outside his research he was a man of little culture – his only pastime appears to have been reading Sherlock Holmes stories. Otherwise he remained obsessive in his attempt to solve nature's crimes, in the form of infectious diseases. Although he was a font of original ideas and techniques, his determination to follow his own ideas at all costs did not always endear him to others. He would frequently divert his energies from the task at hand to follow what appeared to be serendipitous research. But Ehrlich's method of following his nose would soon provide spectacular results.

Ehrlich began experimenting on mice infected with the protozoa trypanosoma, which causes tropical diseases such as sleeping sickness. His previous attempts to dye organisms led him to suspect that this protozoa might be susceptible to coal-tar dyes. In 1904 he found a cure in the form of trypan red, thus discovering the first chemotheraputic agent. However, further tests proved that this chemical was not always effective. The difficulty was to find a chemical which was sufficiently toxic to kill the germs, without killing the host. For instance, disinfectant would certainly kill all germs in the bloodstream, but it would also kill the patient. On the other hand, many dyes simply proved too weak. Ehrlich considered that the effectiveness of trypan red was due to the combinations of nitrogen atoms it contained. He knew that arsenic resembled nitrogen in its properties, but had slightly more powerful poisonous qualities. As a result he began experimenting with similarly configured arsenic compounds.

Ehrlich could be extremely methodical and tenacious when he felt he was on the scent of something, and this proved no exception. By 1907 he and his assistants had systematically experimented with almost a thousand arsenic compounds, yet with no success. It was only then that Ehrlich's team made an almost accidental breakthrough. When a new Japanese assistant called Sahachiro Hata joined the team, Ehrlich told him to start by checking some of their previous results. When Hata reached 'Preparation 606', the arsenic compound dihydroxydiamino-arsenobenzene hydrochloride, he confirmed that it did not affect trypanosomes. He then checked whether it affected the similar bacteria spirochaetes, and this time it did prove effective. Ehrlich at once realized the significance of this. Among the spirochaetes was the bacteria treponema pallidum, the dreaded organism that caused syphilis. It looked as if they had found a cure for one of history's most persistent and grotesque diseases.

By now syphilis was being treated with a chemical concoction of mercury, which only tended to halt the passage of the disease, never curing it. This had led to the bleak witticism, neatly involving the planets, the Greek gods and chemistry: 'One night on Venus, followed by a lifetime on Mercury.' This saying has been attributed to both Baudelaire and Oscar Wilde, two of many who suffered from this 'disease of genius', but it is probably the work of that most varied of all geniuses Anon. However, the cure to which it refers was no witty matter. The effects of prolonged mercury treatment were often almost as bad as the disease itself, for mercury is a cumulative poison which destroys the nervous system. Syphilis itself had three stages, with the tertiary stage liable to rot the nerves, bone or organs and usually reducing the patient to imbecility, catatonia, or other forms of insanity. By the turn of the twentieth century the leading cause of insanity in asylums throughout Europe and America was syphilis; while the pitiful problem of children with inherited syphilis was growing in many large cities.

Ehrlich named his new cure for syphilis salvarsan 606 (the salvation arsenic preparation 606), and immediately embarked upon an exhaustive series of tests, including injecting himself to make doubly sure. Because of the high arsenic content in the drug, it did sometimes have poisonous side effects – but the benefits far outweighed the drawbacks. Ehrlich's high principles and wilfulness were what made him a difficult man in the laboratory, but they would also make him a great man outside it. Having discovered salvarsan, he entered into a tightly negotiated agreement with the German chemical firm Farbwerke-Hoechst by which they would only gain the sole rights to manufacture the drug by first distributing 65,000 units of salvarsan throughout the globe free of charge. Within a few years thousands were being cured of this appalling disease. Syphilis had received its magic bullet.

The chemotheraputic revolution had begun. Ehrlich's method had shown the way forward, and the race was now on to find a chemical cure for each one of the world's major infectious diseases. Yet to the surprise of all, this proved a false start. Despite immense efforts, and the prospect of immense rewards, virtually no progress was made in chemotherapy for over 20 years. Ehrlich's methodology was undoubtedly sound, but it was not producing the expected results. Then a breakthrough was finally made by the German industrial chemist Gerhard Domagk, who was working for the dye firm I. G. Farbenindustrie. Following up the work by Ehrlich, Domagk had been researching the possible antibacterial effects of dyes for several years, but with no success. Then in 1932 he discovered that the bright red dye prontosil appeared to cure a streptococcus infection in mice. Before he could undertake any thorough investigation of this effect, his young daughter Hildegarde fell seriously ill with streptococcus infection after pricking her finger with a needle. As a last resort, Domagk began injecting her with sizeable amounts of prontosil. Almost immediately, this brought about his daughter's recovery. Newspaper reports of this 'miracle cure' spread the name of prontosil far and wide. It received even greater publicity a few years later when it saved the life of F. D. Roosevelt, Jr, the son of the president of the United States.

By now, prontosil had also been found to cure other streptococcal infections such as tonsilitis, scarlet fever and puerperal fever. The effective ingredient of prontosil was a sulphur compound (sulphonamide) which did not in fact kill the bacteria, merely prevented it from reproducing, thus allowing the body's natural antibodies to destroy the infectious agent.

In 1939 Domagk was awarded the Nobel Prize for Physiology or Medicine for his work with prontosil. By now the Nazis had come to power in Germany, and Hitler had forbidden any Germans from accepting the prize, after the 1935 Nobel Peace Prize had been awarded to Karl von Ossietsky, who was at the time in a concentration camp. To ensure that Domagk did not accept his Nobel Prize, the Gestapo raided his home and detained him in jail for a week – though fortunately he was able to collect his prize in 1947, after Hitler and Nazism had both been defeated.

Prontosil was only effective on streptococcal infections, but sulphur-based drugs were soon discovered which were effective against pneumococci, the cause of various types of pneumonia. The sulphonamides passed into widespread use, though they would later be overshadowed by the development of antibiotics. The word antibiotic literally means 'anti biological life', and in medical usage refers to living organisms that kill bacterial life within the body. (The sulphanomides were of course not living organisms.)

The first antibiotic had in fact had been discovered a few years prior to Domagk's breakthrough, but owing to a series of scarcely credible mishaps it would not be developed for use until 1940. This was penicillin, which was accidentally discovered by Alexander Fleming as early as 1928, and then largely ignored. This was due to a combination of circumstance and character. Alexander Fleming was born on a remote hill farm in the lowlands of Scotland in 1881. His father died when he was young, leaving the family in straitened circumstances; and after leaving school at sixteen young Alexander went south to London where he found employment as a lowly shipping clerk. He worked at this for five years, before gaining a scholarship in 1902 to study medicine at London University. Fleming completed his studies at St Mary's, one of the top London hospitals, where he was renowned as a crack scholar and a crack shot. Mainly as a result of the latter, he was given a place in the hospital's inoculation department, and was soon helping St Mary's to retain the coveted Inter-Hospital Shooting Trophy.

The man who was responsible for Fleming's appointment was Sir Almroth Wright, a larger-than-life aristocratic character who had created the inoculation department and would rule over it in autocratic fashion throughout Fleming's career. Wright may have been a man of forthright opinions, but he was also a man of considerable medical skill, who happened to be a personal friend of Ehrlich. In time, Fleming would become Wright's assistant, rising to the rank of professor, yet he would always maintain a self-effacing pose at work, ever respectful of his domineering boss.

Fleming specialized in the treatment of syphilis, and over the years built up a thriving private practice which included several important society and political figures. As a result he soon became a rich man, with a flat in fashionable Chelsea, and later a country house in Suffolk set in extensive grounds with its own fishing stream. When Ehrlich sent Sir Almroth Wright a sample of the newly discovered salvarsan, Wright dismissively passed this on to Fleming. Wright was convinced that 'antibacterial drugs are a delusion' – an opinion which was widely held among the London medical establishment. Fleming tried out salvarsan with some of his patients, found that it worked, and soon became responsible for the new drug being used throughout the country. Yet at the same time he continued to support Wright's views that such drugs were a delusion. As later events will show, Fleming appears to have genuinely believed Wright's claim, despite his anomalous advocacy of salvarsan.

Fleming was a distinctly double-sided character. On his way home from St Mary's, after another long day diffidently endured in Wright's shadow, Fleming was in the habit of calling in at the Chelsea Arts Club. Here he transformed himself into a gregarious man-about-town, very much at home among the convivial artistic members, several of whom were also his patients. Some of these were in the habit of paying him with examples of their work, and in this way Fleming's Chelsea flat and country house soon acquired a fine collection of English contemporary art.

During World War I Fleming served in the Royal Army Medical Corps in France, where he discovered that the anti-septics used to cleanse the wounds of the casualties were largely inadequate. They were often so strong that they in-hibited the body's natural healing processes, and frequently did not even destroy the bacteria causing the infection. Deaths from gangrene were horrendously frequent. After the war Fleming returned to St Mary's, where he set about trying to discover a more effective antibacterial agent. In 1921 he isolated and identified lysozyme, an enzyme found in tears and mucus, which showed promising antibacterial potential. But progress was slow, and after seven years he was still conducting experiments. It was now that a series of astonish-ing coincidences and fortunate accidents brought about the great discovery which made Fleming's name.

During August 1928, London was experiencing a prolonged heatwave, and Fleming was working in his laboratories with the windows open. In the laboratory on the floor below him, they were conducting experiments on how certain types of bacteria spores disperse through the atmosphere. They too were working with the windows open. It was the last day before Fleming left for his summer holiday, and he was preparing a final petri dish of staphylococcus, the bacteria which is responsible for pus in infected wounds and abcesses. In the course of this preparation, the staphylococcus was briefly exposed to the air, during which time some of the spores from the laboratory below fell into the petri dish. For some reason, instead of placing the petri dish in the incubator to encourage the growth of the staphylococcus, he left it on the laboratory bench.

When Fleming returned some weeks later, he found that the staphylococcus in the petri dish had grown. But in amongst this there were specks of mould, around which the staphylococcus had been destroyed. Fleming immediately decided to investigate this interesting phenomenon, and discovered that the specks of mould were *Penicillium notatum*, a mould similar to the blue-green mould that grows on stale bread. Fleming succeeded in isolating the active ingredient of this, which he called penicillin. He then made a culture, and began investigating its properties. He found to his amazement that penicillin not only destroyed staphylococcus but also four other cocci which were responsible for a wide range of bacterial infection (including such virulent diseases as syphilis). Then he discovered that penicillin had no toxic effect on healthy tissue. Penicillin killed bacteria, but was not harmful to human beings.

The accident of the spores entering the window, and then being given two weeks to act upon the staphylococcus, all in exceptionally favourable conditions, had resulted in a remarkable discovery. And these were not the only accidents. Had Fleming placed the petri dish in the incubator, which was maintained at 38°C, this would have killed off the penicillin-bearing spores. Even the hot temperature of the heatwave would soon have done this. But the day Fleming left for his holidays, the heatwave had broken and the temperature had fallen to precisely the most favourable temperature for the *Penicillium notatum* to grow. As Pasteur had maintained: 'Chance favours the prepared mind.' But precisely how prepared had Fleming been? He now encountered his first, minor setbacks. In the course of further experiments he found that although penicillin killed four powerful bacteria, it did not destroy the bacteria which caused bubonic plague or cholera. He also discovered that penicillin was difficult to produce, and even then it was unstable, whereupon he seems to have given up. Astonishingly, it seems he never even thought of testing penicillin on the actual spirochates that cause syphilis.

Fleming wrote up his experiments in a paper, which was published with no indication of any particular importance, in the comparatively obscure *British Journal of Experimental Pathology*. Then he simply returned to his experiments with lysozyme, which was much easier to produce. All he had to do was rub his eye with lemon, and collect the tear drops. Penicillin had been discovered, and almost as quickly it had been forgotten.

Amazingly, this situation would continue for *ten years* – during which countless patients throughout the world died of bacterial infection ranging from gangrene to syphilis. The breakthrough, when it came, would also include some remarkable circumstances. In 1939 the Australian pathologist Howard Florey was working at Oxford, investigating the properties of lysozyme. However, he was not investigating its antibacterial qualities. He knew of Fleming's long and unsuccessful researches into this aspect of lysozyme, and had instead decided to investigate its possible role in combating gastric ulcers.

Florey had been born 40 years previously at Adelaide in Australia, coming to Oxford on a Rhodes scholarship in 1922.

Shortly after this he spent four years doing research in America, where his affable Australian manner ensured him a certain popularity. During this period he made a wide circle of acquaintances, who admired his expert technique as a biochemist and also his ability to enthuse those around him. On his return to England he came to the notice of Sir Edward Mellanby, who had now been knighted for his pioneer work in vitamin research, and was by this stage running Britain's influential Medical Research Council. Mellanby was so impressed by Florey that he put him in charge of a research team at Oxford. One day in 1939 this team was joined by Ernst Chain, a refugee from Nazi Germany who was then in his thirties and according to all accounts bore an uncanny resemblance to Einstein. Chain had been born in Berlin, the son of a Russian businessman who had made his fortune in the chemical industry. His mother had been related to Kurt Eisner, who during the chaotic days following Germany's World War I defeat had briefly established a Bolshevik republic in Bavaria, before being assassinated. Young Ernst Chain had initially been a musical prodigy, before opting to study chemistry with similar virtuosity. When Hitler came to power in 1933, Chain had been forced to flee the country because of his Jewish ancestry. On his arrival in Britain, he had quickly attracted attention. He not only looked like a genius, he was one. Coincidentally, he too had been given a helping hand by one of the pioneers of vitamin research – in this case, Sir Frederick Hopkins, who had also been knighted for his work, and was now president of the Royal Society. It was on Hopkins's recommendation that Chain ended up on Florey's research team at Oxford. The two men quickly established a rapport. Chain's effervescent manner matched with Florey's affability, and may even have penetrated to the essentially friendless lonely man beneath this easy-going exterior.

Unfortunately, by the time Chain arrived at Oxford Florey's research group had run out of money. The world was in the grip of the Great Depression, and there was little funding available for research. Florey had manfully done his best, but now his research account was £500 overdrawn at the bank, a sizeable sum in the days when a working man's weekly wage was £5. By this stage, Florey was not even allowed to buy so much as a glass test-tube. But he had an ace up his sleeve. Through his contacts in America he had heard that the Rockefeller Foundation was interested in setting up ambitious long-term research projects, and he also knew that his American friends would probably back any application he made for funds.

Florey had only achieved inconclusive results with the research into lysozyme as an ulcer retardant, and to keep Chain occupied he asked him to read through Fleming's other research projects in the hope of turning up something similar. Chain came across Fleming's paper on penicillin and brought this to Florey's notice. Florey was interested and decided that they should apply for a grant to make a systematic search of the whole field of antibacterial agents. The application was successful, and the team started to investigate the two most readily available substances – pyocyanase, and a substance obtained from the common fungus actinomycetes. Florey and Chain knew that work was already under way in Germany on pyocyanase, so they chose to start on this. Britain was now at war with Germany, and the discovery of an effective antibacterial agent would prove of inestimable value to any army. Instead of soldiers dying of infected wounds in field hospitals, they could quickly be put on the road to recovery. There was no time to lose.

But Florey's researches into pyocyanase proved disappointing; initial investigations indicated that this antibacterial agent appeared to be highly toxic. There then followed another series of astonishing coincidences. In a corridor of the research building, Chain happened to run into Margaret Campbell-Renton, an acquaintance working on another research project. When he casually mentioned how his own research project had begun after he had read Fleming's paper on penicillin, Campbell-Renton replied that she actually had some culture grown from Fleming's original mould in her laboratory – a remnant of an abortive investigation years previously by her professor. On a hunch, Chain decided to put aside his work on pyocyanase and see if he could get any better results with Fleming's mould. He set to work, and was soon joined by Florey; between the two of them they eventually managed to overcome Fleming's problem and learned how to stabilize penicillin by freeze-drying it. However, this did not overcome an even greater difficulty: isolating the active ingredient from the dissolved mould proved extremely difficult. Initially, all they could obtain was one part of pure penicillin to every two million parts of liquid. Through sheer perseverance they eventually managed to obtain sufficient for an experiment. Eight mice were injected with highly infectious streptococci, then four of them were also injected with penicillin. Next day they found that all four of those injected with penicillin were alive and healthy, while the other four were dead. Even more significantly, they noticed that the urine of these healthy mice had turned brown. Upon investigation, this discoloration was found to be caused by penicillin itself, which had passed right through the body unaltered. This indicated that the penicillin was able to pass into fluids throughout the entire body. Florey and Chain understood at once the significance of this. Not only had they discovered a new extremely powerful antibacterial agent, but this also had practically no toxic effect.

Immediately they set about growing as much of the mould as

possible in any way they could. Milk bottles, saucepans, bed pans and even a bathtub were all pressed into service, until eventually they estimated that they had extracted enough penicillin to carry out a test on a human being. As 20 milligrams of penicillin had proved effective but harmless for a mouse, Florey estimated 'a man is three thousand times the size of a mouse', so 100 grams would be safe yet effective for a human being. Before this hasty calculation could be called into question, they were presented with their first case – an emergency. A policeman had been stricken with staphylococcal septicaemia (extreme bacterial blood-poisoning) after scratching his finger while pruning roses in his garden. The infection had spread rapidly, and he was not expected to live. The policeman was injected at regular intervals with penicillin, and by the fourth day had begun making an almost miraculous recovery. But there was one snag. By this stage they had run so short of penicillin that they were forced to collect the policeman's urine and recycle all they could from this source. Finally, they ran out of penicillin altogether. Almost immediately the policeman took a turn for the worse, and soon he was dead.

Despite this failure, it was evident to Florey that penicillin was one of the most valuable medical discoveries of all time. He immediately set about contacting all the pharmaceutical companies in Britain, using his considerable personal skills to the full in the attempt to get penicillin mass-produced. The question of patenting the new drug hardly even occurred to him. But no commercial firm was able to help. It was now 1940, the darkest days of the war; the Nazis had overrun Europe and Britain was on its own, facing the prospect of an imminent invasion from across the Channel. The Luftwaffe were carrying out a blitz on Britain's industrial cities; meanwhile Britain's lifeline – the convoys across the Atlantic from America – were suffering huge losses from U-boat attacks. At this point, Florey and Chain became so afraid the Germans would overrun the country that they rubbed precious penicillin into the lining of their clothes. If either of them managed to escape the Germans and make it to America, they would be able to carry the secret with them.

Fortunately, this desperate measure proved unnecessary, and in 1941 Florey was able to cross the Atlantic with more orthodox samples of penicillin. Knowing at first hand American laboratory methods, he felt sure that they would soon find a way of manufacturing penicillin more efficiently. His hope proved justified, and chemists at the National Regional Research Laboratory at Peoria, Illinois came up with a method of producing penicillin which was 34 times better than anything Florey and Chain had previously managed. By 1943 the British too were beginning to mass-produce penicillin. Florey travelled to North Africa, where he oversaw its administration in troop hospitals, yet not without facing opposition. The medical authorities on the spot still adhered to Sir Almroth Wright's belief that antibacterial drugs were a delusion and condemned Florey's efforts in no uncertain terms, declaring, 'It's murder.' But Florey was soon able to demonstrate penicillin's effectiveness: it proved particularly effective in eliminating contagious infection and pus from wounds exposed to the flies of the desert.

In 1944 the Russian-American bacteriologist Selman Waksman, working at Rutgers University in New Jersey, succeeded in producing another powerful antibacterial agent streptomycin, which succeeded in destroying bacteria that had proved immune to penicillin, such as the tercule bacillus. The discovery of further antibacterial agents would soon follow – probably the most important being chloramphenicol, which proved effective against typhoid. These drugs soon came to be known collectively as 'antibiotics', and after an initial minor dispute it was accepted that Waksman was the man who first coined this name.

However, a rather less seemly priority battle was now taking place in Britain. When Florey, Chain and his Oxford researchers had published their famous paper in *The Lancet* in August 1940, making public their discovery of penicillin, they had met with a violent riposte from Sir Almroth Wright. He had written to *The Lancet* protesting that penicillin had in fact been discovered in his laboratory at St Mary's as early as 1928, by his assistant Fleming. This letter produced yet another unexpected result. Florey, who had never been shy in his attempts to win friends and influence people, uncharacteristically declined to press claims on behalf of himself and his Oxford team – even though they had unquestionably played the major role in developing penicillin as an antibiotic. Fleming, on the other hand, emerged from his shell. He began revelling in the publicity, taking every opportunity to assert his claim as the discoverer of 'the new wonder drug', as the newspapers now called it. Soon even the press were taking sides in the dispute. Florey was erroneously reported as having made a slighting remark about the British press, whereupon Lord Beaverbrook the powerful owner of the *Daily Express* took umbrage, suggesting that the inevitable Nobel Prize for this historic discovery should be awarded to Fleming alone, rather than any jumped-up Australian and his crew of immigrants. (Beaverbrook was of course an immigrant himself, from Canada, but had now become a naturalized Briton.) Fortunately sanity prevailed in the end, and in 1945 the Nobel Prize for Physiology or Medicine was awarded jointly to Fleming, Florey and Chain. This was one of the quickest Nobel awards ever made: the historic breakthrough and the huge benefits of penicillin in terms of lives, as well as the elimination of suffering and disease, were apparent from the start. And antibiotics would continue to live up to their immense promise through the years to come.

It was only in the last decade of the twentieth century that drawbacks in the use of antibiotics would become apparent. By this time certain bacteria were developing immunity to such drugs, largely through overprescription. In 1987 just 0.2 per cent of strains of pneumococci were found to be resistant to antibiotic drugs; by midway through the following decade this had risen to over 7 per cent. Even more disturbing was the resurgence of tuberculosis, which many had confidently expected to go the way of smallpox and be eliminated from the face of the earth by the end of the twentieth century. Instead, there has been a severe resurgence of this disease, especially in the Indian subcontinent and Russia, from where it has spread to countries of the advanced western world. (As we shall see, AIDS is also partly responsible for this resurgence of tuberculosis, both in the developing world and in the advanced western world.)

However, with regard to overprescription leading to antibiotic resistance we are faced with a problem peculiar to the advanced western world. Scientists have already succeeded in developing half a dozen drugs capable of combating drug-resistant tubercule bacilli, but no pharmaceutical company is willing to take on the task of developing them. This process now costs a massive $200 million, including such things as widespread and prolonged tests, huge insurance costs, and even then the probability of being sued for a fortune in the event of a single failure. Now that we have entered the twenty-first century it seems that when science has solved a problem, this can then pose a problem which remains insoluble to society. As we shall see, this is but one example of an entirely new medical phenomenon confronting contemporary humanity.

16

A NEW FORM OF SURGERY

The rapid development of penicillin was a direct consequence of its utility in war. Other aspects of twentieth-century medicine would also make great advances as a result of war. None more so than surgery, and in particular plastic surgery.

The two leading figures of modern plastic surgery were both New Zealanders. The father of this field is generally recognized as Harold Gillies, who was born in 1882 at Dunedin in the remote and rainy south of South Island, New Zealand. After going to a local school he travelled to England to study at Caius College, Cambridge – William Harvey's former college, which still retained its reputation for medicine. Gillies was an able sportsman and rowed for the university in the celebrated Oxford and Cambridge boat race which takes place on the Thames every year. He was also a popular and highly visible character. It was at Cambridge that he first acquired a characteristic which he would retain, somewhat embarrassingly, throughout his life – namely, his penchant for the student pranks which so characterized this era (chamberpots placed on spires, impersonating foreign dignitaries, and such).

After Cambridge, Gillies completed his medical studies at St Bartholomew's Hospital in London, where he then specialized in otorhinolaryngology (better known as ear, nose and throat). When World War I broke out in 1914, Gillies was 32. He was soon conscripted into the Royal Army Medical Corps and shipped to France. Here he became deeply disturbed by the casualties he encountered. The slaughter in the trenches was horrific, and those who survived often suffered from grotesquely disfiguring wounds. In 1915 Gillies happened across a medical book written by a German surgeon called Lindemann. In this he found descriptions of how to treat jaw fractures and wounds about the mouth, so as to ensure that the patient was left with minimal disfigurement. Gillies felt a deep pang of guilt as he read the pages. He and his fellow surgeons were doing nothing of this nature to their patients; they were simply patching them up as best they could, regardless of any permanent blemishes or outright deformities this might leave. Reading Lindemann's book proved a turning point in Gillies's life. As he put it: 'I felt a tremendous urge to do something other than the surgery of destruction.' He began devoting his considerable energies to petitioning for the establishment of a unit specializing in plastic surgery. As he actuely pointed out, the present situation was actually counter-productive: no surgical work, no anaesthetics, nothing major could be carried out 'when the patient's face looked like a bloody sponge'.

Eventually Gillies's arguments won the day, and in 1916 200 beds at the Cambridge Hospital back in England at the military centre of Aldershot were allotted to a plastic surgery unit. The first patients were soon arriving, shipped across the

Channel from France. With stripped skin and open wounds the patients were at high risk from gangrene. Others suffered from delayed shock, their screaming fits driving entire wards to distraction. Yet worst of all was the despair of those who realized what had happened to their faces. All mirrors were strictly forbidden from the wards; despite this, many committed suicide rather than return to their loved ones and face rejection as living monstrosities. Even Gillies was aware that many of those who left him apparently cured would live out the rest of their lives as shame-ridden recluses hidden away in darkened rooms. He pointedly observed: 'Only the blind kept their spirits up through thick and thin.'

As if the wounds from the trenches were not bad enough, Gillies and his team now began receiving sailors from the Battle of Jutland, many of whom had survived below-decks explosions. In Gillies's words: 'These were wounds far worse than anything we had met before. Men without half their faces; men burned and maimed to the condition of animals. Day after day, the tragic, grotesque procession . . .' Even he himself felt 'appalled and unnerved'.

In 1917 Gillies was promoted and his unit moved to larger and better equipped premises at Sidcup, south of London. In the words of Gillies's biographer Reginald Pound: 'The Cambridge Hospital, Aldershot was the pre-natal clinic of modern plastic surgery. Its birthplace was the Queen's Hospital, Sidcup.' Gillies himself referred to his work as 'a strange new art'. In fact, primitive forms of plastic surgery had been practised intermittently since ancient times, and many of the practices he had learned from Lindemann's book dated from the Renaissance, when plastic surgery had undergone a minor renaissance of its own to deal with the hideous disfigurements of the new syphilis. The main method applied then, and transformed by Gillies, stemmed from rhinoplasty (from the Greek *rhino* 'nose' and *plastos* 'moulded or formed'). In this, a flap of skin was sliced and rolled back from the flesh of the upper arm. The end of this flap was then carefully matched and moulded over the remains of the nose, and then sewn into place. The patient was forced to maintain this awkward position for around two weeks, whilst the end of the skin flap grew itself to the face, all the while nourished by its remaining attachment to the upper arm. This skin-link became known as a 'pedicle': a stalk, serving the same purpose as a stalk in a plant, forming a vital link from the roots to the growing flower.

Gillies was soon performing this, and similar 'autotransplants' of skin and bone tissue from one part of the body to another, upon hundreds of patients a month. Sometimes he had to repeat the process when the grafted skin did not 'take', at other times he would be forced to 'trim' the skin, when it grew faultily. His first concern was always with the patient's ultimate appearance, rather than any astonishing expertise his work might exhibit.

When confronted with sailors who had no facial skin, he developed a technique which involved cutting a long flap of skin and partially detaching it from the abdomen. This was then rolled back over the chest and its end applied to the skinless face, with holes cut for eyes, nose and mouth. Gillies was entering entirely new territory. In his own words: 'I just had to go ahead with the ingenuity of my own mind and the principles of surgery behind it. Little by little principles evolved.' It was the establishment of these principles which made him the founder of modern plastic surgery. His most important discovery concerned pedicles. Whilst cutting the long thin strips of skin he had noticed their tendency to curl inwards on themselves 'as paper curls when heated'. This led to a sudden inspiration: 'If I stitched the edges of those flaps together, might I not create a tube of living tissue which would

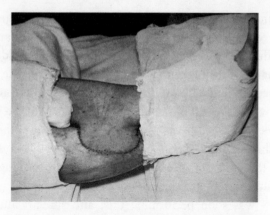

Figure 9a. A cross-flap operation growing the skin from one leg to another

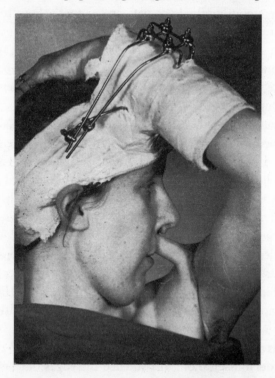

Figure 9b. Shows the tube-pedicle technique developed by Gillies

increase the blood supply to the grafts, close them to infection, and be far less liable to contract or degenerate as the older methods were?' These pipes of living skin he named 'tubed pedicles'.

Gillies soon found that tubed pedicles not only made the entire process of skin grafting much simpler and safer, but it also enabled the operator to work more subtly and effect far better likenesses with the skin graft. At the same time, it enabled him to link more distant parts of the body. Soon his patients were sprouting looped stalks of skin, going from their abdomen or their arm to their lips, their nose, their ears, their forehead, even the crown of their skull. This may have made his patients look like something out of science fiction, but there was nothing fictional about the miraculous plastic engineering it effected.

After the war, the pioneer plastic surgeons who had trained under Gillies at Sidcup would scatter, taking up posts throughout the British Empire and beyond, training up others in this new specialization. In 1920 Gillies published *Plastic Surgery of the Face*, which became the standard textbook, incorporating his famous 'principles'. Meanwhile Gillies himself became a colourful character on the London medical scene. He set up in private practice, and quickly discovered that private plastic surgery for the rich was a highly lucrative untapped source. He bought a Rolls-Royce, which he drove 'like a racing driver'; anyone who overtook him was liable to be chased up the Great North Road until he too was overtaken. Under such circumstances, operations had to wait until the victor returned from his personal 'Grand Prix' – Gillies' operations at the newly established plastic surgery unit in St Bartholomew's Hospital were scheduled on what became known as 'plastic time'. He remained as ever the childish prankster: occasionally with hilarious effect, mostly a cause of extreme irritation and embarrassment. Delivering a public lecture on the new plastic surgery to an audience which included nuns and schoolgirls, he could not resist opening with a series of slides showing the restructuring of a penis.

In 1931 a cousin of his from Dunedin arrived in London. This was Archibald McIndoe, who had just completed a four-year fellowship at the celebrated Mayo Clinic in America, where he had established himself as a first-class abdominal surgeon. Here he had met Lord Moynihan, the president of the Royal College of Surgeons, who was visiting America. Moynihan had encouraged McIndoe to come to England, where he assured him that he would have a great future. Moynihan even promised him work in a new hospital. McIndoe reckoned that he had little left to learn in America, and decided to take up Moynihan's offer. Several months later McIndoe took ship across the Atlantic, accompanied by his wife and young daughter. He arrived in London to find that Moynihan's 'new hospital' had not even been built, and there was simply no other work available. In some desperation he sent a note to his New Zealander cousin, who had now become Sir Harold Gillies. McIndoe was invited to lunch at Gillies's home, where he found himself being served claret by the butler.

There was little family resemblance between the two New Zealand cousins, who were also almost 20 years apart in age. The 52-year-old Gillies was tall and slightly stooped, by now bald, with a round face, greying moustache and a jovial forthright manner. McIndoe wore glasses, had centre-parted dark hair, and a faint shy smile. The bluff middle-aged surgeon encouraged his somewhat intense young cousin to retrain as a plastic surgeon and come into practice with him as a junior partner. Such retraining involved considerable effort on McIndoe's part, and meant abandoning the specialization in which he excelled. When he eventually joined Gillies, there was soon an element of rivalry between them. Gillies could be over-bearing and was prone to make cutting remarks in public about his 'assistant'. McIndoe for his part soon came to regard Gillies's notorious pranks with a distinctly jaundiced eye, seeing through them for what they really were – a childish way of attracting attention to himself.

Their professional partnership also developed strains. Gillies would appropriate all the well-paid jobs, and then take off for a game of golf, leaving McIndoe with the donkey work. Despite these strains, there grew up between them a deep mutual respect where professional expertise was concerned. Gillies may have been the pioneer plastic surgeon, but his young partner quickly established himself as the leading light of the new generation. Together they began developing innovative techniques, also establishing firm guidelines for standard techniques which previously had for the most part been experimental. Where Gillies frequently took time to assess a patient, McIndoe worked with exceptional speed. Although his hands were broad and his fingers stubby ('like a butcher's hands' according to Gillies), he was skilled at sewing skin with utter precision. Also, his ability to draw a freehand incision in skin, so that it exactly matched the area to be covered elsewhere, was little short of miraculous. At the same time, his insistence on the aesthetic finish of his skin grafts was the equal of Gillies's.

The two spurred each other on to ever greater achievements. McIndoe was soon publishing original papers, and by the end of the thirties it was generally recognised that the two New Zealanders now dominated their new speciality. Beside McIndoe's private practice, he also became a consultant plastic surgeon at St Bartholomew's Hospital and consultant to the Royal Air Force. This last appointment was to result in his finest achievement.

In 1939 World War II broke out, and within several months the young spitfire pilots of the Royal Air Force were fighting the German Lufwaffe over southern England in what came to be known as the Battle of Britain. The population watched as the dogfights took place in the sky above them; if this battle was lost, the Germans would be free to invade. For months the British pilots held out against huge odds, but the cost was heavy indeed. Pilots who managed to bale out from their stricken spitfires were often sheathed in burning aircraft fuel. The plastic surgery required on their burns would prove even more drastic than that for the World War I sailors.

At the outbreak of World War II there were just four fully trained plastic surgeons in Britain – the rest were scattered in teaching posts throughout the world. McIndoe was ordered to establish a plastic surgery unit at East Grinstead, 20 miles south of London, and quickly began recruiting a team of surgeons, putting them through a rapid training course. It was now that McIndoe came into his own. Dealing with Gillies had taught him a thing or two about how to succeed and get things done despite being in an inferior position. The RAF top brass had ways of dealing with their junior officers, but McIndoe refused to don a uniform. As a civilian consultant he managed to retain his direct access to the top, and was soon treading on the toes of lesser officers who sought to curb his demands.

McIndoe's plastic surgery unit at East Grinstead soon became a model of its kind. He fought for better conditions, better supplies, and even better sick pay for his injured pilots. He had learned from Gillies that plastic surgery also leaves its psychological scars. He encouraged a camaraderie among his patients, to the extent that they became proud of themselves and took pride in the operations they were forced to undergo. They dubbed themselves 'The Guinea Pig Club' and asked McIndoe to be their president.

In all, over 4,000 airmen would pass through East Grinstead, many so disfigured by high octane aircraft fuel that they would require years of treatment. McIndoe decided that plastic surgery was no longer an adequate term for what he was doing, and renamed his practice 'reconstruction surgery'. There was by now no one to match his skill. Pupils watched in awe as he drew freehand with his scalpel the precise incision necessary to make a match with an area of exposed flesh on another part of the body. By contrast, his gradual reconstruction of an entire face would be undertaken with meticulous planning and in minute detail. Under McIndoe's guiding hand, plastic surgery evolved beyond its heroic pioneer stage and emerged as a fully fledged new branch of medicine.

After the war 'reconstructive surgery' became 'reconstructive medicine' as it moved into even more ambitious fields. From reconstructing the outside of the body, medicine moved to the inside. The field of organ transplants had been pioneered by the brilliant but personally flawed French surgeon Alexis Carrel in America. However, his experiments with animals had in many ways only served to indicate the extreme difficulties inherent in trying to transplant an organ. The frequent rejection of the donor's organ by the host suggested that transplant surgery was facing some as yet undetected biological process.

This process was identified by the London-based Anglo-Lebanese zoologist Peter Medawar in 1951, while he was working on problems connected with skin grafts. Why was it only possible to graft skin from the same body? It had been suggested that soon after birth the cells of a body learn how to distinguish between their own bodily tissue and foreign living matter. Working with mice, Medawar discovered that when a body was confronted with invasive material, its immune system produced antibodies, in the same way as it attacked disease, and thus rejected the foreign matter. He suggested that the way around such rejection was to suppress the immune system by means of a drug such as cortisone.

It was decided that the first human organ transplant should be attempted on a kidney. There were various reasons for this. Firstly, human beings have two kidneys, yet require only one for normal functioning. This meant that a living donor could be used. On top of this, the removal of a kidney is a comparatively straightforward operation; and should complications arise, it is always possible to rely upon a dialysis machine. This performs the function of the kidneys, which is to filter out urea and other waste products from the blood. The first kidney transplant was attempted as early as 1951 in the United States on a patient suffering from terminal Bright's Disease. This is where the damaged kidney not only filters out waste products but also allows the flow of essential protein from the blood into the urine, with the result that the patient gradually wastes away.

The first attempt, and several following, were far from successful; but the intrepid pioneers persisted regardless. In the words of Roy Porter: 'The death rate was so awful that only very courageous, reckless, thick-skinned or far-sighted surgeons persevered.' His choice of adjectives is particularly pertinent for this field, which attracted both maestros and mavericks alike. The reason for their failure soon became clear. For the host body not to reject the donor organ there had to be a precise matching of their tissues, such as is found only in identical twins.

The first attempt at just such an operation was performed by Joseph E. Murray at the Brigham Hospital in Boston in 1954. The 24-year-old Ron Herrick received a kidney transplanted from his identical twin brother Richard. The operation proved successful and the recipient survived for several years. But how to extend such transplants beyond this rare category? During the early sixties Murray succeeded in developing a more successful immunosuppressive drug in the form of azathioprine. This he used in 1961 during an operation involving a kidney transplant from a donor unrelated to the recipient. After several further successful operations he was even able to use a kidney transplanted from a cadaver. Soon many of his patients were able to survive for 20 years. Yet throughout this time there remained the constant problem of infection due to the suppression of the immune system, so necessary to maintain the transplanted kidney.

The advance to attempts at more ambitious transplants, involving other organs, now became inevitable. In 1963 the first successful lung transplant was carried out on a man dying of lung cancer, though he would survive for less than three weeks. The first liver transplant was undertaken in the same year. It soon became evident – for largely unscientific reasons – that the biggest prize of all would be the first successful heart transplant. Popular sentiment still regarded this as the seat of our human life, and the press stoked up popular expectation. But a heart transplant was a different matter altogether. The complications were immense, and went far beyond the problem of rejection (which even so remained a major factor). Experiments in open-heart surgery on animals showed that unlike other organs the heart deteriorates almost immediately following death; it was also impossible to store a heart, and maintain it in working condition. This meant that if a heart were to be transplanted it would have to be removed from the donor and fitted to the patient with extreme haste. Nonetheless it soon became clear that several doctors in America were on the brink of solving these problems.

To the surprise of the world, news of the first human heart transplant came not from America, or Europe, but from South

Africa. In December 1967 at the Groote Schur Hospital in Cape Town, Christiaan Barnard attempted the first successful human heart transplant. He successfully removed the heart of a 25-year-old woman who had been certified brain dead after a car crash. He then prepared to transplant this heart into the body of Louis Washkansky, a 58-year-old Lithuanian-Jewish grocer from Cape Town, who was suffering from a fatal heart disease. In Barnard's own words:

> My moment of truth – the moment when the enormity of it all really hit me – was just after I had taken out Washkansky's heart. I looked down and saw this empty space . . . the realization that there was a man lying in front of me without a heart but still alive was, I think, the most awe-inspiring moment of all.

The operation was to last over five hours, and would involve a team of 20 in the theatre. Afterwards success hung in the balance. Barnard was asked when the danger period would be passed. He replied, 'We don't exactly know. From this point, we are treading in the dark, into new medical territory.'

The operation initially appeared to have been successful, but the medical aspects of this were quickly overwhelmed in a clamour of publicity. These were the years of apartheid in South Africa, which had made the country a leper on the international scene, and it was now keen to trumpet its big achievement to the world. Just four days after his operation a smiling Washkansky was being photographed lying in his hospital bed. At the same time he was also interviewed on live radio by the South African Broadcasting Corporation. 'And how are you feeling, Mr Washkansky?' 'How do you feel to be such a famous man?' 'We have a surprise for you . . .' This turned out to be a visit from his wife.

After 18 days of this, Washkansky died. Suppressed by drugs, his immune system had been unable to combat pneumonia. Soon, 'the man with the golden hands', as Washkansky had called Barnard, was setting off on a world tour to publicize his achievement. Barnard was feted wherever he went, and it was hardly a surprise that fame soon went to the head of handsome 43-year-old Barnard. Further world tours followed, and the man who had suddenly risen from obscurity to become the world's most famous doctor found it impossible to resist the rewards of such fame. Well-publicized affairs with film stars were followed by a well-publicized divorce. Later came the worst blow of all; he began to suffer from arthritis in his hands and was forced to abandon surgery.

Within months of Barnard's astonishing achievement, further heart transplants were carried out in the United States, and later Britain. Many of these suffered from consequent rejections, but this problem was eventually lessened with new drugs and improved techniques. Nowadays this immensely complex and skilful medical achievement is repeated on a regular basis in several countries throughout the world, with ever-improving drugs and techniques, as well as artificial hearts. By the mid-1980s heart transplants were being carried out at the rate of one a day in America. All this is but an indication of the unparalleled advances which were to take place during the last decades of the twentieth century. Heart transplant surgery would be accompanied by the replacement of limbs severed in accidents. The first such operation was carried out as early as 1962. This took place at the Massachusetts General Hospital, when a 12-year-old boy had his severed arm sewn back on again in a comparatively simple fashion. A few months later, after his flesh and skin had sufficiently grafted, an operation to join his nerves was undertaken. This was successful, and within two years his arm had regained many of its normal functions. Such operations would be repeated on an increasingly frequent basis, the main requirement beside the skill of the surgeon being that the severed limb or organ was quickly recovered and frozen.

As early as 1954, the irrepressible 72-year-old Sir Harold Gillies had disregarded medical and ethical advice to perform his final master stroke in plastic surgery: he had undertaken the first sex change operation, transforming a man into a woman. In his view, he was merely correcting 'nature's mistake'. This was to be just the beginning. In time, plastic surgery would add female-to-male sex changes to its accomplishments. However, the most famous of all operations involving the sex organs would occur nearly 40 years after Gillies's pioneering transformation. In 1993 the wife of John Bobbitt of Manassas, Virginia, became so enraged at being constantly subjected to sexual abuse that she cut off his penis with a large kitchen knife. Bobbitt's penis was later found in a nearby dirt lot and sewn back on again to his remaining one-inch stump. The operation was so successful that he later moved to Las Vegas where he made a career for himself in pornographic films, before being sent to jail for taking part in a $120,000 robbery.

17

CURES FOR
THE INCURABLE?

Antibiotics could cure bacterial diseases, but had no effect on viruses, which are so small that they cannot be detected by ordinary microscopes. Viral diseases range from influenza to mumps and measles, from herpes to poliomyelitis (better known simply as polio).

At the end of World War I in 1918 a pandemic of influenza (known as 'The Spanish Flu') began sweeping the world. Eventually this would kill more people than the entire slaughter which had taken place during the preceding four years of the war, making it the most virulent disease to strike the world since the Black Death. In the course of the outbreak, most of the 30–40 million deaths resulted from secondary pneumonia, a bacterial disease. As a result, for many years this flu pandemic was thought to have been caused by a bacteria (*Haemophilius influenzae*). In fact, the bacterial infection only took hold in tissue which had already been severely weakened by the influenza virus. Fortunately this had been realized by 1957, when the potentially worse 'Asian Flu' swept the world and antibiotics hugely reduced the death rate. Influenza epidemics occur regularly every few years, with worldwide pandemics occurring much less frequently. Vaccines against influenza have been developed, but as the influenza virus evolves new strains year by year, these vaccines too must be adapted, in a constant catching up process. The World Health Organization maintains a permanent vigilance against the spread of new forms of influenza, which originate in the Far East and are thought to spread from pigs living close to human habitation.

This vigilance would pay dividends with the arrival of the first pandemic of the twenty-first century, which was caused by SARS (severe acute respiratory syndrome). This viral disease was first reported in a southern province of China in February 2003, from whence it quickly spread. The disease was passed on by person-to-person contact, especially from airborne droplets expelled by sneezing. The illness began with high fever, accompanied by many flu-like symptoms, and after seven days respiratory difficulties frequently required the patient to be placed on an 'iron lung' (artificial respirator). Pneumonia usually followed. At one stage, SARS victims were reported to be suffering a death rate of almost 20 per cent in some locations.

Owing to the speed, frequency and interpenetration of modern air travel, SARS was soon being reported in over two dozen countries across four continents. For the first time entire modern cities were seriously affected – in this case, Hong Kong and Toronto (alarmingly, on opposite sides of the globe from one another). International collaboration, coordinated by the World Health Organization, was soon operating worldwide. Toronto simply closed down; the entire population of Hong Kong was issued with face masks.

The effect of these draconian measures eventually became apparent. By the end of July 2003, within six months of the first reported cases in remote Chinese villages, no further cases were being reported in the affected countries throughout the entire world – from Singapore to the United States, from Vietnam to Britain. By this time 8,098 people had caught the disease, with 774 people dying. Had the battle not been so quickly won, the consequences might well have been apocalyptic – it would be some months after this before a vaccine was developed. (Six months later a further single case was reported in southern China; it was also discovered that this disease probably originated from civet cats.)

The battle against SARS was short and acute. The earlier battle against other viral diseases required time and ingenuity, and proved a lot less cooperative. Indeed, the attempt to produce a vaccine for polio resulted in one of the most acrimonious disputes in medical history.

The earliest outbreaks of severe polio were noticed in the nineteenth century. Cases were recorded in England (1835), Louisiana (1841) and the remote south Atlantic island of St Helena (1844). Such far-flung and apparently unrelated incidents gradually settled into more regular occurrences. By the twentieth century this 'summer plague' was striking down as many as 30,000 a year in the United States alone. Polio was not a great killer, but its effects were highly distressing. It tended to attack young children, resulting in serious and permanent paralysis. Normally healthy infants were crippled, reduced to wearing metal braces to support their useless limbs, and sometimes life could only be maintained on an iron lung.

In 1908 researchers discovered that polio was caused by a virus which affected the nervous system or other tissues. Yet still there remained no cure, and by 1916 9,000 cases were being reported annually in New York City alone, with almost 2,400 deaths. Bafflingly, this was not a disease of the overcrowded immigrant slums; it seemed to strike regardless of class or social circumstances. No one knew what to do. The authorities wrung their hands, and medical science seemed powerless – until the situation was resolved by a typically American solution. Franklin D. Roosevelt was struck down by polio in 1921. Despite being seriously disabled and for the most part reduced to a wheelchair, he was elected mayor of New York, and in 1932 became president. Whereupon, a National Federation for Infantile Paralysis was set up; a 'March of the Dimes' was organized, encouraging even the poorest to contribute; and soon tens of millions of dollars were pouring in.

By 1935 two different vaccines had been prepared. One was a weakened virus solution, prepared in the manner recommended by Pasteur for bacteria vaccines. The other was a 'killed virus' vaccine, for which the virus was treated chemically so that it was no longer capable of causing the disease, but was still capable of provoking an immune response which produced antibodies. The vaccines were tested on 17,000 children, but the result was a disaster. A dozen children developed polio, and a further six died.

The struggle to find a remedy resumed with renewed vigour. The charity balls continued to be held at the White House on the president's birthday, and the National Foundation continued to donate large sums for research. It had been thought that the polio virus entered the body through the nose and the respiratory system, but in 1939 it was shown to enter through the mouth and the digestive tract; faecal matter from infected patients was evidently a principal transmitter of the disease. This was an important finding, for it meant that when an outbreak occurred all swimming pools were closed and the local health department mounted a hygiene campaign – thus minimizing the contagion.

Even so, it was another ten years before the long-anticipated major breakthrough. This was achieved by John F. Enders and his team at the Harvard Medical School. Enders was an unusual man to be making a major medical discovery. Born in 1897 in Hartford, Connecticut, he was the son of a wealthy banker. After studying English literature and Celtic languages at Yale, he left to became a pioneer pilot, and then a flying instructor, in the US Navy Reserve at Pensacola, Florida. On his discharge after the end of World War I he went into real estate, but soon found that he had not inherited the family talent for business and abandoned this to take up graduate studies in English literature at Harvard. Here he found himself sharing a boarding house with a number of medical students, one of whom showed him the work he was doing in the bacteriology labs. Enders was immediately hooked. Amazingly, he had not only discovered a subject which totally enthralled him, but one at which he seemed to be uniquely adept. He finished a PhD on immunology in 1930, and by the time America entered World War II just over a decade later he had been appointed a civilian consultant to the US War Department. He continued to hold this post after the war, while he worked in his laboratory at the Children's Hospital in Boston.

It was here that he achieved the breakthrough which would one day make a vaccine for polio possible. As Koch and Pasteur had discovered, bacteria could be cultivated in a test tube with a broth of nutrients. Viruses, on the other hand, were parasites which could not exist apart from their host. They could only grow in the living nerve tissue of humans or monkeys. Where monkeys were concerned, such experiments were both highly expensive, wasteful and cruel. For a simple speculative test of uncertain outcome, literally scores of primates were required. And to discover a vaccine, let alone carry out tests on it, would require innumerable such tests. Under these circumstances, progress towards a vaccine was severely hampered. Then a technique was found for cultivating viruses in smaller organisms, such as chick embryos. But in such cases the viruses would quickly be overwhelmed by bacteria, making it impossible to separate the two. Enders took this one step further, when he attempted to grow mumps virus on mashed up chicken embryos mixed with nutrient blood. He soon found a technique that succeeded in growing viruses, thus establishing that the organic tissue did not have to be complete or intact. Mumps virus could be grown on simple tissue.

But there still remained the problem of separating the virus from the bacteria which grew at the same time. However, Enders soon realized that this no longer presented an insurmountable difficulty. With the recent development of penicillin, he now had a means of eliminating the bacteria. The virus, which was not affected by the penicillin, would remain intact. Ironically, what had been the problem with viruses – their resistance to penicillin – would now provide a solution. In 1949 Enders obtained tissue from stillborn human foetuses, on which he managed to cultivate polio viruses; these were then cleansed of bacteria with penicillin. At once the way was open. Polio viruses which affected human tissue could now be cultivated in large quantities, and widespread tests could be carried out in the search for a vaccine. (Enders would not play a leading role in this endeavour, though years later in 1965 he would discover a vaccine against the measles virus, and in 1970 he would receive a Nobel Prize for his pioneering work with polio viruses.)

The next advance came from another American, this time one whose talent was equalled by his overweening ambition. Jonas Salk was born in a tenement in the East Harlem district of New York in 1914. His parents were Polish-Jewish immigrants who worked in the garment industry. Jonas showed exceptional talent at school and won a scholarship to study at New York

University College of Medicine. During World War II he helped develop a vaccine against influenza, whose widespread occurrence was sapping the US Army war effort. This vaccine was of the 'killed-virus' type, which orthodox medicine still regarded with some suspicion, not least because of the 1935 polio vaccine debacle. In 1949 Salk was appointed professor of bacteriology at the University of Pittsburgh. Here he was approached by the National Federation for Infantile Paralysis which asked him to work on research into a polio vaccine. Salk leaped at this opportunity, well aware that solving this problem would bring lasting recognition. His general ebullience of manner was soon upsetting more senior researchers working in the field, such as Albert Sabin at the nearby University of Cincinnati. Salk was convinced that the killed-virus vaccine approach would prove effective, while Sabin favoured the weakened-virus approach pioneered by Pasteur.

Making full use of the technique developed by Enders, Salk managed to produce a killed virus by soaking polio viruses in formaldehyde. He calculated that with this method there was just a one in a thousand billion (10^{12}) chance of each batch containing a live virus. In 1952 he decided to test this on two children who had recovered from polio, and thus should have been resistant to the disease. To his delight, he found that his killed-virus vaccine brought about the required increase in antibodies in the children's blood. It worked! Next he tried his vaccine on some children who had not suffered from polio, and again it produced antibodies. After further successful tests – including on himself and his own children – large quantities of the vaccine were manufactured. In April 1955, before the assembled newsreel and television cameras, as well as 150 journalists from the national press, it was announced that a succesful vaccine against polio had been discovered. The announcement was broadcast live on public address systems and church bells rang out through the nation. Ten days later President Eisenhower in the White House Rose Garden conferred on Salk a citation 'for his extraordinary achievement'.

Unfortunately these celebrations proved somewhat premature. A few batches of vaccine prepared at a laboratory at Berkeley in California had not entirely eliminated the live polio virus. When injected, these vaccines eventually resulted in 204 cases of polio, most of which suffered paralysis. Eleven of them died. An enquiry was called, at which Enders warned Salk that his killed-virus technique was not foolproof as there was always the possibility that his vaccine contained some live virus. But Salk and the authorities chose to ignore this possibility: the chances of it occurring were a thousand billion to one – so minimal as to be practically non-existent. As soon as the faulty batches of the vaccine from the laboratory at Berkeley were traced and eliminated, the programme of vaccination continued, and over 9 million people were injected with the 'Salk Vaccine', as it came to be called. The results were hugely impressive. In 1954 the number of polio cases per 10,000 of population was 13.9. By 1969 it had been reduced to just 0.5. The Salk Vaccine came to be seen as one of civilization's great achievements, and Salk himself was soon being compared to Churchill and Gandhi.

Others were less impressed, including Albert Sabin, who still maintained that the killed-virus vaccine method was far from foolproof. There were two reasons for this: first, it had not yet been proved that the killed-virus vaccine would continue to work and provide immunity for years to come; and second, it was not completely safe because it could contain a live virus. A public battle royal now took place between Salk and Sabin, who also happened to be developing his own vaccine.

Ironically, Albert Sabin was from the same Polish-Jewish background as Salk. He had been born in 1906 in Bialystok in a part of Russia that is now Polish. At the age of 13 he had emigrated to the United States with his parents. He too had gained a medical degree at New York University. During the 1930s polio outbreak in New York, he had been an intern at the city's Bellevue Hospital. Ten years before Enders, he too had attempted to grow polio virus on tissue; but at the time penicillin had not yet been developed, so he had found it impossible to eliminate the accompanying bacteria. Once Enders had succeeded in this, Sabin understood that it was only a matter of time before a polio vaccine was developed. He chose to believe in the weakened-virus vaccine, insisting that the killed-virus vaccine would not produce sufficient antibodies to remain successful over a long period.

By 1956, a year after Salk, Sabin had developed his own vaccine. This was taken by mouth, so that the weakened living virus was absorbed into the body where it continuously multiplied, ensuring that the body continuously produced antibodies. Its effect was thus permanent, it only required one dose, and was easy to administer. Salk's vaccine, on the other hand, was administered by injection, as well as requiring multiple shots and a booster.

But Sabin's vaccine was not taken up. By this time the American public was not in the mood to be subjected to a further set of polio vaccine tests (and scares). Sabin was forced to try out his vaccine on prison volunteers. But he too was determined to achieve success with his vaccine. In the end he pulled off a spectacular coup, managing to persuade the Russian authorities to use his vaccine, whereupon it proved a huge success, banishing polio throughout the entire Soviet Union. This was followed by further successes in countries ranging from the Congo to Britain. By the 1960s orthodox medical opinion in the United States was beginning to swing in favour of Sabin's vaccine, which proved highly popular when it was administered in the form of cherry-flavoured vaccine on a sugar cube. Between 1962 and 1964 over 100 million vaccines were administered free of charge on 'Sabin Sundays'.

However, the continuing vitriolic public controversy between Salk and Sabin had won neither of them many friends. Sabin referred scathingly to Salk's scientific methods: 'You could go into a kitchen and do what he did,' and declared that Salk 'had never had an original idea in his life.' Such breaches of scientific decorum quickly backfired. On the other hand, Salk's greed for the limelight had known few bounds, and he had done little to discourage his vaccine being called the 'Salk Vaccine', although its discovery had in fact involved a team of dedicated researchers. When the rival Sabin vaccine sought a licence for public use in the United States, Salk declared this to be 'unnecessary and ill-advised', mentioning that in his view the weakened virus would certainly lead to some developing full-blown polio. He lost few opportunities to make disparaging remarks about Sabin and his vaccine, and many accused him of neglecting to mention the leading role played by Enders in the development of the polio vaccine.

The latter accusation was largely untrue, but Salk was his own worst enemy. His divorce and consequent marriage to the glamorous Françoise Gilot, former mistress of Picasso, did not help matters. Nor did his avid intellectual self-promotion. Having been loosely compared to other celebrated benefactors of humanity such as Gandhi and Churchill, he took such estimations at face value and began promoting himself as a philosopher, writing pseudo-scientific articles on 'the survival of the wisest' and the 'anatomy of reality'. His arguments were a subtle blend of the abstruse and the absurd, claiming that through the 'merging of intuition and reason' humanity was undergoing a 'major transformation' to a higher plane, with the aid of social 'error-correcting mechanisms' similar to enzymes which rectified chemical faults 'in our genetic code'. However, such harmless hyper-egoism can be forgiven when placed alongside his more solid achievement.

Although both Salk and Sabin eventually waived their patent rights, donating their discoveries to the world, both became rich men. Salk put his fortune to good use, founding an institute for biological reasearch at La Jolla, on the coast outside San Diego in southern California. The Salk Institute, as it inevitably became known, soon began attracting a number of maverick geniuses who would produce ground-breaking work. These would include Leo Szilard, the brilliant Hungarian physicist who first conceived of (and patented!) nuclear fission, the Nobel Prize-winning immunologist Gerald Edelman, and Francis Crick the co-discoverer of the structure of DNA. Such a feat could not be matched by Sabin, whose acquiescence to a more sober public persona eventually led to his reinstatement in the esteem of his professional colleagues, though by then the damage had been done. Neither Salk nor Sabin ever received the full professional recognition they deserved – only Enders's role would be marked by the Nobel Prize. Towards the end of his life, Salk would ruefully remark: 'The worst tragedy that could have befallen me was my success.' Doubtless Sabin would have agreed.

In the decade after the discovery of the first polio vaccine, preventive medicine presented the world with another coup, one which would transform society like no other medical discovery before or since. This was preventive medicine of a very different kind, in the form of the contraceptive pill. As with so many modern discoveries, this was the work of several scientists, and even several different teams. However, the man who made the crucial breakthrough, who is generally recognized as 'the father of the pill', is Carl Djerassi, a chemist of Austro-Bulgarian descent.

Djerassi was born in Vienna in 1923. His Austrian mother divorced his Bulgarian father when he was a child, and he enjoyed a middle-class Jewish upbringing with his mother in a fashionable apartment overlooking the Danube. In 1938 the Nazis took over Austria, and a year later the 15-year-old Djerassi and his mother managed to flee. They arrived off the boat in New York with just $20, only to be relieved of this by the taxi driver who took them the short distance to their cousin's apartment.

The young Djerassi spoke good English with a slight accent, and decided that he needed a good education. So he took the unusual step of writing to Eleanor Roosevelt, the wife of the president: 'Dear Mrs Roosevelt . . . I must have a scholarship to finish my schooling.' His astonishing audacity paid off, and the first lady arranged for him to take up a scholarship at a Presbyterian college in the Midwest. Here he exercised his 'agnostic Jewishness' by secreting the *Reader's Digest* inside his Bible during the daily services he was obliged to attend, and was soon earning money giving talks in nearby churches about 'The European Situation'. He quickly learned to spice these with personal reminiscences, adding witticisms adapted from magazines. (He took to describing Balkan Revolutions as 'abrupt changes in the form of misgovernment'.)

When war broke out, Djerassi missed conscription because of a lame knee, caused by a childhood skiing accident on winter holidays in Bulgaria. Sophisticated, self-consciously brilliant and highly ambitious, by the age of 22 he had completed his PhD thesis in chemistry at the University of Wisconsin. He dreamt of an academic career, but the needs of wartime along with academic anti-Semitism meant that instead he joined the pharmaceutical company CIBA of New Jersey. Here he soon proved himself by helping to synthesize one of the earliest antihistamines, the drugs which block allergies.

After this he wanted to try and synthesize cortisone, one of the steroid hormones which control the internal chemistry of the human body. (Medawar would later suggest its immune-suppressive properties for transplant surgery.) CIBA were unwilling to embark upon such an ambitious project, so in 1949 Djerassi left and joined Syntex, a small new company set up by European immigrants in Mexico City. This was an exceptionally bold move. In his own words: 'At the time the idea of doing any chemical research in Mexico seemed preposterous: "serious" chemistry supposedly stopped at the Rio Grande.' But in Mexico he had the freedom to exercise his talents as he saw fit. At the time, cortisone could only be produced outside the human body by extracting it from cattle bile, an expensive process which cost $200 a gram. Djerassi and his team at Syntex set about trying to extract cortisone from a species of wild Mexican yam. Within two years they had succeeded, beating several well-funded American teams to the prize. Syntex retained the patent rights, but by now Djerassi had invested some of his own money to keep the company going. His only profit was the modest increase in his investment.

Djerassi then began investigating the steroid hormone progesterone. This had been termed 'nature's contraceptive': its presence in the female body once pregnancy has begun prevents male sperm from fertilizing female eggs (by stopping menstruation and the release of more eggs). Unfortunately progesterone proved too weak to inhibit ovulation when taken by mouth; instead, it had to be injected. Like cortisone, this also could only be extracted with difficulty from obscure sources such as bulls' testicles and sows' ovaries, making it too extremely expensive. Within a year, Djerassi and his team had succeeded in producing a synthetic version of progesterone. Although this meant that its availability increased, it still suffered from the drawbacks of naturally produced progesterone. Yet any attempt to alter its chemistry so as to increase its potency was doomed to failure because steroid hormones were known to be structure-specific. This meant that as soon as their structure was altered, they lost their specific potency. But Djerassi was aware that some recent experiments on another steroid hormone, which acted as a cardiac stimulant, had shown that this was not always the case.

Working on an inspired guess, Djerassi began attempting a similar structural alteration to progesterone, with the aim of increasing its potency. The result was a modified form of progesterone known as norethisterone. This not only proved a highly potent progestational agent, but also remained so when taken orally. Despite being well aware of its properties, Djerassi modestly confesses: 'Not in our wildest dreams did we imagine that this substance would eventually become the active progestational ingredient of nearly half the oral contraceptives used worldwide.' They duly filed their patent application in November 1951.

Djerassi and the Syntex team sent their new drug for tests at the Worcester Foundation in Massachusetts. This was run by Gregory Pincus, who had long been seeking an ovulation inhibitor which might act as a contraceptive. He soon realized the potential of norethisterone. A series of exhaustive tests were carried out on women in Brookline, Massachusetts, as well as in Haiti and Puerto Rico. All proved successful, and in 1962 the drug finally received Federal approval under the name Ortho-Novum.

Djerassi had received his coveted academic appointment as early as 1951, and in 1959 he was appointed professor of chemistry at the prestigious Stanford University in California. Here he established himself by introducing original research methods, as well as original teaching methods. On one occasion, after delivering a course on steroid chemistry he asked each student to propose a question for the exam, promising that each of them would then be allotted one of these questions. When he gave the students their allotted question, one after another began protesting that there had been a mistake: they had been given back their own question. Only gradually did they realize the subtlety of Djerassi's method. Determined to demonstrate their brilliance at the expense of another by the difficulty of their questions, each of the students now found that they had placed themselves in the hot seat.

Despite these subsequent appointments, Djerassi had always retained his original investment in Syntex. This eventually made him rich beyond the dreams of avarice. He bought a spectacular 1,200-acre estate, consisting of redwood forests and canyons in the Santa Cruz Mountains overlooking the Pacific (next door to rock star Neil Young). This he named SMIP (Syntex Made It Possible), and here he eventually settled down to write novels and an autobiography.

Djerassi's pill, 'The Pill' as it came to be called, would transform modern western society. Within seven years of its introduction almost one in four American women would be using it; by the turn of the century, 85 per cent of American women had used it. The first effects were seen in the wild sexual liberation of the sixties; more lasting effects came with the ongoing social liberation of women. Yet the effects of modern contraception in the world at large have yet to be realized. The most welcome medical benefits which the First World has passed on to the Third World are modern medicine and hygiene, which have brought tragedy in their wake in the form of a population explosion. (India alone has 35,000 births per day.) This was 'the introduction of death control without the introduction of life control,' as the physicist Victor Weisskopf succinctly put it. Even present-day birth control pills have not so far proved effective, for reasons ranging from cost to lack of education, from Catholic doctrine to problems of distribution.

Once again we are faced with the prohibitive cost and difficulty of developing a cheap, effective new drug. Owing to the genetic diversity of human beings, even the safest drug will always affect some people adversely. This may not show up in tests involving 10,000 people, but will affect measurable numbers among millions of users. Despite this, a few new contraceptive drugs have been developed and are in use. Depo-provera, which requires an injection every three months, is available in an increasing number of countries; and now there is Norplant, involving a surgical implant which releases synthetic progestin and can bring contraception for five years. But perhaps the last word here should be with Djerassi: 'The overwhelming fact is that at my birth there were 1.9 billion people in this world. Now there are 5.8 billion, and at my 100th birthday there are likely to be 8.5 billion. That has never before happened in human history – that during a person's lifetime, the world population more than quadrupled. That can never happen again.'

Alongside this battle to prevent lives, the battle to save lives goes on as never before. By the 1960s informed medical opinion was firmly convinced that the age of pandemics and plagues was over. Indeed, in 1969 no less a figure than the US Surgeon General solemnly announced: 'the book of infectious disease is now closed.' Yet towards the end of the twentieth century, the world suddenly found itself faced with what appeared to be potentially the worst pandemic in human history – namely, AIDS (acquired immunity deficiency syndrome). This is caused by a virus known as HIV (human immunodeficiency virus) which over a period attacks a variety of white blood cells essential to the body's immune system. When this system finally breaks down, the body is powerless to defend itself against attack by opportunistic diseases, including cancer and pneumonia, until it is overwhelmed and the victim dies.

The historical origins of AIDS remain something of a mystery. It appears likely that chimpanzees in the jungles of the Congo basin had long been carriers of a virus genetically similar to HIV, but remained unaffected by it. Sometime around 1970, this virus evolved into HIV, which was transferred to humans who hunted and ate these chimpanzees. (Retrospective examination of Central African blood samples reveal no evidence of HIV before 1971.) From there it spread, at first largely unnoticed.

However, there is some curious evidence that appears to contradict this hypothesis. Retrospective tests indicate that a British seaman died of AIDS in Manchester as early as 1959. Another case has been traced to a young adolescent from Missouri who died in 1968. Also, there were outbreaks of diseases now known to be AIDS-related in Central Africa during the 1950s. All this indicates that HIV may initially have crossed into humans much earlier than 1970, and then either died out or lain dormant.

In 1981 doctors in New York and San Francisco began reporting cases of young and active homosexual men dying from Kaposi's Sarcoma, a rare type of skin cancer which usually occurrs after a breakdown in the immune system. Other types of death resulting from immunodeficiency then began occurring with alarming frequency, and the medical profession realized that it was faced with a new and highly dangerous infectious disease, which it named AIDS. As panic spread, others began calling it 'the gay plague', while fundamentalist preachers declared that it was the wrath of God descending on the inhabitants of the licentious bathhouses of San Francisco and other sinks of homosexual iniquity. But soon reports of AIDS began coming in from countries world-wide, and it became clear that this was not a disease limited to homosexuals. In sub-Saharan Africa, the disease had spread along the main highways running east and west, transmitted by male lorry drivers to the female prostitutes along their routes. By 1984 50 per cent of Kenya's prostitutes were HIV positive. By the following year 10,000 people in the United States alone were infected, and the majority would die within two years of being diagnosed. The disease spread through all levels of society, taking a particularly heavy toll on the artistic and intellectual community. In France, the philosopher Michel Foucault died of AIDS in 1984. Later, the film star Rock Hudson would be the first well-known American figure to declare publicly that he had AIDS shortly before he died in November 1985.

By now considerable research had been carried out into AIDS. It had been discovered that the disease was spread through the transmission of sexual fluids or blood. It could enter by way of cuts or abrasions, particularly those caused in the sensitive tissues of the sexual organs and the anus. Another prevalent way of passing on the disease was the shared use of syringes by drug abusers. Pregnant women could pass on HIV to their foetuses by way of their bloodstream, and even after birth HIV could be passed on through the mother's milk. It was also found to be passed on to people requiring blood transfusions, such as haemophiliacs – there was still no test which could detect the HIV virus in blood samples. However, despite all the hysteria it was soon understood that the disease was not passed on by normal social contact, or even deep kissing; and 'safe sex' (involving careful use of a condom) also prevented possible contamination.

HIV was found to be a retrovirus that affected the white blood cells known as Helper T cells which were essential to the body's immune system. Alarmingly, after the initial infection there was a long period during which the patient showed no symptoms of illness whatsoever. This asymptomatic period could last for months, or even years, with the infected person unaware that he was HIV positive, while at the same time passing on the virus. During this stage Helper T cells were attacked by the HIV virus and gradually reduced from their normal density of 1,000 per microlitre to the critical point around 200 per microlitre, when the patient suffered from immune deficiency (AIDS). As a result he or she would be exposed to illnesses from tumours to diseases of the nervous system, and at the same time also be liable to suffer from such distressing symptoms as personality changes, memory blanks and dementia. On top of this, viruses which had long lain dormant in the body were no longer suppressed and became active. This latter aspect contributed to the rise in tuberculosis around this period.

The quest for a vaccine to combat AIDS began early, but major difficulties soon became apparent. The HIV virus was found to be capable of mutating into new strains even more rapidly than the influenza virus. Normally a vaccine would only be capable of combating a single strain. On the other hand, anyone who did come up with a successful vaccine would be assured of worldwide gratitude, to say nothing of the unimaginable fortune which the patent rights would bring.

Two front runners in the race to develop a vaccine soon emerged – the American Robert Gallo and his team at the National Institutes of Health in Maryland, and a French team at the Pasteur Institute under Luc Montagnier. To begin with Gallo and Montagnier cooperated, maintaining constant and friendly contact. Gallo would even dine with Montagnier in Paris, when they would each reveal their latest developments. But differences of personality and national approach soon emerged. In the words of Randy Shilts, the leading historian of AIDS: 'Montagnier and Gallo were as dissimilar as two human beings can be, and each made the other vaguely uncomfortable. While Gallo was chummy, aggressive and charismatic, Montagnier held himself aloof and was frequently described as doughty and patrician.'

Gallo was born of Italian immigrant parents, and had strong reason to be involved in research into diseases of the blood. At the age of 11 he had watched his younger sister die of leukaemia: 'I saw her emaciated, jaundiced, covered with bruises . . . When she smiled I saw only caked blood over her teeth . . . It was the last time I would ever see Judy . . . It remained the most powerful and frightening demon of my life.'

Montagnier had grown up in provincial France, near Poitiers, where he happened to be taught medicine by the father of the philosopher Michel Foucault. Moving to Paris, one of his formative experiences was reading in the library of the Pasteur Institute, which he considered 'the Mecca of microbiology'. Later he would conduct research in Britain, at London and Glasgow. He dreamed of going to California, but returned to Paris, where he ended up heading a team of researchers at the Pasteur Institute. Early in 1983, just months after starting his AIDS research, Montagnier isolated a new retrovirus, which was a possible candidate for causing AIDS. This he later named LAV. Towards the end of the same year, Gallo also isolated a new retrovirus, which he named HIV. Some weeks later, he found what he believed was conclusive evidence that this was the causative agent for AIDS, whereupon he announced that HIV was the cause of AIDS, rather than the French retrovirus LAV. It was then discovered that LAV and HIV were in fact identical, and that the sample in which Gallo had discovered HIV had originated from Montagnier's laboratory. All hell now broke loose. Accusations of theft from

Montagnier were countered by accusations of incompetence by Gallo, and the brickbats began to fly. In fact, it now emerges that Gallo had acted in all innocence. Yet his insistence that he had been the first to demonstrate that HIV/LAV was the cause of AIDS did little to calm things down. Then things got worse.

Early in 1984 the US Secretary of Health Margaret Heckler made a highly publicized announcement that Gallo and his team at the National Institutes of Health would have a vaccine ready for testing in two years time. Here the hapless Gallo was a victim of political manipulation by the Reagan government, which was anxious for some good news on the health front. Gallo had insisted that a vaccine would take years to develop, but in an unguarded private moment had admitted that if they got lucky they might even have a vaccine in as little as two years. The administration had seized on this. Montagnier was derisive, and Gallo was duly chastened. However, he did succeed in redeeming himself somewhat. At the press conference Secretary of Health Heckler had also said that Gallo would have a successful blood test for the HIV virus within six months. This would prevent innocent haemophiliacs from being infected by blood transfusions. Fortunately, by this stage Gallo had produced sizeable quantities of the HIV virus, and to the surprise of many he did manage to develop a blood test for HIV within six months.

But the battle between the two camps had by this stage become a matter of national pride. The French had in fact developed a strictly limited blood test for LAV some years previously, but the Americans had chosen not to recognize this. Consequently, the French authorities (though not Montagnier) now decided to take tit-for-tat measures against Gallo's blood test, which was refused recognition by the French authorities. This led to a disaster. While the French continued with their efforts to develop their own general blood test, over 300 French haemophiliacs died from AIDS as a result of infected blood, and many more became HIV positive. It subsequently emerged that there was another reason for the French not accepting the American blood test. They had large stores of blood products ready for sale on the international market. If these were held back for tests, a sizeable portion might turn out to be worthless, and many buyers might well turn elsewhere to a more reliable source. Someone stood to lose a lot of money. Consequently, four French health workers were tried and jailed – yet the suspicion remains that these were scapegoats for much more senior figures in the French administration. As if to confirm this, similar scandals soon emerged in Germany and Japan.

Inevitably, the disputes between Gallo and Montagnier led to the courts. After four years, and huge expense, the case between them still dragged on. At this stage a miraculous resolution was effected by a man even more experienced in acrimonious scientific dispute than Gallo and Montagnier – none other than Jonas Salk. It was finally agreed that Gallo and Montagnier should be recognized as codiscoverers of the HIV virus. The French HIV blood test had by now been developed to the same standard as the one developed by Gallo – so it was decided that patent rights on the blood tests should also be shared. So divisive were the international repercussions of this dispute that the final agreement ending it was signed by President Reagan and President Mitterand.

By this stage, gay activists had begun taking matters into their own hands. Their forceful championship of their desperate cause had begun to question the paternalistic attitude of the medical profession. Who was to say that an anti-AIDS drug was effective, or even safe? Why should dying people be made to wait until drugs had been 'properly' tested? Gay activists began privately importing untried anti-AIDS drugs manufactured in laboratories abroad, especially in Mexico. They also began contesting the validity of the HIV blood test. Anyone testing positive was liable to become a social outcast: losing his or her job, losing partner and friends, as well as being dropped by insurance companies. Instead, many turned to the leading Californian virologist Peter Duesberg, who denied the entire HIV theory of AIDS. In his view, AIDS was not caused by HIV, it was not a viral disease at all, instead it was caused by poverty, aberrant behaviour or drug abuse.

Meanwhile, through the ensuing decades the search for a vaccine against HIV continued in earnest. At the time of writing, no cure or vaccine has yet been found. Though treatments have been discovered, such as ZDU, which acts as a retroviral inhibitor. This does not cure the patient of the HIV retrovirus, but stems the rate of its advance, thus prolonging the patient's life. Even more effective is HAART (highly active antiretroviral therapy), which combines a number of inhibitors – necessary because HIV can quickly evolve strains resistant to any single inhibitor. HAART halts the replication of the HIV virus, permitting the immune system to rebuild itself, and has resulted in a lowering of the mortality rate by as much as 80 per cent. However, HAART is expensive and has side effects. It also involves a highly complex regime, with the patient expected to take combinations of some 24 or more pills or liquids daily. Failure to ingest just one of these can result in a serious setback – hardly a satisfactory state of affairs for a patient who has lost everything that made his or her life worth living. Despair and meticulous self-discipline are not easy companions.

Despite this, AIDS continues its grim passage around the globe. After a slight downturn in the early 1990s, it then returned with a vengeance. By the end of the century, AIDS was reliably estimated to have caused over 20 million deaths throughout the world. At the same time, 36 million were estimated to be HIV positive. Almost three-quarters of these were living in sub-Saharan Africa. In some of these countries, such as Botswana, almost 50 per cent of the adult population are now infected with the HIV virus.

International response has varied. Some countries – such as Germany, Canada and Denmark – have passed laws requiring all cases of HIV infection to be registered. Some poorer countries – such as Brazil and South Africa – have begun taking matters into their own hands: openly flouting the international drug patent laws, they have begun producing their own cheaper versions of anti-HIV drugs. Other countries have responded less actively. China, as well as some Catholic and some Muslim countries, have refused to offer special treatment to prostitutes, drug abusers and homosexuals, being unwilling to give official approval to these illegal lifestyles.

Most agree that the epidemic is gradually being brought under control in many advanced western countries, whereas it is undeniably out of control in Africa and many Third World countries. For how long this bipartite state of affairs can continue is uncertain. However, one thing is certain: similar diseases will continue to appear at more or less lengthy intervals. In the blind process of natural selection, human beings are far from being alone in their struggle for survival on this planet. In order to survive, viruses too will evolve and discover their own methods of adapting to circumstances. Yet in discovering how to overcome AIDS, finding a vaccine against such an elusive virus as HIV, humanity may well discover the means to win these battles to come.

18

THE SECRET OF LIFE?

The effects of the latest, and almost certainly the greatest, discovery to influence medical science are still unfolding; and the ultimate consequences for humanity of this discovery remain unclear. The first step in this process was the discovery in 1953 by Crick and Watson of the structure of DNA. This also had more than its fair share of controversy and high drama.

The discoverers themselves were an unlikely pair. Francis Crick was born in 1916 in Northampton in the English midlands. His father ran a shoe manufacturing firm which went bankrupt during the recession. The family moved to London, where Francis won a scholarship to Mill Hill, an English public school. Crick ended up by taking a modest degree in physics at University College, London. During World War II he worked on research into underwater mines for the British Admiralty. Around this time he read *What is Life?* by the

Nobel prize-winning Austrian physicist Erwin Schrödinger. Though little longer than a pamplet, this book persuaded Crick to abandon physics in favour of studying 'the division between the living and the non-living . . . the chemical physics of biology'. This was the field which would eventually become known as molecular biology, and one of its central problems concerned the nature of the gene, which appeared to hold the key to how human life was passed on from one generation to the next. Crick's newfound enthusiasm for this subject transformed him from a talented physicist into a bumptious biologist bubbling with ambitious ideas – not least of his own intelligence. However, these still remained largely unfulfilled when he arrived as a researcher at the Cavendish Laboratory in Cambridge in 1949 at the comparatively late age of 33.

Two years later he was joined at the Cavendish by a somewhat gauche and immature young American called James Watson, who also happened to be convinced of his own intellectual pre-eminence. As a child prodigy Watson had starred in the 'Chicago Quiz Kid Show'. By the age of 22 he had a PhD in biochemistry, and then left on a Merck Foundation fellowship for Europe. Around this time he too discovered Schrödinger's *What is Life?* and was immediately convinced by Schrödinger's thesis that the key to the transmission of life lay in the gene. He decided that here was the subject for him, and as a result he made his way to the Cavendish, where he encountered Crick.

Watson and Crick hit it off from the word go: their supreme self-confidence and ambition serving as a mutual spur rather than introducing any negative element of competitiveness. They quickly found that their original fields of expertise ideally complemented one another, as together they blundered enthusiastically into the unknown territory of molecular biology. They agreed at once that the 'genetic code' referred to by

Schrödinger must somehow lie in the structure of the gene. The vital factor here appeared to be the immensely complex molecule deoxyribonucleic acid (DNA), which consisted of over 30,000 molecules and atoms. Over pints of beer at The Eagle, a pub around the corner from the Cavendish, they began testing their ideas on one another. As Crick put it: 'It is one of the requirements for collaboration of this sort that you must be perfectly candid, one might almost say rude, to the person you are working with.' Fortunately both proved suitably thick-skinned, and despite a few tempestuous episodes the partnership held. Gradually they began piecing together in the Cavendish the immensely complicated model of a DNA molecule. This had to be capable of containing all the necessary information for a human embryo, and also be capable of replicating an evolved version of itself to pass on to the next generation.

Much of the evidence on which they would base their work came from the crystallographer Rosalind Franklin, a woman of forbidding intellectual and emotional reputation. You crossed Dr Franklin at your peril. Even her boss at King's College, London, the New Zealand-born Maurice Wilkins who had previously worked on the atomic bomb, entered her laboratory with some trepidation. Crick and Watson travelled down from Cambridge and blundered in with innocent self-confidence. When Franklin showed them her ground-breaking X-ray diffraction pictures of DNA, they quickly decided that these first blurred shapes indicated some kind of helix-like structure. Franklin, a painstaking and dedicated experimentalist, dismissed this idle theorizing out of hand. It was impossible to judge on such slim evidence. In her eyes Crick and Watson were just a couple of chancers. The undaunted duo returned to Cambridge and set about trying to build a helix-like model of DNA.

Basic experimental analysis of DNA's chemical components

had revealed that it was a macromolecule consisting of over 30,000 different constituents. Assembling these in anything like a workable structure would be an extremely intricate and demanding task. After several months Crick and Watson ground to a halt, overcome by the sheer enormity of their task. There seemed to be no way of matching all the molecules and atoms to the structure they had in mind. Franklin had obviously been right: it wasn't a helix.

Then late in 1952 came some sensational news from California. Linus Pauling, the finest chemical mind of the twentieth century, had published an article describing the structure of DNA. Crick and Watson realized they had been scooped; and to make matters worse, when they read the article they discovered that Pauling was suggesting a helix-like structure for DNA. But Pauling's model differed from theirs. Instead of their tentative twin helix, it consisted of a three-chain helix. Yet the more they read on, the more they began to suspect that there was something wrong. Then they spotted it. In paying meticulous attention to detail, Pauling had somehow overlooked the fact that DNA (deoxyribonucleic acid) was an acid. He had made a schoolboy mistake – the overall structure which he described was not an acid! Crick remained downcast; it was only a matter of time before Pauling spotted his blunder and rectified the structure. But Watson was ecstatic; even the great Pauling thought that DNA had a helix-like structure.

Watson decided to pay a visit to London, and danced gleefully into Rosalind Franklin's lab to announce the news. Whereupon Rosie exploded: there was still no evidence whatsoever for a helical structure. Incandescent with rage, she stormed around the laboratory bench, seemingly intent upon physical assault. The chance arrival of Wilkins at the door was the only thing which enabled Watson to escape. Wilkins assisted the shaken young Watson back to his office, where he showed him Rosalind Franklin's latest brilliant X-ray plates. Watson was astonished: the helical structure seemed unmistakable. How could she still insist that there was no evidence? Indeed, in his view the images were now so clear that it might even be possible to calculate precisely how many interlocking chains the helix contained. By the time Watson had arrived back in Cambridge on the train that night, he had calculated that the structure of DNA definitely contained two interlocking helices. Crick was quickly convinced, and the two of them set about constructing a new model from scratch.

DNA had a double-helix structure, like two entwined spiral staircases (see diagram on following page). The two interlocking helices were linked by 'steps'. Each of these contained base pairs of the form AT or CG. These combinations contained the genetic information. Replication took place when the two helices unravelled, with the 'steps' breaking and each side retaining one base. These then joined to another unravelled helix strand to form a new double helix, with its own unique set of joined base pairs, resulting in 3 billion pieces of information. Here were the building materials for each human being. From hair colour to fingerprints, from cranial structure to susceptibility to disease, this was the blueprint for each unique individual person. This was the 'code' which Schrödinger had predicted.

Crick and Watson hurriedly began assembling their model, racing against the clock. Speed was now of the essence. Wilkins and Franklin in London would surely soon accept the unmistakable helical structure. And in California Pauling only had to spot his simple mistake . . . This time it fell into place – the double helix worked!

The newspapers hailed Crick and Watson's success as the discovery of the 'secret of life'. This was hardly an exaggeration. The discovery of the structure of DNA may yet prove to

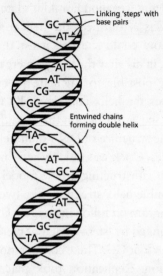

Linking 'steps' with base pairs

GC
AT
AT
AT
CG
GC

Entwined chains forming double helix

TA
CG
AT
GC

AT
GC
GC
TA

Figure 10a. A section of the final DNA molecule discovered by Crick and Watson

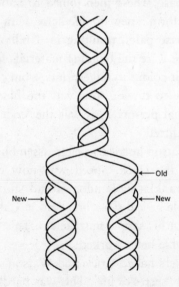

Old

New →   ← New

Figure 10b. DNA replication

be the most significant knowledge humanity has ever acquired. In time, this led directly to the launch of an ambitious project to map the entire sequence of the human genome. The human genome consists of the 3 billion letter alphabet contained within the DNA helices. Typed out single-space on A4 paper this alphabet would cover 750,000 sheets. These letters form the coded instructions which combine to produce each single characteristic of a particular human being. They control every inherited aspect of that individual's existence, from whether it will be male or female, to whether he or she will be prone to certain types of cancer.

In June 2000, it was announced that the Human Genome Project, as it had come to be known, was finally complete. In fact, it wasn't – quite. This was a public relations exercise intended to paper over the dispute between the two rival projects racing to achieve the final goal. Crick and Watson had worked on a shoestring – or, more accurately, a fragile model made out of clamped tin plates and sprouting spindles of metal. Their aim had been glory. And in 1962 they were duly awarded the Nobel Prize, along with Wilkins, whose participation had proved so crucial. (Rosalind Franklin, whose work had been even more crucial, had died of cancer in 1958 and was thus not eligible for the prize.) The prize for winning the race to map the human genome would be both more spectacular and more mundane. The first to map any gene sequence could patent it. Those genes which played a role in disease could be of immense value – monetary and otherwise – to medical science.

Along with the Human Genome Project we are learning increasingly sophisticated techniques for manipulating human genes. Sheep and cats have been successfully cloned; more ambitious projects are well under way. Several years ago James Watson himself predicted: 'Within the next ten to twenty years, I anticipate that there will be doctors and scientists who will correct faulty genes in living patients through the introduction of DNA.'

In fact, gene therapy – the correcting of faulty genes – is now reality. Four months *before* the announced completion of the Human Genome Project, doctors at the Necker Hospital in Paris attempted gene therapy on a baby boy born with a defective immune system. Prior to this operation, the baby was doomed to certain and imminent death. Even its 11-month survival so far had been regarded as something of a medical miracle. Permanently isolated from all outside contact in the germ-free, clinically sterile atmosphere of an airtight bubble, the ailing underweight infant was already suffering from telltale disfiguring skin blotches, and constant diarrhoea, its enfeebled strength gradually ebbing away. Doctors Alain Fischer, Marina Cavazzana-Calvo and Salima Hacein-Bey decided to attempt gene therapy as a last desperate measure. Over a number of days bone marrow cells were removed from the child. Healthy genes were then manipulated into these cells: a complex and extremely skilful process of uncertain effect. The bone marrow cells were then placed back in the child. The latter was a comparatively simple operation taking half an hour, and involving an infusion of just 25 millilitres of fluid. The first effects became apparent after only two weeks. The disfiguring red skin blotches began to recede, the diarrhoea abated, and the child began to breathe more regularly. It even began to put on a little weight. Within three months of being treated, the ailing underweight infant who could only survive in an infection-free airtight bubble had developed into a normal healthy child. The boy's astonished parents were able to take him home, where he now lives the rough and tumble life of a typical youngster.

This is only the beginning. W. French Anderson, director of

gene therapy at the University of South California, echoes the opinion of many in this new field: 'By the year 2030 I anticipate that there will be gene-based treatment for every disease.' Yet this is just one side of the coin. From here it is only a step to embarking upon the programme of eugenics, the ill-fated science which sought to 'improve' human beings through selective breeding by using only the 'finest specimens'. As French Anderson fears: 'the downside of this powerful technology might be that eugenics will be practised on a scale far larger than any "selective breeding" policy could accomplish.' This is no scaremongering. If the human genome can be engineered to eliminate 'faulty' genes, it can also be transformed in more questionable ways. Moral debate continues to range back and forth over this territory. Is 'human life', with all its faults, in any way 'sacred'? The genes which made us what we are contain the seeds of our humanity. They have evolved slowly, over millions of years. In eliminating at a stroke susceptibility to diseases from our genetic structure, we might also be transforming our humanity into something unforeseen, something essentially different from what we are at present. Medicine, and our medical susceptibility, may yet prove to be a fundamental part of our human condition.

Here medicine is turning full circle – becoming embroiled in the very philosophy from which Hippocratic medicine originally sought to distance itself almost 2,500 years ago. Yet such involvement would now seem inevitable. In so many ways, medicine has become the victim of its own success. Perhaps the most glaring example of this is public medicine, which has been transformed beyond recognition by the recent technological advances. This book has been about the development of medicine as a science, but these achievements are nothing if they cannot be delivered. Cost and public expectation have

risen in accord with the rapid advances of the late twentieth
century. The results of this are visible in hospitals throughout
the western world. News reports speak of spilling wards and
patients left in corridors. But it is the images which accompany
these reports which tell the full story. Where wards were once
filled with neat uncluttered rows of beds, we now see beds
amidst banks of expensive equipment. The patients left in the
corridors are overwhelmed by the latest apparatus.

Once again, this leads to philosophical questions. Can such
expensive medicine remain available for all? If not, for whom?
Must public medicine be drained of its finest resources by
those who can afford to pay for such services? These are
philosophical questions which do fall within the Hippocratic
realm. Hippocrates' oath required a doctor to swear 'to use my
power to help the sick to the best of my ability'. Yet Hippocrates, and his disciples, needed payment in order to survive.
The unresolved question of how to reconcile the practice of
medicine, and those who cannot afford to pay for it, is as old as
medicine itself. Whether Hippocrates always provided precisely the same standard, attention and thoroughness of treatment to both the ailing rich and the more widely ailing poor is
a moot point. How we, in the twenty-first century, choose to
deal with this anomaly is decided by another ancient Greek
notion which Hippocrates would have considered to be beyond the realm of medicine – namely, democracy.

Another idea which is as old as medicine itself may also
determine its future conduct. The entire process of diagnosis
may soon be revolutionized by breath analysis. Hippocrates
stated that a patient's breath could give hints to identifying
illness. However, it was not until 1971 that the great chemist
Linus Pauling undertook a thoroughgoing chemical analysis of
the contents of human exhalation. He was surprised to find
that our breath contains as many as two hundred separate

compounds. Some years later, Pauling's work came to the attention of Australian researcher Michael Phillips: 'I thought: if all these compounds are there, they must be signifying something.' This idea was not in itself novel. Breath tests for the presence of the bacterium *Helicobacter pylori* – which indicates ulcers and other diseases – are routine. But Phillips had a more ambitious idea. He dreamed of a machine which could test for conditions across the board – from cancers to heart transplant rejection. His quest would take years, but its inspiration was close to hand: his wife was a survivor of breast cancer. Phillips's optimism was grounded on solid theory. Many diseases produce an excess of molecules with 'free radicals' (unpaired electrons). Free radicals damage certain tissues, giving rise to a higher than normal amount of volatile organic substances, which are expelled in exhalation. Phillips's aim was to analyse these by means of a mass spectrometer. The spectral 'fingerprints' of volatile organics other than those present in a normal healthy human being could then be identified. Critics claim that some of these 'disease fingerprints' are bound to be caused by pollutants in the atmosphere, such as hydrocarbons from traffic. Phillips, who is now a professor at New York Medical School and runs his own Menssana Laboratory on Staten Island, is confident that he can overcome these problems. He is already designing tests to detect the effects of external toxins, as well as tests identifying markers of biological ageing and angina. If breath tests prove successful, this method may replace more cumbersome and invasive methods such as biopsy, which involves the removal and analysis of bodily tissue.

Finally, we come to the future of medical discovery. The aims are obvious. Cures for the likes of cancer, AIDS, Alzheimer's disease and many other scourges are all being sought with great urgency and at great cost. The breakthroughs have been long awaited, but will certainly come. Yet will they be cures, or will they be mere palliatives, which simply check the progress of the disease (like HAART for AIDS)? How can we cure a disease such as cancer, when we are seemingly still as far as ever from discovering its cause at a molecular level? Surprisingly, this is not an insurmountable problem. As the medical writer Paul W. Ewald points out: 'In the mechanistic sense, a concensus on causation exists for only about half the diseases listed in current medical textbooks.' As we have seen, Jenner discovered the efficacy of vaccination while having no conception of viruses. Semmelweis understood what to do long before Pasteur pinpointed bacteria. Even the discoverers of antibiotics did not understand *how* they worked. Some researchers are beginning to look at such afflictions as cancers, heart attacks and Alzheimer's through new eyes. What if these are the infectious diseases of the modern world, a consequence of viruses which cause tissue deterioration, which then manifests itself as a cancer or Alzheimer's? As we discover more about the workings of the human genome, we will certainly discover more about propensity to disease, and be able to remedy this. Many modern diseases also show unmistakable signs of being caused by our modern surroundings and lifestyle: could a new ecological therapy arise within regions of transformed environment? Any one of these avenues of enquiry could well produce an entirely new understanding of disease, and its discoverer will be hailed as the new Pasteur. If ever medicine was ripe for the appearance of such a hero, it is now. Whether or not such a figure does appear, there can be no doubt that exciting times lie ahead. In line with the twenty first-century world we live in, medicine appears to be poised for a metamorphosis, one which is liable to bring about the greatest transformation in its history.

So how will this come about? The use of new technology

will certainly play a role here. The medical profession now has a vast array of diagnostic machinery at its disposal. This has been, and certainly will be, aided by new developments in computer technology, such as CAT (computerized axial tomography) scanning. Nuclear science is likely to bring even greater advances than PETT (positron emission transaxial tomography) scanning. Meanwhile other aids such as MRI (magnetic resonance imaging), lasers and ultrasound are yielding insights (both literal and theoretical) as never before.

When considering the prospects for the twenty-first century, it is worth remembering that our ability to see into the human body involves science in realms which we did not even know existed at the turn of the twentieth century. What lies ahead is equally unimaginable. What seems certain is that this will in some way involve gene therapy. Here the entire notion of medical cure takes on new meaning. Our ability to alter the most fundamental element of our physical humanity – our DNA – opens up a Brave New World which we may indeed wish to remain unimaginable.

Similarly, public health finds itself faced with scourges which were also unknown at the turn of the twentieth century. We have seen what BSE (bovine spongiform encephalopathy), new Asian flus and SARS can do. Such scourges will doubtless return, as will similar new scourges. Meanwhile AIDS threatens to ravage Africa as the Black Death ravaged Europe seven centuries ago. All of these diseases are the subject of intense efforts to find cures, with research budgets running into millions (billions, in the case of AIDS). These efforts will certainly bear fruit one day, if past experience is anything to go by. The history of medicine may be a history of varied and hideous sufferings, but it is also a history of our solutions to these problems.

On a less apocalyptic note, public health campaigns have

changed our lifestyle. Previous generations were taught the value of such fundamentals as outer cleanliness, in the form of social and personal hygiene. Now that such matters have become habitual, the emphasis has shifted to a more inward focus. We may be what we eat, but what we do to ourselves also determines what we are. Public health campaigns have transformed our attitudes to smoking, exercise and diet. As a result, lung cancer, heart disease and obesity all seem set to decrease.

Here medicine found it comparatively easy to sway public opinion. In other matters, the public has not been so readily convinced. More controversial is the debate concerning vivisection and animal experiments. The latter in the cause of cosmetic research is justly condemned. However, the use of both these methods in the pursuit of appropriate cures is also seen as problematical. Luddite resistance and violence is aimed at laboratories which are subject to the most stringent legislation. If laboratories are closed down, such research is liable to be carried out in countries where there is no such legislation. Consciences in the First World will be clear, but at what cost? Medical research using such methods will certainly continue – its benefits, both medical as well as financial, are too great to remain ignored. For understandable reasons, the Third World is literally crying out for such research.

The difference between the First and the Third World is particularly acute in the medical field, often in grotesque fashion. As Roy Porter put it: 'the role and scope of medicine in advanced states seems destined to change in the twenty-first century as the accent shifts from overcoming disease to the fulfilment of lifestyle wishes, bodily enhancement and further extensions of life.' Meanwhile developing countries require more than liposuction and breast enhancement. Such disparities will probably be solved in medicine much as they are in economics. But what is it to be – 'trickle-down' or welfare hand-outs? For different reasons, neither of these tend to have effect where they are most needed. Inadequate economic infrastructure and corruption can render an entire society ill. As with economics, so with medicine. The export of expertise and technology will prove more effective than hand-outs or hand-downs. But this export of practical and theoretical know-how must be a two-way process, involving the import of grant-aided students and the creation of a new generation of medical professionals ready to return to their country and take over.

A two-way process has also been advocated for the pharmaceutical industry. The multi-national giants of this industry are naturally keen to reap the rewards resulting from their inordinately costly research (which has no guarantee of successful outcome). When their products are ripped off, regardless of international patents, and sold at cut price in developing countries the pharmaceutical companies inevitably protest. However, with the aid of suitable tax incentives these same companies could themselves be encouraged to set up cheap manufacturing plants in these very countries – thus guaranteeing the integrity of their product in all ways.

Some such solutions will inevitably be found. It is not false optimism to believe that many of our present medical problems will be overcome in the near future. In the words of Charles Horace Mayo, co-founder of the Mayo Clinic: 'Medicine is about as big or as little in any community, large or small, as the physicians make it.' Like it or not, we now live in a global community. It is up to us, and our physicians, to make medicine large enough for this community.

SOURCES

Because this is intended as a popular work, I have not included footnotes and an exhaustive list of sources. Where appropriate, the sources of most direct quotes have been indicated in the text. The following is a list of suggested further reading, for those who wish to follow up on the main subjects included in each chapter.

Prologue: Reading Amid the Battle

Keynes, Geoffrey, *The Life of William Harvey*, Oxford, 1966.
This is still the standard biography, despite its comparative age. It contains a wealth of details and many informed speculations.
Aubrey, John (ed. Oliver Lawson Dick), *Aubrey's Brief Lives*, Penguin, 1980.
Contains only a few pages on William Harvey, but these are highly vivid and further brought to life by the author's personal involvement.

Chapter 1 – Out of the Darkness: First Light

Goldberg, Herbert S., *Hippocrates: Father of Medicine*, Watts, 1963.

A good short introduction to the father of medicine, his life and times, and how the science of medicine came into being.

Jouanna, Jacques, *Hippocrates*, Johns Hopkins, 1999.

The latest in a long line of biographies which cover the same few acts. This also contains selections of the works.

Gillispie, Charles C. (ed.), *Dictionary of Scientific Biography*, Scribners, 1970.

This indispensable 16-volume work covers all the major, and many of the lesser, figures of science since its inception. The 30-page entry on Aristotle is particularly good, and contains an entire section on his anatomy and physiology. Also has a useful bibliography for further study. This work also contains useful entries (and bibliographies) for Herophilus and Erasistratus.

Chapter 2 – A Tradition is Born

Sarton, George, *Galen*, Kansas, 1954.

This is still the standard biography of Galen. Highly readable and contains a wealth of details which place his life in the context of its times.

Chapter 3 – Figures in a Dark Landscape

Flanagan, Sabina, *Hildegard of Bingen*, Routledge, 1998.

A good short biography which covers all of Hildegarde's many achievements and interests.

Berger, Margret, *Hildegard of Bingen: On Natural Philosophy and Medicine*, Brewer, 1999.

Concentrates on her various medical works, with selections and some closely argued commentaries. Scholarly but also readable.

Chapter 4 – A Fresh Start

Hartmann, Franz, *The Life and Doctrine of Paracelsus*, Health Research, 1998.

A good account of this never less than fascinating character and his ideas.

Chapter 5 – Blueprint for a Science

O'Malley, Charles Donald, *Andreas Vesalius of Brussels*, California, 1964.

Gives a good idea of medical life in the sixteenth century, as well as providing such details as are available of Vesalius himself.

Chapter 6 – Harvey the Circulator

Again, by far the best source is:

Keynes, Geoffrey, *The Life of William Harvey*, Oxford, 1966.

This is still the standard biography, despite its comparative age. It contains a wealth of details and many informed speculations.

Chapter 7 – Explorer of an Invisible World

Dobell, C., *Antony van Leeuwenhoek*, New York, 1958.

Tells the tale of this often overlooked character and his intruiguing exploration of the world of 'animalcules'.

Chapter 8 – An Era of Medical Enlightenment

Von Haller, Morgagni, and the Chamberlens can be seen in the context of their time and contemporary medical development in the excellent encyclopaedic history of medicine:

Porter, Roy, *The Greatest Benefit of Mankind*, Fontana, 1999.

Chapter 9 – A New Cure for an Old Scourge

Fisher, R. B., *Edward Jenner 1749–1823*, Deutsch, 1991.

Covers the sympathetic life of this quiet genius, as well as the controversies which his great discovery caused.

Cook, Trevor M., *Samuel Hahnemann, the Founder of Homeopathic Medicine*, Thorsons, 1981.

Another controversial life, which divides people to this day. Was he a genius or a charlatan? Read and decide for yourself.

Chapter 10 – Giants of Physiology

Olmsted, J. M. D., *Claude Bernard: The Experimental Method in Medicine*, Schuman, 1962.

A difficult, but curiously touching life of this man whose field continues to excite violent controversy to this day.

Carter, K. and B., *Childbed Fever: A Scientific Biography of Ignaz Semmelweis*, Greenwood, 1994.

Recognized as a hero, but too late.

Chapter 11 – Eliminating the Surgeon's Enemy

One of the best accounts of this fascinating tussle and its scandalous characters is the ever readable:

Friedman, Meyer, and Frieland, Gerald, *Medicine's 10 Greatest Discoveries*, Yale, 1998.

Chapter 12 – The Pioneer Women

There are many biographies of Florence Nightingale, ranging from the gushing to the dismissive.

Baly, Monica E., *Florence Nightingale and the Nursing Legacy*, Routledge, 1988.

A good, readable text.

Strachey, Lytton, *Eminent Victorians*, Continuum, 2002.

This book may be 80 years old but its swingeing chapter on Nightingale still reads as wittily as if it were written today.

Holmes, Rachel, *Scanty Particulars*, Viking, 2002.

This biography of 'James Barry' attempts to tell us how she got away with it.

Chapter 13 – Pride and Prejudice

A character such as Pasteur is bound to inspire contradictory feelings.

Debré, Patrice, *Louis Pasteur*, Johns Hopkins, 1998 (trans. from French)

Gives the accepted story.

Geison, Gerald L., *The Private Science of Louis Pasteur*, Princeton, 1995.

Gives us the alternative version, making use of lab notebooks.

Chapter 14 – Medicine for the World
Fisher, Richard B., *John Lister*, Macdonald, 1977.
A worthy study of a worthy man.
Brock, Thomas B., *Koch*, Madison, 1988.
A detailed account of a difficult life.

Chapter 15 – The Start of the Modern Era
Strathern, Paul, *Röntgen and X-rays*, Arrow, 2000.
A brief history of the man and his idea which changed the world.
Newton, James D., *Alexis Carrel*, Harcourt, 1987.
Despite all the controversial opinions, he did make an important
   contribution – and here is his story.
Wilson, D., *In Search of Penicillin*, Knopf, 1976.
Recounts this never less than astounding story.

Chapter 16 – A New Form of Surgery
Pound, Reginald, *Gillies: Surgeon Extraordinary*, Joseph, 1964.
Tells the story of this larger-than-life figure.
Barnard, Christiaan, *One Life*, Bantam, 1971.
Tells his side of the story.

Chapter 17 – Cures for the Incurable?
Gould, Tony, *A Summer Plague: Polio and its Survivors*, Yale,
   1995.
Shilts, Randy, *And the Band Played On*, Viking, 1988.
Despite its age, this remains by far the best historical account of
   AIDS.

Chapter 18 – The Secret of Life?
Watson, James, *The Double Helix*, Penguin, 1998.
One of the greatest stories of science, by one of those who took
   part in it. There is even an introduction by Steve Jones which
   attempts to set the record straight.
Wyke, Alexandra, *Twenty-First Century Miracle Medicine*, Ple-
   num, 1997.
From robo-surgery to the quest for immortality, the unimaginable
   future.

INDEX

Page numbers in **bold** refer to main entries.